Endoscopic Facial Plastic Surgery

Endoscopic Facial Plastic Surgery

Gregory S. Keller, M.D., F.A.C.S.
Assistant Clinical Professor
Department of Surgery
Division of Head and Neck Surgery
University of California
Los Angeles, California
Private Practice
Santa Barbara, California

Mosby

St. Louis Baltimore Boston Carlsbad Chicago Naples New York Philadelphia Portland
London Madrid Mexico City Singapore Sydney Tokyo Toronto Wiesbaden

Mosby
Dedicated to Publishing Excellence

A Times Mirror
Company

Publisher: Anne S. Patterson
Editor: Robert Hurley
Developmental Editor: Christine Pluta
Project Manager: Linda Clarke
Production Editor: Julie Cullen
Associate Production Editor: Andrew Hall
Composition Specialist: Camillo M. Gonsalves
Designer: Carolyn O'Brien
Manufacturing Manager: William A. Winneberger, Jr.
Cover Photos: PhotoDisc, Letraset Phototone

Printed in the United States of America
Composition by Mosby Electronic Production, Philadelphia
Printing/binding by Walsworth Publishing Company

Mosby–Year Book, Inc.
11830 Westline Industrial Drive
St. Louis, Missouri 63146

Library of Congress Cataloging in Publication Data
Endoscopic facial plastic surgery / [edited by] Gregory S. Keller.
p. cm.
Includes bibliographical references and index.
ISBN 0-8151-5192-6
1. Facelift. 2. Face—Endoscopic surgery. I. Keller, Gregory S.
[DNLM: 1. Face—surgery. 2. Surgery, Plastic. 3. Surgery, Endoscopic. WE 705 E56 1996]
RD119.5.F33E53 1996
617.5'20592—dc21
DNLM/DLC
for Library of Congress 96-45493
CIP

97 98 99 00 01 / 9 8 7 6 5 4 3 2 1

Associate Editors and Contributors

ASSOCIATE EDITORS

M. Sean Freeman, M.D.
Director
Plastic Surgery and Laser Center
Charlotte Eye Ear Nose & Throat Associates
Charlotte, North Carolina

H. Devon Graham III, M.D., F.A.C.S.
Clinical Assistant Professor
Department of Otolaryngology–Head and Neck Surgery
Tulane University
Department of Plastic and Reconstructive Surgery
Ochsner Clinic
Ochsner Medical Foundation
New Orleans, Louisiana

CONTRIBUTORS

William H. Beeson, M.D.
Clinical Assistant Professor
Department of Otolaryngology–Head and Neck Surgery and Department of Dermatology
Indiana University
Indianapolis, Indiana

W. Gregory Chernoff, M.D., F.R.C.S.C.
Clinical Assistant Professor
Indiana University
Private Practice
Chernoff Plastic Surgery and Laser Center
Indianapolis, Indiana

Grady B. Core, M.D., F.A.C.S.
Private Practice
Birmingham, Alabama

Julene E. Cray, R.N.
Private Practice
Aesthetic Laser Consultants
Los Angeles, California

Terence M. Davidson, M.D.
Professor of Surgery
Division of Otolaryngology–Head and Neck Surgery
University of California
San Diego, California

Douglas Dedo, M.D.
Clinical Assistant Professor
Department of Otolaryngology–Head and Neck Surgery
University of Miami
Attending Physician
Good Samaritan–St. Mary's Hospital
Wellington Regional Hospital
Jackson Memorial Hospital
West Palm Beach, Florida

Robert Hutcherson, M.D., F.A.C.S.
Associate Clinical Professor
University of California
Senior Surgeon
St. John's Hospital and Heath Center
Los Angeles, California

Nancy Jurek, R.N.
Director of Nursing
De La Vina Surgicenter
Santa Barbara, California

Wayne F. Larrabee, Jr., M.D.
Clinical Professor, Department of Otolaryngology–Head and Neck Surgery
University of Washington
Staff
Swedish Hospital
Seattle, Washington

Kathleen H. Makielski, M.D., F.A.C.S.
Associate Professor
University of Washington
Chief, Otolaryngology–Head and Neck Surgery
Pacific Medical Center
Seattle, Washington

Mark M. Oyama, M.D.
Private Practice in Facial Plastic and Reconstructive Surgery
Beverly Hills, California

David H. Perrott, D.D.S., M.D., F.A.C.S.
Associate Professor
Harvard School of Dental Medicine
Unit Chief and Resident Director
Massachusetts General Hospital
Boston, Massachusetts

Larry D. Schoenrock, M.D., F.A.C.S.
Clinical Professor
Division of Facial Plastic Surgery
Department of Otolaryngology
University of California
San Francisco, California

Ashley Shobe
Surgical Technologist
De La Vina Surgicenter
Santa Barbara, California

Ronald W. Strahan, M.D.
Assistant Clinical Professor
Division of Otolaryngology–Head and Neck Surgery
Martin Luther King/Drew School of Medicine
Los Angeles, California
Clinical Associate Professor
Department of Stomatology
Division of Oral Maxillofacial Surgery
Northwestern University Dental School
Chicago, Illinois

Jonathan Sykes, M.D.
Assistant Professor, Department of Otolaryngology–Head and Neck Surgery
University of California, Davis Medical Center
Sacramento, California

This book is dedicated to my wife, Paula, without whose support it could never have been written; to my children, Bret, Reid and Tara, who have had less of my attention because of it; and to my parents, Martin and Elizabeth Keller.

I would also like to dedicate this book to the teachers of my formative years at the University of Illinois and their excellent Department of Otolaryngology and Division of Facial Plastic Surgery (among them, Gene Tardy, Ralph Levin, Drs. Soboroff and Kodros, and all the other dedicated and unselfish members of the department), as well as to those facial plastic surgeons, plastic surgeons, dermatologists, occuloplastic surgeons, engineers, scientists, and cell biologists who have since contributed to my knowledge.

Preface

It is always difficult to stop writing about a developing field. To curtail the writing and send this book, in particular, into actual production required intense coercion on the part of the editorial staff at Mosby-Year Book.

Since my first presentation in the field of endoscopic facial plastic surgery in 1991 at the American Academy of Cosmetic Surgery meeting in Scottsdale, I have believed that this field would constantly evolve. The temptation to recruit yet another author to write yet another chapter in this text reflects that belief.

I believe that we have covered the techniques of minimally invasive forehead and necklifting quite well. These are the procedures that are currently acceptable to most surgeons and are the procedures that should be covered in a textbook. The goal of this book (and the AAFPRS ad hoc endoscopic committee) was to portray accepted procedures and background principles of endoscopic facial plastic surgery with quality endoscopic photography and illustrations so that other surgeons could understand the procedures. Another goal was to provide an introduction to less universally applied procedures. I feel that the authors have achieved these goals admirably.

Endoscopic mid-facelifting, endoscopic use of "biomaterials" (such as hydroxyapatite) and implants, and endoscopic reconstructive surgery are discussed here, but were not as advanced at press time as they have recently become. Concurrent or staged use of laser resurfacing to contract skin is also currently being debated.

Aiache, Toledo, Isse, Graham, Byrd, Hester and many others have, since this book's completion, produced new concepts that could not be summarized and written about in time for this edition. Some of their procedures will never be acceptable to most surgeons performing facial plastic surgery and, perhaps, should not be covered. Others may, it is hoped, evolve, become universally acceptable, and become chapters in future endoscopic textbooks.

Automation, "robotization," and remote control of endoscopy will evolve and become practical. Most importantly, new procedures will be proposed, the knowledge base will expand, and future authors and editors will face the same challenge of when to stop writing and publish.

Acknowledgments

An incredible amount of work and effort goes into the production of a book. Equally extensive is the amount of labor and "people power" required in the development of a new field.

For the book, I would like to acknowledge the efforts of the staff at Mosby-Year Book: Bob Hurley, Chris Pluta, and Julie Cullen, who managed to turn ideas into reality. Their vision and abilities were essential.

I would like to thank my office and surgical staff for their tolerance of the time that it took to develop these procedures. Julene Cray, my friend and associate, was instrumental in shepherding this book and the endoscopy project in general through every step— from concept to organization to course development. Ashley Shobe and Nancy Jurek are especially to be acknowledged for their patience and input during this time. Jeannine Monarrez, Gretchen Ostergren, Donna Holzwarth, Laura Andreas, Rosanna Andrade, Connie Davis, Susan Robuck, and the rest of my office and surgical team were key to the data collection and assembly of material. Barbara Daly, a nurse and photographer, was responsible for photodocumentation.

This project could not have been completed without the Karl Storz Endoscopy team, particularly Paul Hensler, Ellen MacDonald, and Jeff Kritzer, who provided the technical support and unlimited backing during the development phase of my portion of the endoscopy adventure. Sue Smith and the others at Laserscope are also to be thanked for their help. Mona Green, Cliff Morrow, Michael Slatkin, Ben Givli, Michael Kochmann, Yasha Sutton, Karen Amburgey, Tom Paulino, and the staff at Sharplan provided laser technical assistance and support.

The artists Barbara Seide, Kate Sweeney, Kathy Makielski, and Vince Quaranta (On-Q Productions) are to be recognized for their ability to turn obscure concepts into visual reality. Bob Locke at Imagemanager is acknowledged for his help in obtaining the quality endoscopic digital images.

Most of all, the authors and co-editors of this text are to be acknowledged for their unselfish contributions of knowledge and effort. Thanks to Wayne Larrabee for his anatomical work in the evolution of our field. This book is largely an endeavor by the former Ad Hoc Committee on Endoscopic Surgery of the American Academy of Facial Plastic and Reconstructive Surgery, although many interdisciplinary experts provided support and knowledge.

Contents

introduction

The Future of Endoscopic Facial Plastic Surgery: Why an Endoscope?

Terence M. Davidson, MD

Not very long ago medical diagnoses were made by history and physical examination. The desire to improve the examination led to improvements, and one of those improvements is the endoscope. The endoscope began with metal pipes and candles. Mirrors were added to peer around corners and ground glass improved optics and added magnification. Electricity, light bulbs, and fiber-optic technology improved the lighting and by the second half of the twentieth century diagnostic endoscopy was being performed via virtually every human orifice.

In otolaryngology we began with bronchoscopy and nasopharyngoscopy. The ear was and still is examined and operated on with a binocular microscope providing 6× to 40× magnification. Telescope enhanced bronchoscopy, and 70- and 90-degree telescopes greatly improved office laryngoscopy.

The facial plastic surgeon requiring magnification employed 2× to 6× loopes. Nasal, laryngeal, and bronchotrachael examination made a quantum improvement with flexible fiber-optic endoscopes. Rhinologists use 2.7-mm and 4-mm glass rod endoscopes to examine the nose. With the advent of endoscopic sinus surgery, the endoscope became a new and important tool for examination and surgical intervention. At the same time, urologists used endoscopes to examine and operate on the genitourinary tract and orthopedic surgeons developed their own tools for arthroscopic examination and surgery. The gynecologists and general surgeons utilized rigid endoscopes first to examine and then to operate inside the abdominal cavity.

Today we are faced with a whole new application called endoscopic facial surgery. The advantages are smaller incisions, the ability to operate 5 cm, 20 cm, or more from the incision, and improved magnification. Glass rod endoscopes provide excellent illumination and 6× magnification.

As of this writing endoscopic forehead surgery is developed to a degree where it is easy to perform and provides clear advantage over other approaches (e.g., direct brow lift with forehead lifts, pretrichial and coronal forehead surgery). While I firmly believe that the endoscope will play an important role in other aging face surgeries, the techniques and applications are not yet developed to a point where they offer significant advantages over other approaches.

It is my projection that soon we will use endoscopes to repair many facial fractures, specifically those requiring screw and plate fixation. There will be applications for face-lift, particularly those benefiting from deep plane dissection. Ultimately, I predict applications for tumor excision, beginning with excision of submandibular glands and lymph nodes.

Extirpative surgery will temporarily remain the province of open surgery, because here a small incision provides little benefit. Endoscopic surgery will generally take longer to perform than previously used open techniques because it is microsurgery; when the surgeon can see better dissection is meticulous and time consuming. Patients will request endoscopic surgery because there is less scarring, less pain, and they will perceive a benefit of "new" advanced technology.

What are the techniques that will enhance endoscopic surgery? The first is the television camera. Operating by viewing a television screen has several advantages. The surgeon can stand or sit with his or her back straight and not have to bend over to peer through the ocular. Surgery performed directly through the scope is boring to everyone in the operating room; with a camera and television everyone present can watch and participate. The interest level is much higher and the entire operating room team becomes involved because they know what is happening and what is needed. The disadvantages of the camera are its weight, its color replication, and its cost. Improving technology is producing smaller, lighter cameras. While one-chip camera technology provides sufficient color replication, the three-chip camera is even better. As cost and weight decrease it will be interesting to see if the multiple-chip camera replaces the single chip or if other technology supercedes. As the chip decreases in size it can be positioned at the patient end of the endoscope thereby eliminating the need for fiber-optic cables; the endoscope will house electric wires, maneuvering wires (if required), and light cables. This technology is now available for large endoscopes like the gastroscope. It will be miniaturized and ultimately it will be available for the 5-mm, 4-mm, and 2-mm endoscopes used for the head and neck.

Some argue that operating through the scope is superior because it provides better optics and a three-dimensional feel and orientation. These are surgeons who have not taken the time to learn the mechanics of operating off a monitor. Almost everyone who has mastered the monitor finds it superior.

One disadvantage of endoscopic surgery is that there is no stereo-optic field depth. This appears to be a minor disadvantage, but it too will soon be remedied with burgeoning three-dimensional technology. The current three-dimensional cameras are too heavy for endoscopic facial surgery, but the technology will be improved and miniaturized so that this perception can be added.

Virtual reality (VR) technology adds yet another dimension. VR headsets provide a monitor that is mounted on the headband. The visual quality is far less than that offered by the standard cathode ray television, but everyone has his or her own headpiece. This technology is driven by the entertainment industry's desire to develop increasingly realistic video games—telemedicine is a fortuitous spin-off. With VR display instrument control, a surgeon in Washington, DC, could operate on a patient in Los Angeles, Africa, or outer space. While I doubt that the advantage of operating while sitting in your office or at home will drive the VR industry, the telemedicine requirements for military, space, and rural medicine will provide the impetus to advance this technology. Much of the VR technology will have significant spin-off from endoscopic facial surgery.

The next important step is the evolution of robotics. The first robotic arms are already in clinical practice. They can hold and manipulate tissue retractors and endoscopes. The use of robotics has three advantages. It frees the surgeon to hold a suction device or second instrument, it holds an endoscope with a "heavy" camera with no tremors or vibrations, and with appropriate control the endoscope can now be micromanipulated by the surgeon or an assistant. The next generation of robotic arms will operate and direct instruments, such as a sucker, suction cautery, laser beam, or surgical instrument.

Current developments in neurosurgery, spine surgery, and paranasal sinus surgery are using the image-guided technology. This technology utilizes magnetic resonance (MR) for soft-tissue targets and computed tomography (CT) for bone-related surgery. CT is better for bone surgery and it is cheaper than MR, but it exposes the patient to radiation; MR is faster, but more expensive and it is not applicable if the body contains magnetic metals. For sinus surgery a traditional sinus CT is used, and orientation of the CT is accomplished with standard location points such as the nasion and external auditory canals. For example, a patient is placed in a headband and the instrument, in this case an endoscope, has a locator at its tip. The locator is zeroed for position by placing it on the forehead and calibrating the CT computer. A monitor displays the coronal and/or axial and/or sagittal CT scans. As the endoscope is inserted into the nose, the CT changes, at all times localizing the endoscope position.

In more expensive paradigms the patient is positioned in a fast CT scanner or MR imager and new scans or images are taken to locate the endoscopes and instruments and to provide updated information about the patient's anatomy. For facial plastic surgery, we may use CT to check bony orientation and xeroradiographs for soft-tissue position.

Perhaps the most amazing developments are the experimental robotics applications. Several centers (such as Johns Hopkins University) and companies (such as Computer Motion of Santa Barbara) across the country have set up remote control surgery sites where aspects of surgery are actually performed by remote control. There is little doubt that technology will continue to advance.

chapter one

Surgical Anatomy for Endoscopic Facial Surgery

Wayne F. Larrabee, Jr.,
Kathleen H. Makielski, and Jonathan Sykes

Endoscopic surgery of the face is rapidly expanding its boundaries. Although currently used primarily for face-lift surgery, particularly in the forehead, endoscopic surgery may in the future become the method of choice for such procedures as revision rhinoplasty, repair of facial fractures, as well as other potential applications. There have been excellent books written on the anatomy of the face; therefore, in this chapter we will attempt to emphasize only those aspects of facial anatomy that are particularly relevant to endoscopic surgery as currently practiced. Specifically, it is important to understand the various fascial layers and the clefts between the layers where the endoscope can be passed. It is also necessary to know the functions of the specific muscles that can be treated endoscopically to create changes in the surface anatomy. We will not discuss the fine anatomy of the nose, lips, ears, or eyelids, because those topics are either not particularly relevant to endoscopic surgery at this time or are extensive and well covered in other books.

SYSTEMS AND CONCEPTS

Skin and Subcutaneous Tissue

The skin and immediately underlying subcutaneous fat form a complex organ that provides soft-tissue coverage for the hard-tissue foundation of the face. The intervening fascial layers create complex connections between hard- and soft-tissue layers. The surface of the face can be divided into facial aesthetic units. Within each unit, the skin is consistent in color, texture, thickness, and mobility. This principle of facial units has been refined in recent years by the subunit principle. Subunits are topographic units that have a predictable contour from person to person. By placing incisions at the boundaries of facial units or subunits, final scars are minimized visually because the eye is expecting a contour change. Our concept of the aesthetic facial units is demonstrated in Figure 1.1 and has been expanded upon in *Principles of Facial Reconstruction* (Larrabee and Sherris, 1995).

The skin is subdivided into the thinner, more superficial epidermis and the more fibrous dermis. The epidermis is stratified squamous epithelium, which varies greatly in depth, ranging from the thickness of the scalp to the delicate skin of the eyelid, which, at 0.04 mm, is the thinnest skin on the body. The dermis, composed primarily of connective tissue, also contains nerves, blood vessels, muscles, lymphatics, sweat glands, and pilosebaceous glands. The more superficial and thinner dermis is termed the papillary dermis. The deeper and thicker dermis is the reticular dermis. The dermis is composed primarily of collagen.

The dermis contains a superficial vascular plexus and a deep vascular plexus. The superficial plexus, also known as the subepidermal or subpapillary plexus, runs in the papillary dermis just beneath the epidermis, where it sends an arcade of capillary loops into each dermal papilla. The deep plexus, or dermal plexus, surrounds the skin appendages in the reticular dermis and is composed of larger vessels.

Subcutaneous fat varies greatly in thickness and texture among individuals and in different regions of the face. It is thickest in the concavities of the cheeks, temples, and neck. Lobules of subcutaneous fat are divided

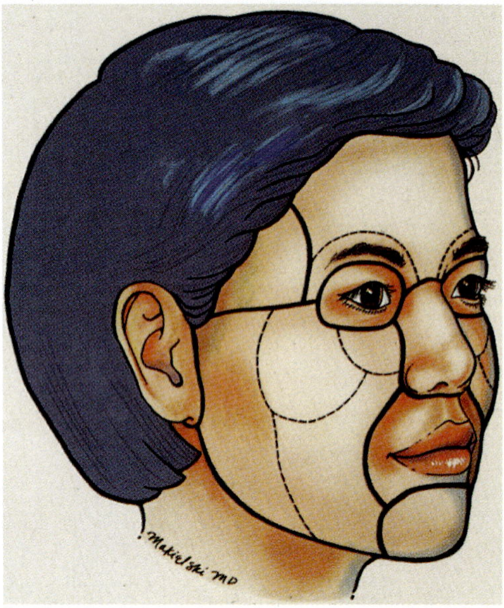

FIG. 1.1. Facial aesthetic units. The forehead, temple, cheeks, nose, periorbital area, lips, and chin each constitute a facial aesthetic unit that shares skin contour characteristics. Incisions that cross the unit boundaries should be avoided when possible. The forehead and the cheek have additional areas of variation in skin thickness that are indicated by dotted lines. *(From Larrabee W and Makielski K: Surgical anatomy of the face, Philadelphia, 1993, Raven.)*

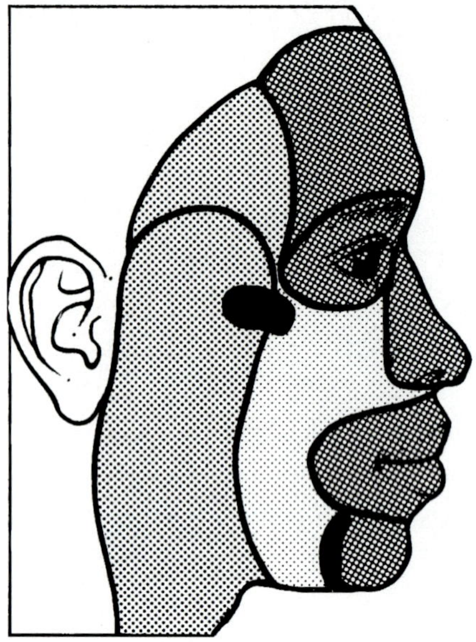

FIG. 1.2. The relative strength of attachments in the fibromuscular superficial musculoaponeurotic system and the dermis.

by fibrous septae, which contain vessels, nerves, and lymphatics. These septae represent a fibrofatty layer of subcutaneous tissue, which, in some areas of the face, connects to the fibromuscular layer of the superficial musculoaponeurotic system (SMAS). The fibromuscular layer consists of fibrous tissue, which envelops the muscles of facial expression. The connections between the fibrofatty and fibromuscular layers are variable throughout the face. They are quite strong in the lip, nose, forehead, scalp, and eyelids (Figures 1.2 and 1.3). They are almost nonexistent in the midcheek, and are of intermediate strength over the parotid, temples, and neck. The fibrous connections between the skin and deeper structures are important, particularly in face-lift surgery.

Fascia and Their Relationships

SMAS. The SMAS is a fibromuscular layer investing and interlinking the muscles of facial expression (Figure 1.4). The SMAS provides a conceptual framework to understand the fascial layers of the face. Although the SMAS as a structure exists in the neck, face, and scalp, it is distinctly different in each of these regions. The SMAS is essentially discontinuous at the zygoma (Figure 1.5). The fibrous galea aponeurotica is much stronger than the thin tenuous SMAS of the midcheek. Thus, particularly with endoscopic surgery, it is important to know the relative attachments and strengths of the SMAS in each area.

The SMAS concept was introduced by Tessier, and later defined by Mitz and Peyronie in 1976. The term "musculoaponeurotic" refers to the occasional muscular fibers seen in the fascia over the parotid and elsewhere in the face. The major vessels and nerves have consistent relationships to the SMAS within each region of the face. An understanding of these relationships can help the surgeon protect key structures and delineate correct dissection planes for the endoscope.

The characteristics used by Tessier and his students to describe the SMAS include: (1) it divides the subcutaneous fat into two layers; (2) fibrous septae extend from the dermis to the SMAS; (3) fat without septae lies between the deep facial muscles and the SMAS; (4) major vessels and nerves are initially deep to the SMAS and the smaller branches that perforate it, whereas the subdermal plexus is superficial to it; (5) the network of the SMAS acts as a distributor of force for the various facial muscles—a concept that has held up well, although there have been some areas of disagreement. In the original definition, the SMAS below the zygoma corresponds to the superficial fascia of classical anatomy, and thus is superficial to the parotid fascia. Jost and Levet (1984) described cadaver and clinical studies to support their view that the true SMAS layer in the cheek includes the parotid fascia. These authors believe that the parotid fascia, as a remnant of the primitive platysma, represents the structurally important layer of the SMAS in this area. They describe it as continuous with the platysma below and extending to the zygoma above. Wasset (1987) reported an anatomic study that confirms this position. His meticulous dissections revealed the parotid fascia to be essentially one

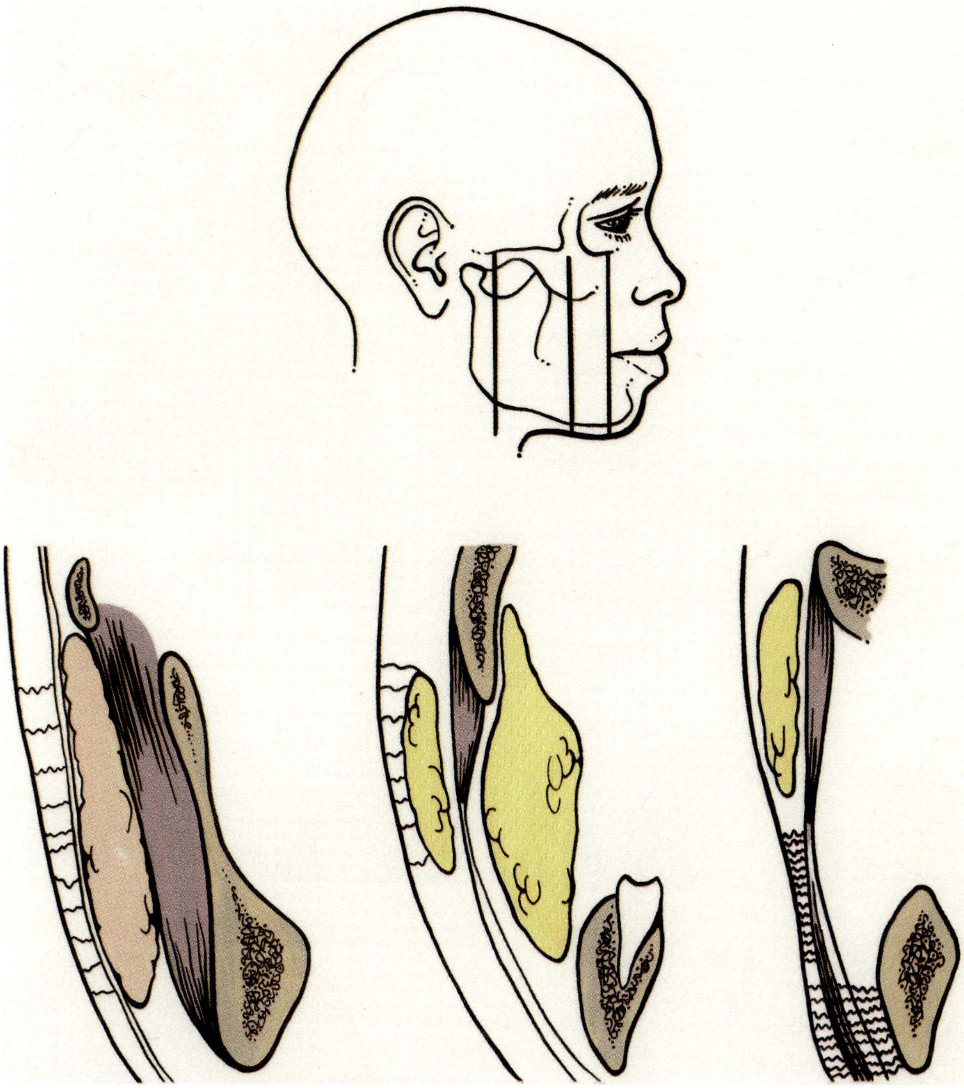

FIG. 1.3. Fascial attachments at the sequential facial planes. The attachments of the skin to underlying SMAS over the face. They are quite firm over the forehead, eye, nose, lip, and chin area. They are of intermediate strength over the cheek and neck area. They are relatively loose over the cheek and temple. The zygomatic masseteric ligaments and mandibular cutaneous ligaments are particularly strong and involve some attachments to the periosteum.

and the same as the SMAS. He believes that the platysma muscle, parotid fascia, and fibromuscular layer in the anterior cheek represent the same layer. This layer is analogous to the primitive platysma in other mammals. Wasset (1987) also states that the superficial layer of the orbicularis oris muscle, where the dermis is directly attached to the underlying muscular tissues, represents the SMAS. In the midface, the fibromuscular SMAS extends from the parotid and envelopes the facial muscles, including the zygomatic major muscle. Because of this firm attachment to the zygomatic major muscle, which has bony attachments, posterior tension on the SMAS cannot significantly affect the contour of the cheek anterior to this level.

Part of the complexity of these fascial layers is due to the difference in embryologic development between the muscles of the lower face and those of the midface and upper face (Figure 1.6). The muscles of the lower face and neck derive from the embryonic primitive platysma, including the true platysma, the risorius, the depressor anguli oris, the posterior auricular muscles, and the parotid fascia. The muscles of the midface and upper face derive from the embryonic sphincter colli profundus muscle, including the muscles of the skull and the muscles grouped around the orbit and upper mouth. Of interest, the muscles derived from the primitive platysma have limited bony insertions, whereas those derived from the sphincter colli profundus have strong bony insertions.

The SMAS above the zygoma is a more substantial layer than the fragile fibrous network seen in the midface. There is a discontinuity of the SMAS at the level of the zygoma because of attachments of the various fascial layers at the zygomatic arch. In the scalp, the SMAS is represented by the fibrous galea aponeurotica, which then splits to ensheathe the frontalis, the occipitalis, the procerus, and some of the periauricular muscles. In the temporal region, the SMAS, the superficial temporal fascia, and the temporoparietal fascia are synonymous.

There are important regional variations in the relationship of the SMAS to neurovascular structures. In the lower face, the facial nerve branches are always deep to the SMAS and innervate the facial muscles on their undersurface. The vessels and sensory nerves in the lower face similarly arise deep to the SMAS and remain at that level, except for their terminal branches. These structures are thus protected if dissection is superficial to the SMAS. In the midface, the facial nerve branches are pro-

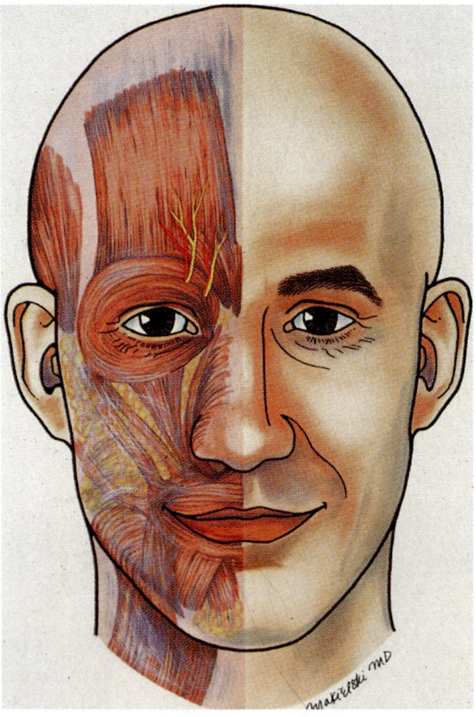

FIG. 1.4. Full-face view of the SMAS. The SMAS constitutes a fibromuscular network that interconnects the muscles of facial expression. In addition to its usefulness as a deep layer to tighten in face-lift surgery, it serves as a guide to the depth of key neurovascular structures in the lower face, and the facial nerve branches enter the muscles of facial expression on their deep side and are always deep to the SMAS. Similarly, in the lower face, vessels and sensory nerves originate deep to the SMAS, and their terminal branches run with it superficially. In the upper face, the important neurovascular structures arise from their deeper origins and course within the SMAS. The infratrochlear and supratrochlear neurovascular pedicles lie within the SMAS over the frontalis muscle. *(From Larrabee W and Makielski K: Surgical anatomy of the face, Philadelphia, 1993, Raven.)*

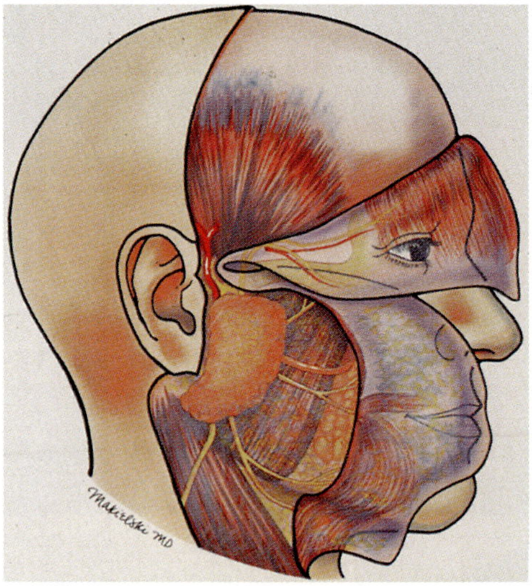

FIG. 1.5. The SMAS reflected. The SMAS is somewhat discontinuous at the zygoma. Below the zygoma, the SMAS is substantial over the parotid and the neck but becomes a more tenuous "meshwork" over the anterior cheeks, lips, and nose. The facial nerve branches and the parotid duct are seen deep to the SMAS and superficial to the masseter and the buccal fat pad. Above the zygoma, the SMAS is a more consistent layer that envelops the frontalis muscle and then forms the galea aponeurotica. The temporal branch of the facial nerve runs with the SMAS in the temple and is particularly vulnerable over the zygoma, where it lies quite superficially just beneath the subcutaneous fat. *(From Larrabee W and Makielski K: Surgical anatomy of the face, Philadelphia, 1993, Raven.)*

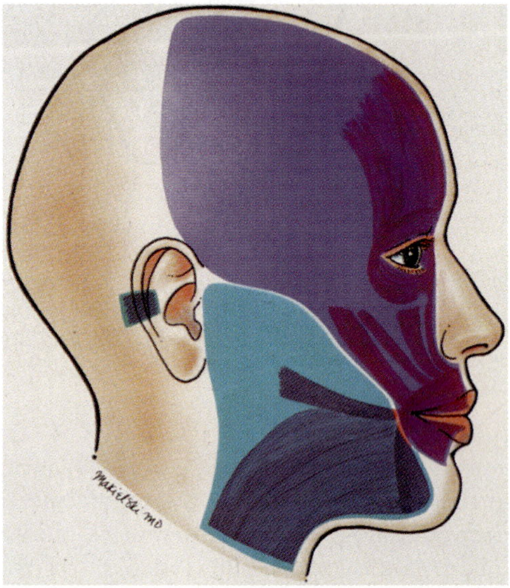

FIG. 1.6. Muscular derivations of the SMAS. The upper face and associated SMAS develop from the sphincter colli profundus. The SMAS in the lower face is derived from the primitive platysma. The frontalis muscle, superficial temporal fascia, orbicularis oculi muscle, elevators of the lip and the orbicularis oris muscle constitute the upper division. The lower division includes the true platysma and its fascia, risorius muscle, depressor anguli oris muscle, and posterior auricular muscle. The muscles derived from primitive platysma have limited bony insertions in contradistinction to those derived from the sphincter colli profundus. *(From Larrabee W and Makielski K: Surgical anatomy of the face, Philadelphia, 1993, Raven.)*

tected if the dissection is superficial to the muscles of facial expression (e.g., the zygomaticus major muscle).

In the temporal area, the temporal branch of the facial nerve emerges from its position deep within the parotid just inferior to the caudal border of the zygomatic arch. At the arch level, it closely approximates the periosteum and lies deep to the temporalis fascias. Once the nerve has crossed the arch, it emerges from the deeper fascia and lies within the fatty tissue on the deep surface of the temporoparietal fascia (SMAS) until it enters the undersurface of the frontalis muscle. In the upper face, the vessels and sensory nerves arise from their origins (bony foramina or notches) and penetrate the SMAS. Here, they run within the superficial aspects of the SMAS or on its surface. Examples are the supraorbital and supratrochlear neurovascular bundles that arise from their respective foramina (or a joint notch), penetrate the SMAS, and then course along the superficial aspect of the frontalis muscle. The sensory nerves emerge from deep to superficial with a common pattern (Figure 1.7). The more medial branches of the nerves emerge from the submuscular to the subcutaneous plane almost immediately after leaving the orbit; the more lateral branches traverse superiorly before making this change to the subcutaneous plane. Similarly, the superficial temporal vessels course with the auriculotemporal nerve along the SMAS (temporal parietal fascia or superficial temporal fascia) for a few centimeters before entering the subcutaneous fat.

The Temporalis Fascia

The temporalis fascia is a key landmark to various endoscopic procedures. The terminology in this area has always been somewhat confusing and has become more so with the advent of various deep plane, subperiosteal, and endoscopic techniques. Some surgeons have suggested redesignating these layers with a more logical nomenclature. Table 1.1 represents some of these alternatives. Although it is possible to design new systems, at this point in time they are confusing and we believe it is preferable to retain traditional terminology. For example, the superficial temporal fascia or temporal parietal fascia is an extension of the SMAS in the lower face. We prefer to call this layer the "temporal parietal fascia" so it is not confused with the layers of the deep temporalis fascia. Similarly, we suggest calling the fatty layer, which lies just deep to the temporal parietal fascia above the zygomatic arch, the "temporal parietal fat pad." This differentiates it from the superficial temporal fat, which lies between the superficial and deep layers of the deep temporal fascia.

The temporalis muscle is covered by a dense tough fascia, the deep temporalis fascia, which is continuous with the periosteum of the skull at the temporal line. A few centimeters above the zygomatic arch at approximately the level of the superior orbital rim is the temporal line of fusion, where the deep temporalis fascia splits into its superficial and deep layers, which then insert into the superficial and deep surfaces of the zygomatic arch at its superior surface (Figures 1.8 and 1.9). Between these two layers is found the wedge-shaped superficial temporal fat pad, which sits on the superior surface of the zygomatic arch. As discussed previously, there is a more tenuous fatty layer (temporal parietal fat pad), which is used as a key landmark in endoscopic procedures that is superior to the arch, superficial to the superficial layer of the deep temporal fascia, and deep to the temporal parietal fascia; it is contiguous with the subaponeurotic plane. The middle temporal artery, which arises from the superficial temporal artery at the level of the zygomatic arch, enters the deep tem-

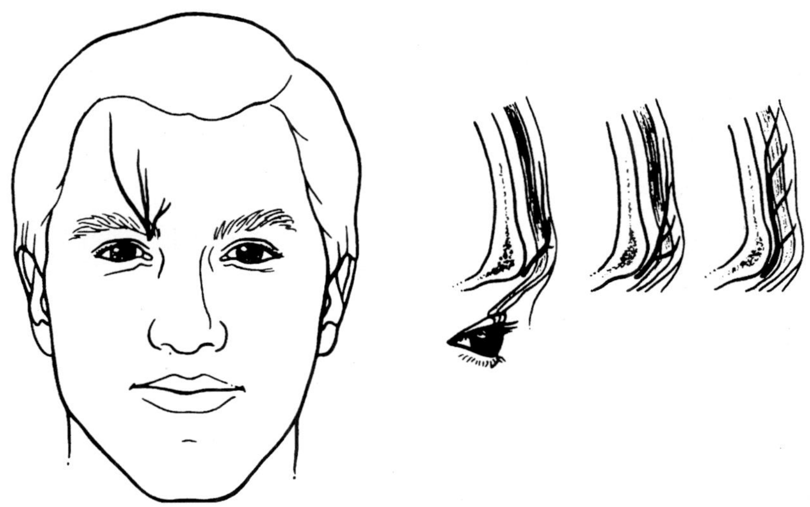

FIG. 1.7. The more lateral branches of the sensory nerves of the forehead penetrate the frontalis muscle in a more superior plane. *(From Larrabee W: Facelift anatomy, Facial Plastic Surgery Clinics of North America, Nov. 1993.)*

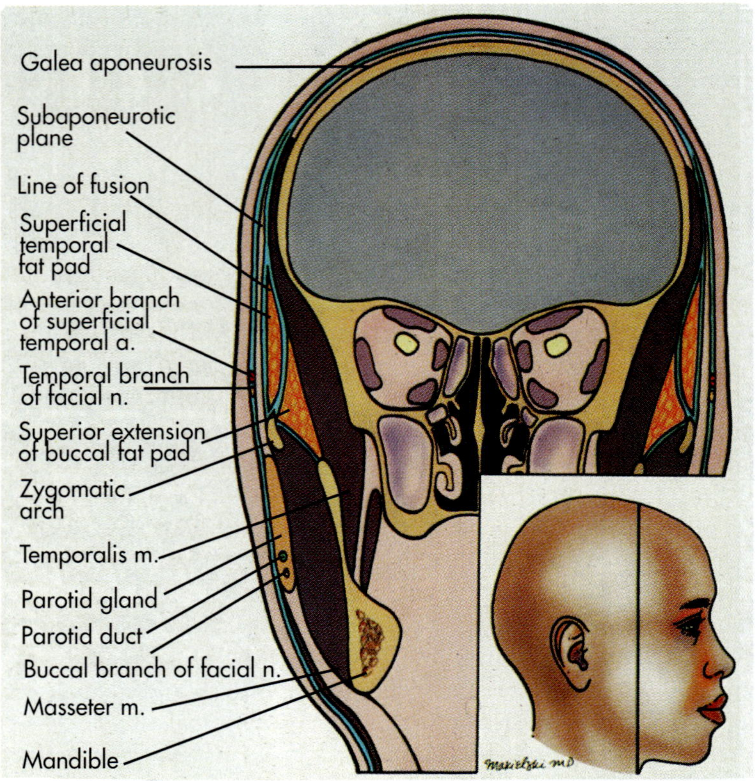

FIG. 1.8. Coronal section demonstrating the SMAS. The fibrous galea aponeurosis divides anteriorly and posteriorly to ensheathe the frontalis and the occipitalis muscles. In the coronal plane, the galea aponeurosis extends to the temporalis muscle, where it thins and covers the temporalis fascia as a layer of the SMAS (alternatively called the superficial temporal fascia or the temporoparietal fascia). In the temple above the zygoma, the temporal branch of the facial nerve and the anterior branch of the superficial temporal artery run within this layer of the SMAS. The deep temporalis fascia splits at its line of fusion into deep and superficial layers. Both attach to the zygoma, and between them lies the superficial temporal fat pad. The superior extension of the buccal fat pad lies deep to the deep layer of the temporalis fascia. Inferior to the zygoma, the SMAS covers the parotid gland and becomes contiguous with the platysma. In this plane, the parotid duct and the buccal branch of the facial nerve lie within the parotid. The muscles of mastication surround and insert into the mandible. *(From Larrabee W and Makielski K: Surgical anatomy of the face, Philadelphia, 1993, Raven.)*

TABLE 1.1
SOFT-TISSUE LAYERS IN THE TEMPORAL AREA

Layers	Alternate Names
Skin	None
Subcutaneous fat	None
Temporal parietal fascia	SMAS Superficial temporal fascia
Subaponeurotic plane	Subgaleal fascia Innominate fascia Aereolar fascia Loose areolar tissue
Temporal parietal fat	Superficial temporal fat (Ramirez, 1991)
Superficial layer deep temporal fascia	Intermediate temporal fascia (Ramirez, 1991)
Superficial temporal fat pad	Intermediate temporal fat (Ramirez, 1991)
Deep layer deep temporalis fascia	Deep temporal fascia
Deep temporal fat pad	None

poralis fascia immediately above the zygomatic arch, supplies the fascia and the superficial temporal fat pad, and gives off branches to the temporalis itself.

Superficial to the deep temporalis fascia is the temporal parietal or superficial temporalis fascia. It lies immediately deep to the dermis, and is continuous with the galea aponeurotica above and the SMAS of the face below. The superficial temporal artery and its anterior and posterior branches lie within the fascia and the accompanying vein lies immediately

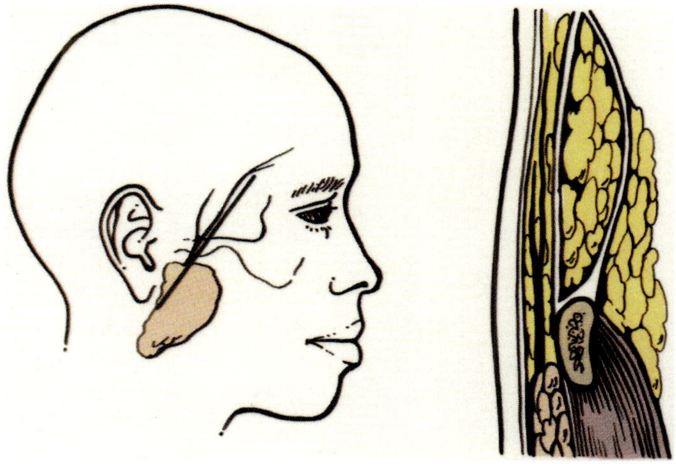

FIG. 1.9. Relationship of the frontal branch of the facial nerve to the zygomatic arch.

superficial to it. The superficial surface of the temporal parietal fascia is attached loosely to the subdermal tissues. The temporal branch of the facial nerve lies within and then immediately deep to the fascia, 1 to 2 cm posterior to the lateral orbital rim in a thin layer of fat. The surgeon is more likely to recognize the superficial temporalis fascia after passing through it, thus putting the nerve at risk. A surgical approach that goes deep to the superficial layer of the deep temporalis fascia inferior to the line of fusion is the safest way to avoid the nerve, although this can cause some fat atrophy.

Both the deep and superficial temporalis fascial layers have axial blood supplies that are provided by the middle temporal artery and the superficial temporal artery, respectively.

A very important plane (or layer) lies between the temporal parietal fascia and the superficial layer of the deep temporal fascia. We prefer the term "subaponeurotic plane," but it has also been termed the "innominate fascia," "areolar fascia" (or plane), "submuscular aponeurotic fascia," and "subepicranial fascia." Anteriorly, this plane is continuous with the eyebrow fat pad or retro-orbicularis oculi fat (ROOF). Inferiorly, it extends to the temporal parietal fat pad and then the zygomatic arch. It is well supplied by vessels from the superficial temporal artery. In endoscopic surgery this layer, which contains the temporal parietal fat pad, the eyebrow fat pad (ROOF), and by analogy the suborbicularis oculi fat pad (SOOF), has become important as a landmark and occasionally as a mechanical support structure.

FACIAL MUSCULATURE

The muscles of facial expression are of primary interest to the endoscopist. These mimetic muscles move the skin of the face and scalp and act as sphincters for the eyes, nose, and mouth (Figure 1.10). They are innervated by the facial nerve, the motor nerve of the second branchial arch. There is considerable individual variation, and frequently these muscles blend into one another.

Forehead

The frontalis and corrugator supercilii muscles are the primary muscles of the forehead. The frontalis muscle courses vertically and inserts into the galea aponeurotica (Figure 1.11). It raises the eyebrows and produces transverse forehead wrinkles. A paralysis of the temporal branch of the facial nerve, which innervates the frontalis muscle, causes a unilateral brow ptosis and loss of forehead motion. The corrugators arise from the medial orbital rim just above the nose and insert into the frontalis muscle and skin of the eyebrows. These paired muscles act to pull the eyebrows together and to produce glabellar frown lines. The corrugator, procerus, and orbicularis oculi muscles (with the depressor supercili muscles) act in concert to close the eyes and create transverse and oblique glabellar lines (Figure 1.12).

The frontalis muscle forms the frontal belly of the occipitofrontalis muscle. Each quadrangular segment of the frontalis muscle is wider and taller than the opposing occipital muscle and contains muscle bundles that are more delicate than those of the occipital muscle. The frontalis muscle has no bony attachments. Superiorly, it inserts into the galea aponeurotica. Inferiorly, it merges with the procerus muscle, corrugator muscle, and the orbicularis oculi muscle.

Orbicularis Oculi

The orbicularis oculi surrounds the orbit and extends into both eyelids. It originates from the periosteum of the medial orbital margin and the medial canthal tendon. Its attachments are all medial to the supraorbital neurovascular bundle. The muscle surrounds the orbit and is arbitrarily divided into orbital, palpebral, and lacrimal portions.

The palpebral portion of the orbicularis muscle is commonly divided into preseptal and pretarsal parts: the preseptal part overlies the orbital septum, and the pretarsal part overlies the tarsal plate. The preseptal portion arises from two heads: a deep head attached to the lacrimal fossa and posterior crest, and a superficial head arising from the medial canthal tendon. Laterally, the preseptal muscles join at the lateral palpebral raphe. The pretarsal part also originates from two heads: a deep head termed the "tensor tarsi" (Horner's muscle) and a superficial head from the medial canthal tendon. The superficial heads of the preseptal and pretarsal muscles in essence become the medial canthal tendon. The medial canthal tendon has a close relationship to the lacrimal sac. The sac lies between the anterior and posterior limbs, and contraction of the tendon creates a pumping action in the sac.

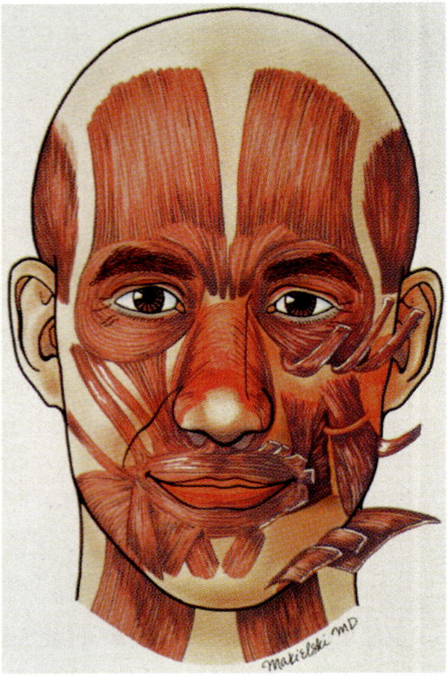

FIG. 1.10. Musculature of face. The risorius, the major and the minor zygomatic, and the levator labii superioris muscles on the face's left side have been reflected to show the underlying levator anguli oris and the buccinator muscles. *(From Larrabee W and Makielski K: Surgical anatomy of the face, Philadelphia, 1993, Raven.)*

Laterally, the pretarsal muscles join to form the lateral canthal tendon, which inserts on the periosteum of the orbital tubercle approximately 5 mm behind the rim.

The medial superior fibers of the orbicularis depress the medial brow. These fibers can be more or less separate from the remainder of the orbicularis and are named the depressor supercilii muscle. The orbicularis oculi muscle merges at the periphery with the surrounding muscles to include the frontalis, procerus, and corrugator. Inferiorly, the orbicularis is superficial to the muscles of facial expression, including the levator muscles of the upper lip and the zygomatic major muscle.

Nose

The nasal muscles are the procerus, nasalis, and depressor septi (Figures 1.13 and 1.14). The procerus is

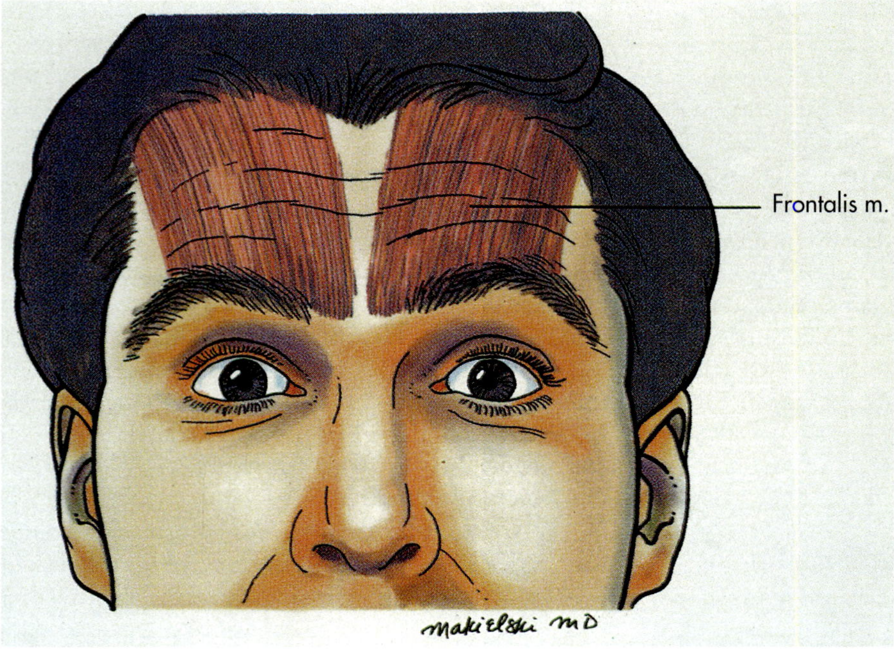

FIG. 1.11. Frontalis muscle. The frontalis muscle elevates the brows and creates the horizontal forehead creases. The lateral extent of the frontalis muscle corresponds to the extent of the forehead creases. *(From Larrabee W and Makielski K: Surgical anatomy of the face, Philadelphia, 1993, Raven.)*

the most superior of this group, arising from the nasal bone and upper lateral cartilage and inserting into the forehead skin. The procerus pulls forehead skin down and may cause transverse creases between the brows.

There are two parts to the nasalis muscle. The upper, transverse part attaches to its counterpart across the dorsum of the nose and acts to compress the naris—hence its other name, compressor naris. It continues into the lip area where it becomes confluent with the orbicularis oris and attaches to the anterior nasal spine and premaxilla. The second part is the alar portion, or dilator naris, so named because it elevates the lower lateral cartilage to flare the nostril.

Cheek

The buccinator muscle (bugler's muscle) arises posteriorly from the pterygomandibular raphe and the alveolar processes of the maxilla and mandible, deep to the buccal fat pocket, and extends anteriorly to attach to the mouth at the orbicularis oris muscle. The buccinator functions to keep food between the teeth during chewing and maintains air pressure during blowing.

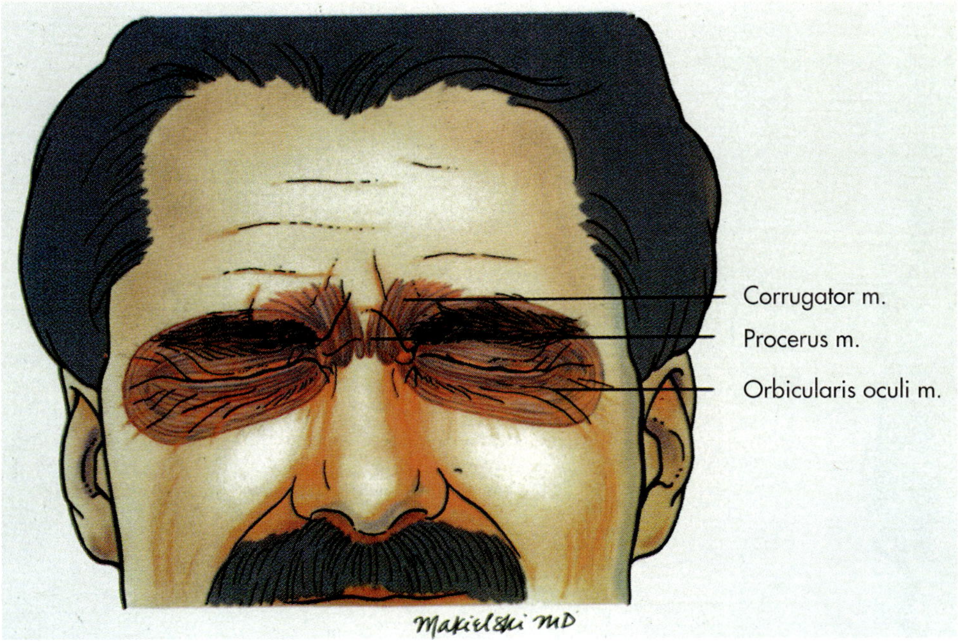

FIG. 1.12. Orbicularis oculi, procerus, and corrugator muscles. These muscles act as a unit to close the eyes and create facial expressions such as a "squint." *(From Larrabee W and Makielski K: Surgical anatomy of the face, Philadelphia, 1993, Raven.)*

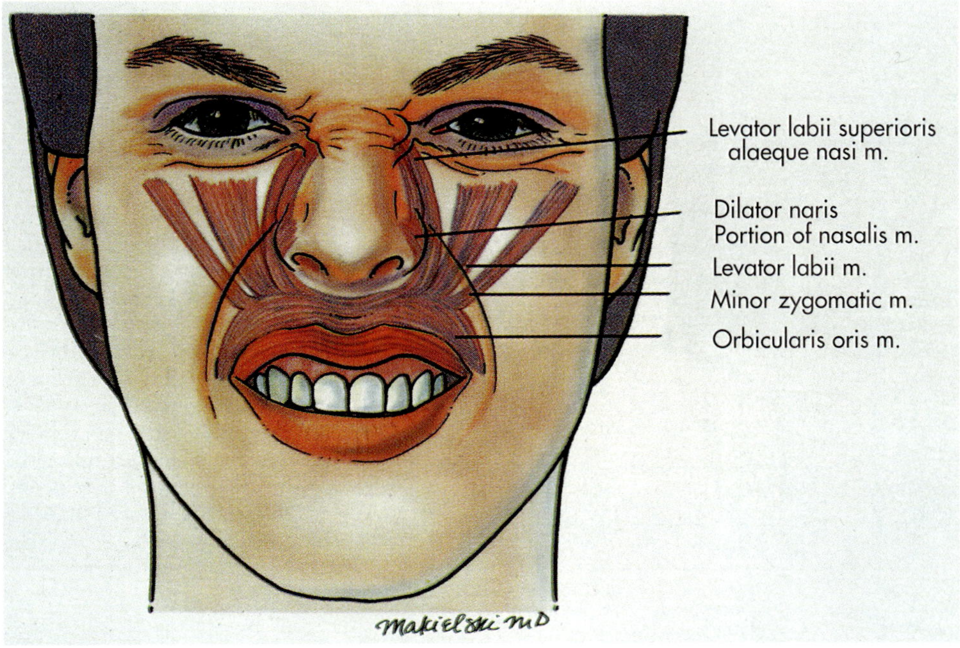

FIG. 1.13. Upper lip and nasal musculature. The orbicularis oris muscle is primarily a sphincter essential for oral competence, speech, and social expression. Its contraction is opposed superiorly by the action of the major lip elevators: the nasalis, the levator labii, and the minor zygomatic muscles. *(From Larrabee W and Makielski K: Surgical anatomy of the face, Philadelphia, 1993, Raven.)*

Mouth and Lips

The anatomy of the perioral musculature is extremely complex (Figure 1.15). Although the orbicularis oris does have a simple sphincter function, it is composed of various layers of muscular filaments with different directions of pull. It is, in essence, a confluence of various mimetic muscles, which can be roughly divided into elevators and depressors of the lip. The deeper muscles include the buccinator mentioned previously, which inserts into the modiolus at the commissure. At the next level toward the skin lie the levator anguli oris (caninus) and the depressor anguli oris (triangularis). These cross each other and run respectively into the lower and upper lip. At the next more superficial level, one sees from lateral to medial the major zygomatic major, the zygomatic minor, the levator labii, and the levator labii superioris alaeque nasi muscles (Figure 1.16). The zygomaticus major muscle arises from the zygomatic bone near the zygomaticotemporal suture. Its most superior part is covered by the obicularis oculi muscle. It inserts at the modiolus of the mouth and interdigitates with the levator anguli oris, the buccinator, and the depressor anguli oris. The origin of the zygomaticus major muscle can be found at the inferior aspect of the malar bone where it is crossed by a line drawn from the lateral canthus to the angle of the mandible. From lateral to medial over the lower lip are the risorius muscle, which moves the corner of the mouth, and the lip depressors, which include the depressor labii inferioris with variant contributions from the

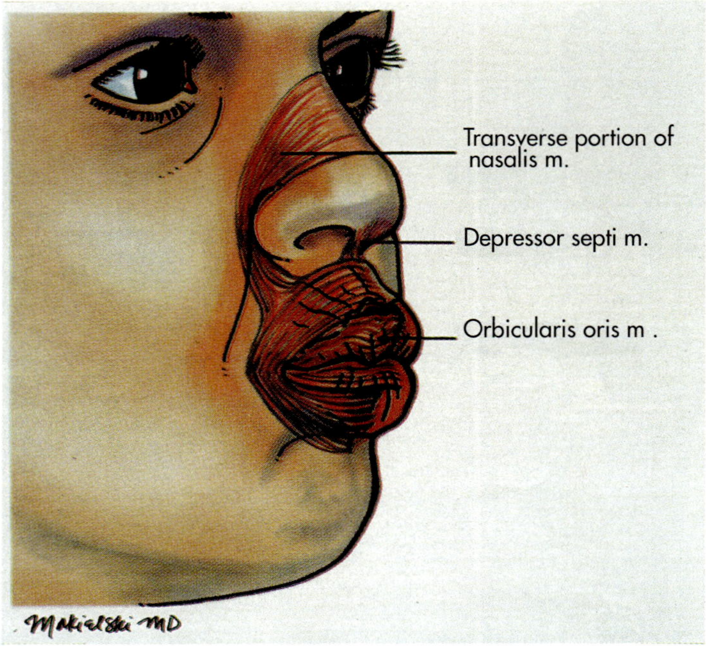

FIG. 1.14. Orbicularis oris and nasal musculature. The nasalis and the depressor septi muscles interdigitate with the orbicularis oris muscle. A strong depressor septi muscle depresses the nasal tip with smiling and can be interrupted during rhinoplasty surgery to decrease active tip depression and help maintain tip position. *(From Larrabee W and Makielski K: Surgical anatomy of the face, Philadelphia, 1993, Raven.)*

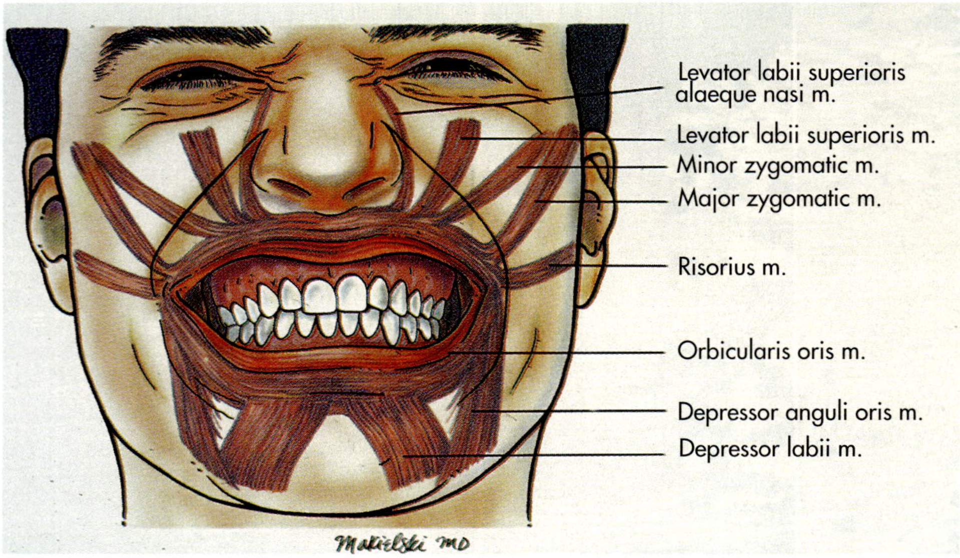

FIG. 1.15. Musculature of mouth and lips. The multiple functions of the lips (oral competence, speech, social expression) require a complex set of motions facilitated by the antagonism between the circular contraction of the orbicularis oris and the radial action of the lip elevators and depressors. *(From Larrabee W and Makielski K: Surgical anatomy of the face, Philadelphia, 1993, Raven.)*

platysma itself (Figure 1.17). The mentalis muscle attaches from the soft tissue inferior to the lip to the mandible and is responsible for elevating and protruding the lower lip.

All of these muscles work in a complex fashion for facial expression, speech, and other functions of the lips. The risorius pulls the angle of the mouth primarily laterally, whereas the depressor labii inferioris has a primarily inferior and slightly lateral pull on the lower lip. The depressor anguli oris also depresses the angle of the mouth primarily inferiorly. The zygomatic major pulls the angle of the mouth superiorly and somewhat laterally. The levator labii superioris elevates the upper lip and pulls it slightly anteriorly. The levator labii superioris alaeque nasi has two slips; one elevates the lip, and one dilates the nares. The levator anguli oris muscle, the buccinator muscle, the corrugator supercilii muscle, and the deeper segments of the orbicularis oris muscle constitute a foundation of the perioral musculature. The remainder of the muscles discussed, including the superficial portions of the orbicularis oris, are more superficial.

Platysma

The platysma muscle is a flat muscle whose thickness varies widely among individuals; men generally have a thicker platysma than women. Inferiorly, this muscle inserts into the subcutaneous tissues of the subclavicular and acromial regions; superiorly, it inserts into the chin at the commissures of the mouth and into the anterior one third of the oblique line of the jaw. The platysma is a depressor of the lower lip innervated by the cervical branch of the facial nerve. Posteriorly and superiorly, the fibers form an S and pass posteriorly to the angle of the mandible. Medially, the fibers usually interdigitate and form an inverted V at the chin, 1 to 2 cm below it (most common), or at the level of the thyroid cartilage (Cardosa, 1980). Deep to the platysma are the

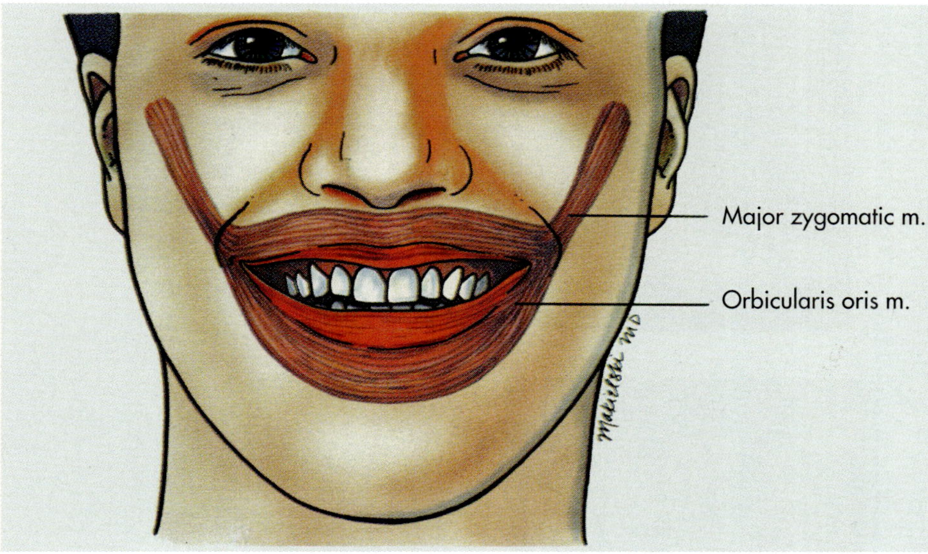

FIG. 1.16. Smile muscles. The major zygomatic and the orbicularis oris are the main muscles used to smile. Other muscles contribute to the subtle lip movements needed for the vast range of facial expression. The major zygomatic muscle contracts in approximately the same vector as that desired for the temporalis muscle when it is transferred for facial reanimation. *(From Larrabee W and Makielski K: Surgical anatomy of the face, Philadelphia, 1993, Raven.)*

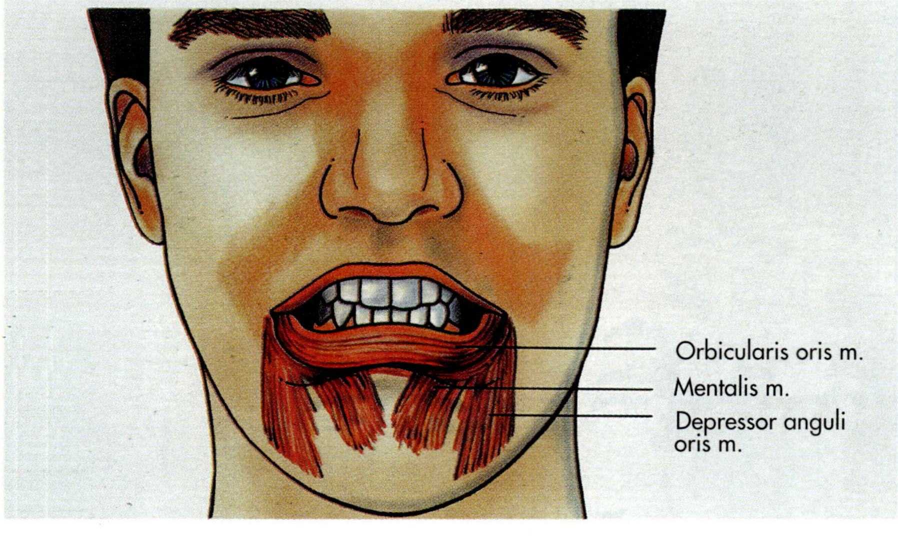

FIG. 1.17. Lip depressors and mentalis. These muscles are innervated by the marginal mandibular branch of the facial nerve. Unilateral paralysis of this branch results in the typical facial asymmetry seen with smiling, in which the counteraction of the orbicularis oris muscle creates an elevation of the lip on the paralyzed side. (Depressor labii inferioris has been removed to better show the mentalis muscle). Mentalis muscle elevates and protrudes the lip. *(From Larrabee W and Makielski K: Surgical anatomy of the face, Philadelphia, 1993, Raven.)*

submandibular glands, the facial nerve, and facial artery. Laxity of the platysma with age creates "platysma banding" and can accentuate submandibular gland ptosis.

Muscles of Mastication

Among the muscles of mastication, the masseter and temporalis muscles have the greatest surgical relevance (Figure 1.18).

The masseter. The masseter muscle arises in two portions from the zygomatic arch. Its superficial part arises from the lower border of the anterior two thirds of the arch, whereas its deep part arises from the inner surface of the arch and its posterior third. The fibers of the superficial part run inferiorly and posteriorly, whereas the deep fibers run almost directly inferiorly. The muscle as a whole inserts into the entire lateral ramus of the mandible. The nerve supply is the masseteric nerve from the mandibular division of the fifth cranial nerve (V), and the arterial supply is the masseteric artery from the maxillary artery. The neurovascular bundle runs through the coronoid notch to enter the deep surface of the muscle, where it arbor-

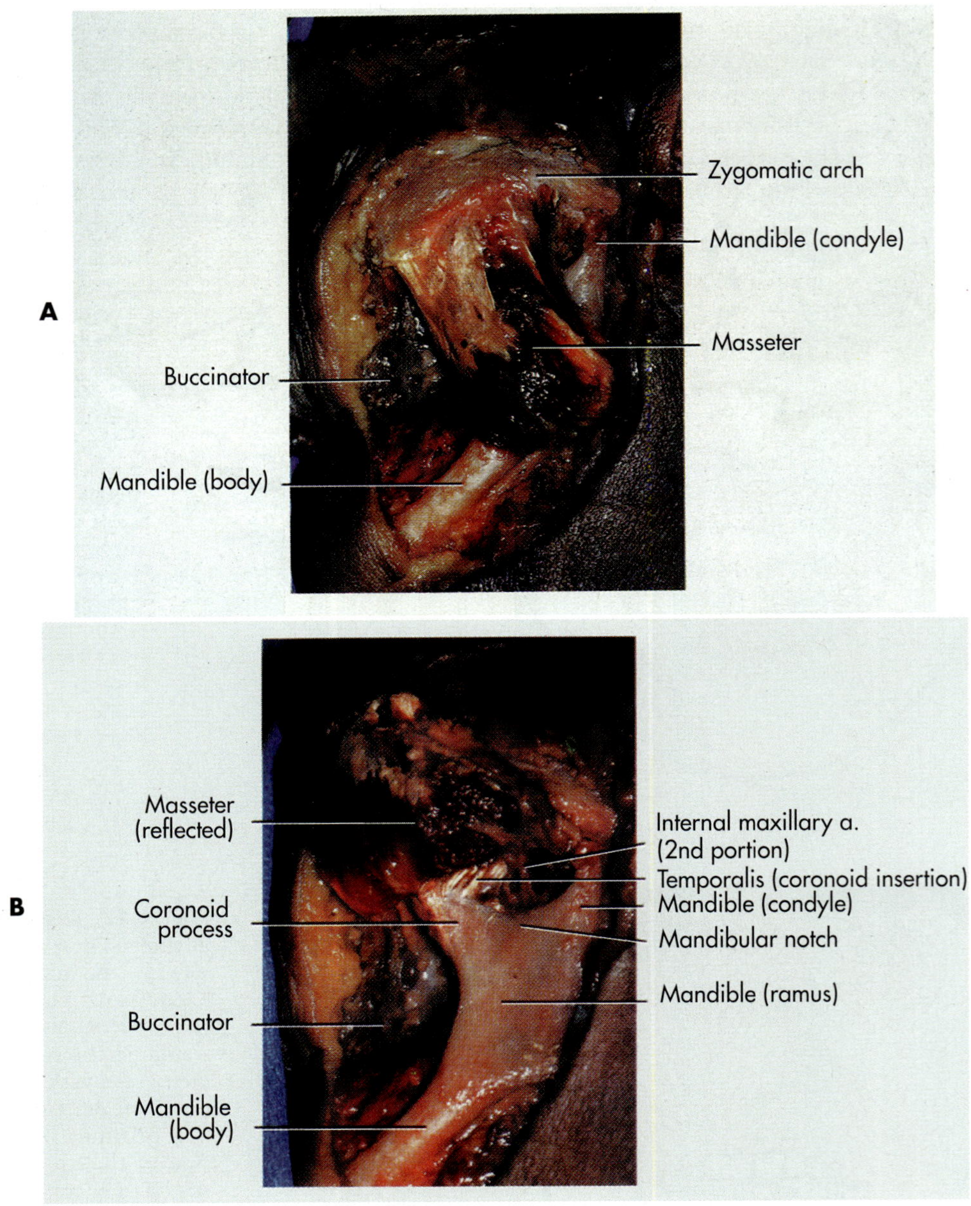

FIG. 1.18. Deep relationships of masseter and temporalis muscles. **A,** The masseter has been reflected from the ramus of the mandible to show the vascular supply. The insertion of the temporalis on the coronoid process is demonstrated, and the contents in the mandibular notch are clearly visible. **B,** The superficial temporal fascia and superficial layer of the deep temporal fascia have been removed to the line of fusion, revealing the superficial temporal fat pad.

Continued.

izes in an oblique anteroinferior direction (Castro and Zani, 1973).

The parotid gland overlies the posterior portion of the masseter, and the buccal branches of the facial nerve are closely applied to the anterior muscle body by the parotid-masseteric fascia (Figure 1.19). The buccal fat pocket lies just deep to its anterior edge.

The temporalis. The temporalis is a broad, fan-shaped muscle originating from the temporal fossa on the side of the skull. Its fibers converge into a tendon, which inserts into both the medial side of the ramus of the mandible and the entire coronoid process. The temporal extension of the buccal fat pocket lies on the temporalis tendon, which separates it from the zygomatic arch, and then continues around the anterior edge of the muscle along the lateral orbital wall. The innervation of the temporalis is from the mandibular branch of the trigeminal nerve via two (usually) deep temporal nerves, the anterior and the posterior. The blood supply is from the temporal branches of the maxillary artery. The blood vessels and nerves travel together from the infratemporal fossa to enter the deep surface of the temporalis.

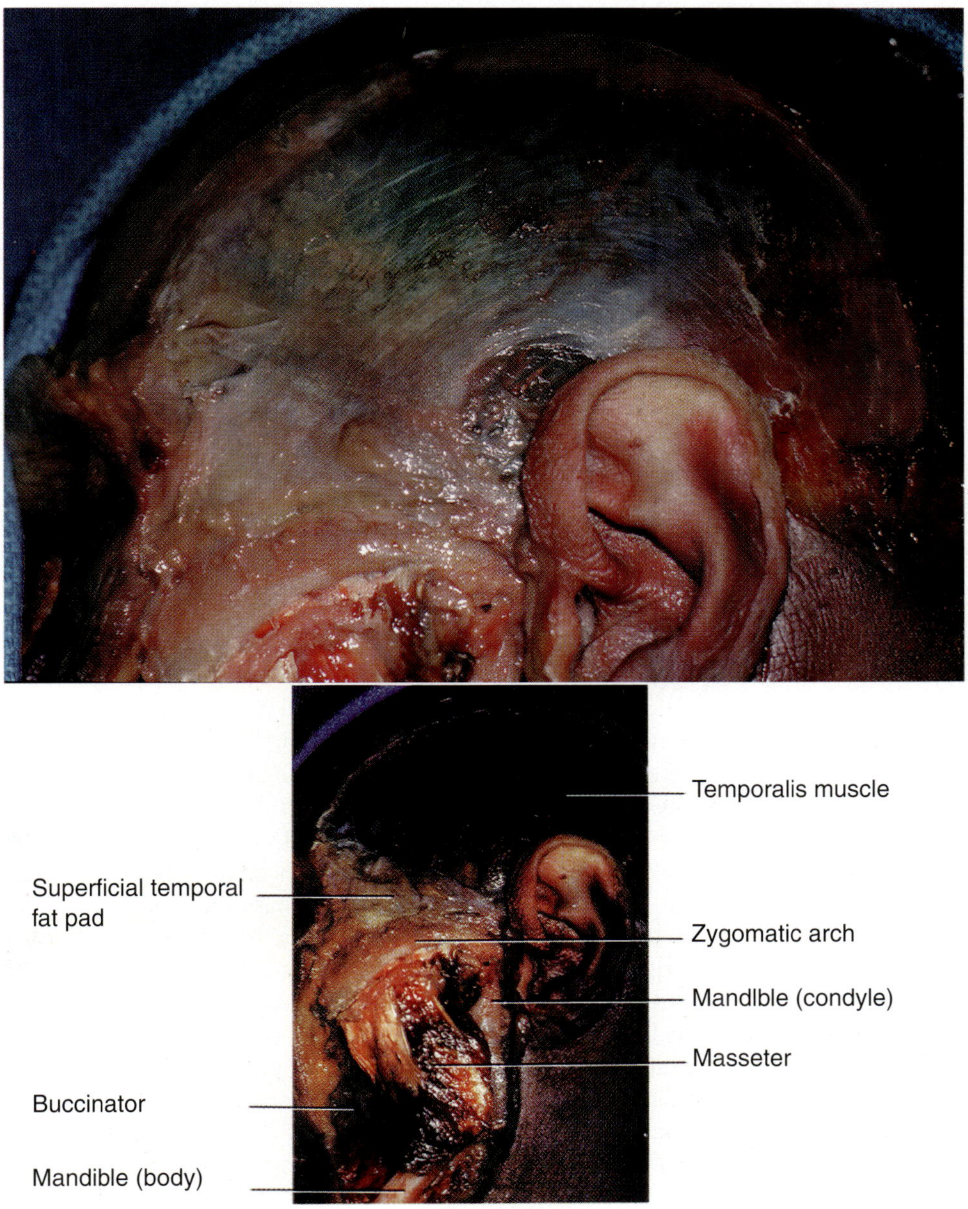

FIG. 1.18, cont'd. C, The superficial layer of the deep temporal fascia has been removed. The deep layer of the deep temporal fascia has been preserved and is shown underlying the superficial temporal fat pad. **D,** The superficial temporal fat pad has been removed, which demonstrates the insertion of the temporalis on the coronoid process of the mandible. *(From Larrabee W and Makielski K: Surgical anatomy of the face, Philadelphia, 1993, Raven.)*

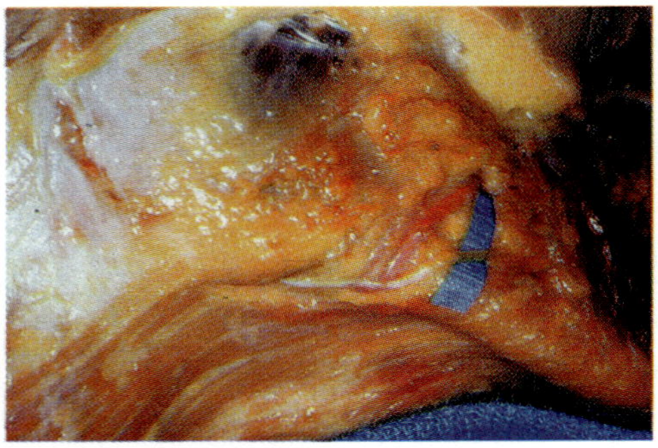

FIG. 1.19. Masseter muscle with facial nerve branches. Buccal branches of the facial nerve course over the masseter within the fascia after they exit the parotid gland. *(From Larrabee W and Makielski K: Surgical anatomy of the face, Philadelphia, 1993, Raven.)*

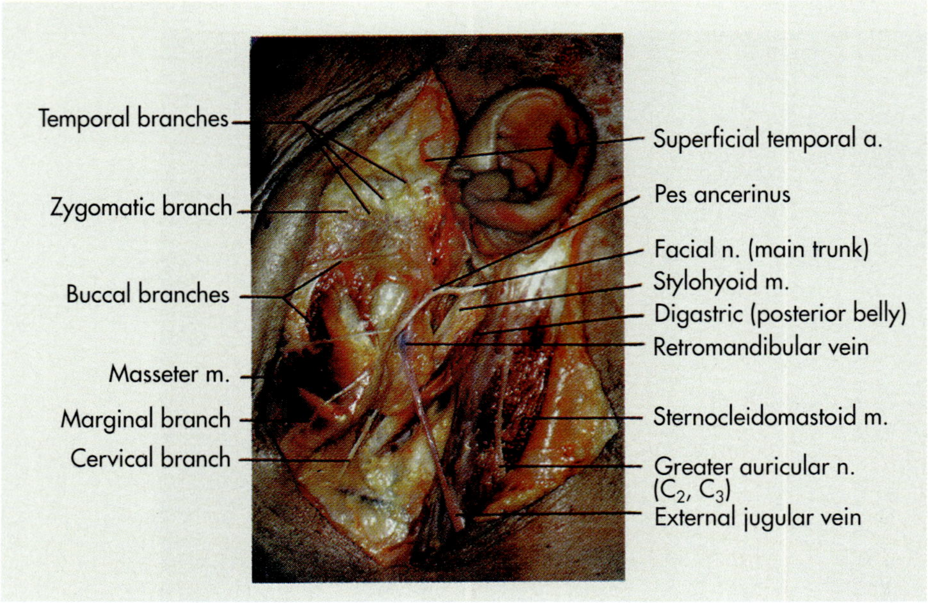

FIG. 1.20. Facial nerve after a total parotidectomy. The facial nerve exits the stylomastoid foramen and divides into inferior and superior segments at the pes ancerinus. In this case, note the multiple temporal branches and the relationship of the nerve branches to the posterior belly of the digastric. The buccal branches overlie the masseter. The greater auricular nerve courses over the sternocleidomastoid muscle. *(From Larrabee W and Makielski K: Surgical anatomy of the face, Philadelphia, 1993, Raven.)*

FACIAL NERVE

The pathways of the facial nerve from the stylomastoid foramen to the undersurface of the muscles it innervates are quite variable. A knowledge of the landmarks for the common branching patterns and the depth of the nerve in specific regions is essential for safe and effective endoscopic surgery.

The main trunk of the nerve exits the stylomastoid foramen and immediately enters the parotid gland. The five commonly listed major branches of the facial nerve are the temporal (or frontal), zygomatic, buccal, marginal mandibular, and cervical rami. In reality, the main trunk usually divides within the parotid into superior (temporofacial) and inferior (cervicofacial) divisions, but the branching patterns then become quite variable. Davis and colleagues (1956) classified these patterns into six types; although of interest, this type of classification is not of much practical benefit. A cadaver dissection shows a typical configuration. There are frequent anastomoses between the buccal and zygomatic branches. The cervical branches are somewhat at risk with subplatysma dissection (Figure 1.20). In 4% to 5% of the population, the cervical branch innervates the depressors of the lip; in these patients, damage to the cervical branch can give a pseudomarginal paralysis. The temporal and mandibular branches are usually terminal branches without anastomotic connections. The buccal branches are at risk during surgery where they cross over the masseter muscle and the buccal fat pad.

The temporal branches of the facial nerve have perhaps the most complex anatomy, both in terms of horizontal branching patterns and in their relationship to fascial and muscular layers. The literature is somewhat contradictory, particularly concerning surface landmarks that determine the course of the nerve.

The path of the temporal branch of the nerve was described during the discussion of the SMAS. In summary, it emerges just beneath the zygomatic arch from the parotid, crosses over the periosteum of the zygomatic arch, and then becomes more superficial and runs on the deep surface of the temporal parietal fascia (SMAS) before entering the undersurface of the frontalis muscle (Figure 1.21). The nerve branches are

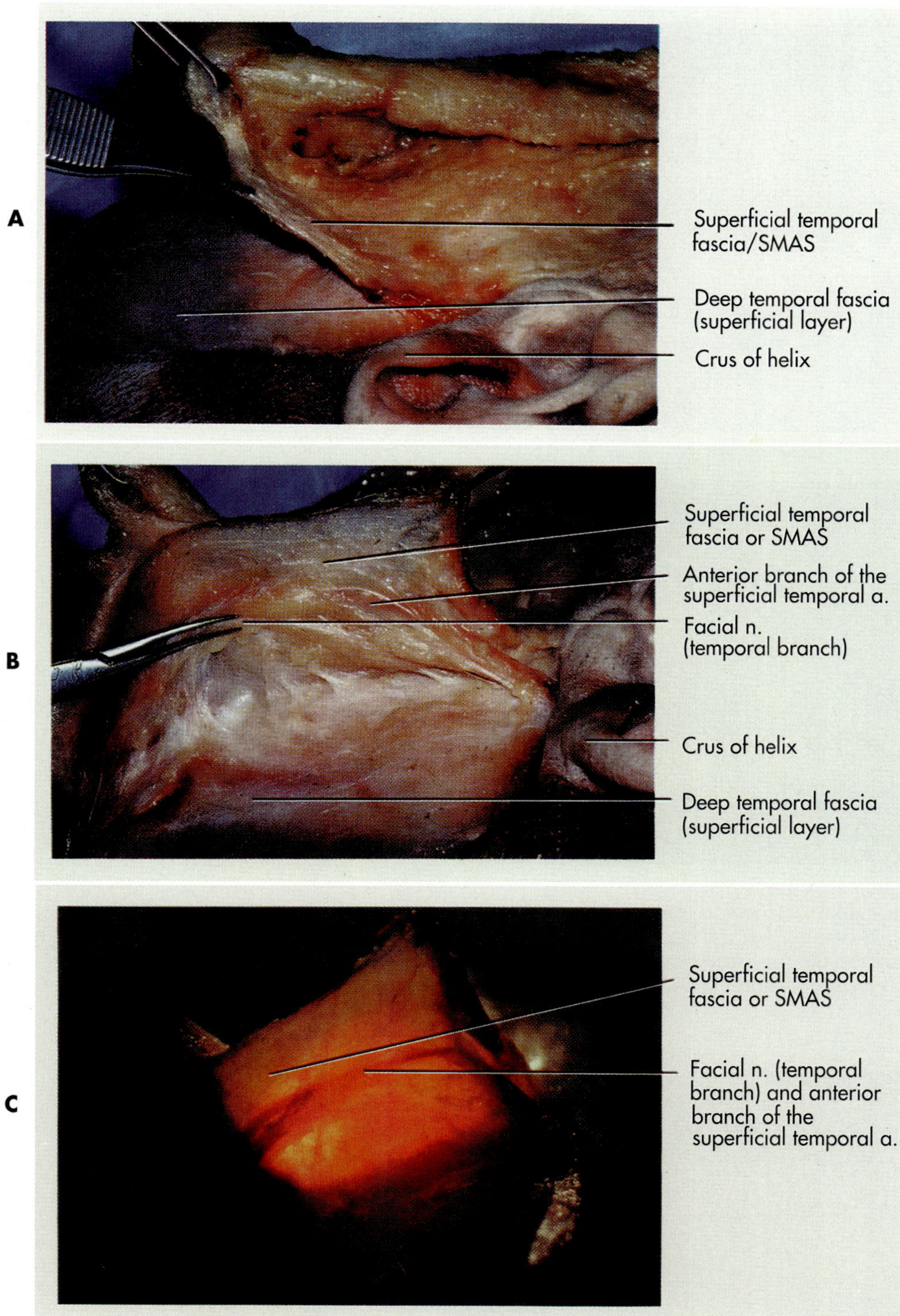

FIG. 1.21. Relationship of the SMAS, temporalis fascia, and frontal branch of the facial nerve. **A,** A bicoronal flap has been elevated in the subgaleal plane. Over the temporalis muscle, dissection is deep to the superficial temporal fascia, which carries the temporal branch of the facial nerve. A skin flap has been elevated inferiorly. The superficial temporal fascia, which is continuous with the SMAS inferiorly, is seen posteriorly (retracted with clamps). **B,** The same dissection is seen from above, which demonstrates the temporal branch of the facial nerve (hemostat) running in the SMAS with the anterior branch of the superficial temporal artery. **C,** The SMAS is transilluminated to demonstrate the temporal branch of the facial nerve and accompanying artery. *(From Larrabee W and Makielski K: Surgical anatomy of the face, Philadelphia, 1993, Raven.)*

superficial to both layers of the deep temporalis fascia. Thus, to avoid injury to the temporal branch of the nerve when elevating flaps, one should undermine either in the immediate subcutaneous plane or deep to the temporal parietal fascia immediately adjacent to the superficial layer of the deep temporal fascia (Figure 1.22). Particular care is required over the zygomatic arch, where there is fusion of the fascial layers.

Familiarity with the location of the marginal mandibular nerve is essential when operating in the lower face (Figures 1.23 and 1.24). If the marginal mandibular nerve is injured during surgery, the resulting paralysis of the muscles, which depresses the corner of the mouth, is quite deforming. Dingman and Grabb (1962) noted in a large cadaver study that posterior to the facial artery, the marginal mandibular nerve passed

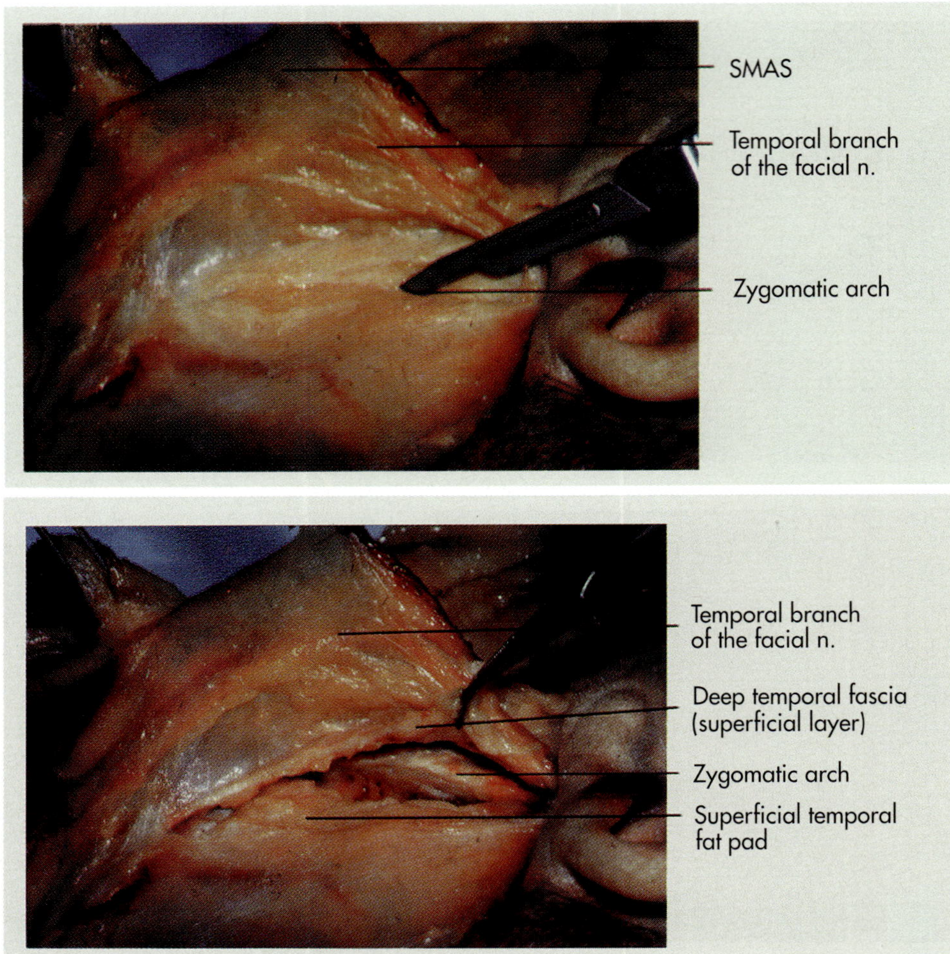

FIG. 1.22. Coronal approach to the zygoma. **A,** The temporal branch of the facial nerve is at risk as the coronal flap is elevated over the zygoma. **B,** The nerve can be protected when approaching the zygoma by incising the superficial layer of the deep temporal fascia inferior to the plane of the fusion. *(From Larrabee W and Makielski K: Surgical anatomy of the face, Philadelphia, 1993, Raven.)*

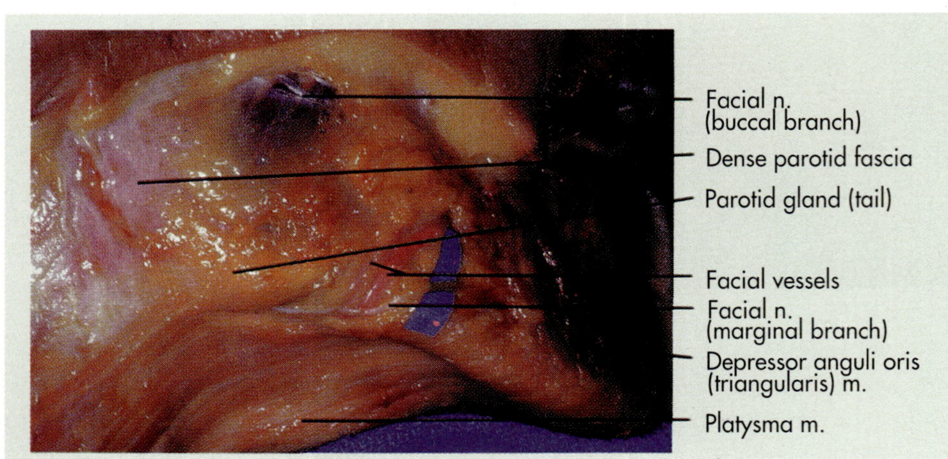

FIG. 1.23. Dissection of the marginal branch of the facial nerve, which shows the relationship of platysma and facial vessels. The marginal branch of the facial nerve is seen as it emerges along the anterior border of the parotid gland. The nerve crosses the inferior border of the mandible lateral to the facial vessels to supply the muscles of the lower lip and chin. *(From Larrabee W and Makielski K: Surgical anatomy of the face, Philadelphia, 1993, Raven.)*

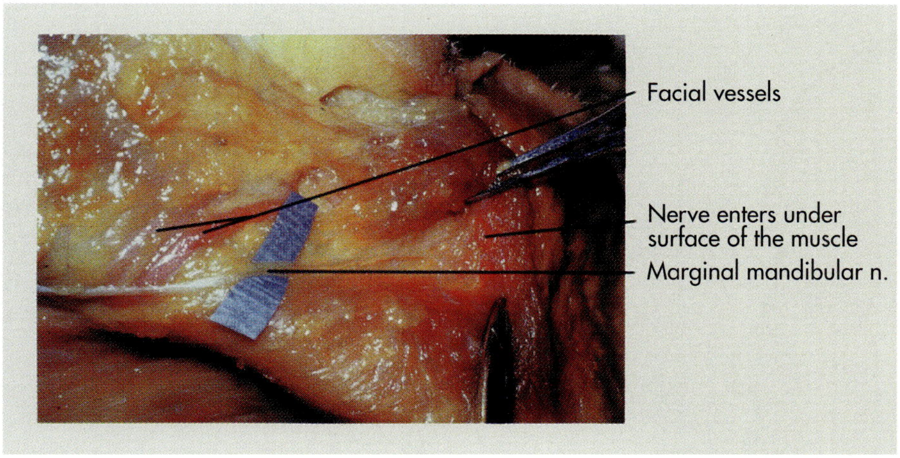

FIG. 1.24. Detailed dissection of marginal nerve. The marginal nerve is seen entering the undersurface of the depressor muscles. *(From Larrabee W and Makielski K: Surgical anatomy of the face, Philadelphia, 1993, Raven.)*

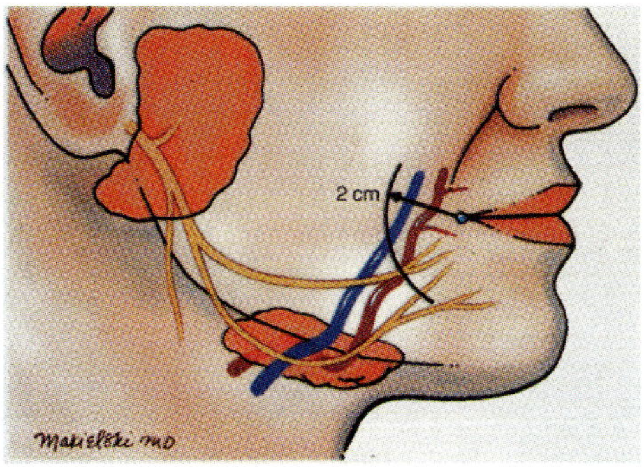

FIG. 1.25. Landmarks for marginal mandibular branch of the facial nerve. The mandibular branch is located deep to the platysma until it reaches a point about 2 cm lateral to the corner of the mouth. At this point, the nerve becomes more superficial and penetrates the undersurface of the facial mimetic muscles. Thus, in a face-lift or other skin-flap procedure, the mandibular nerve is fairly well protected if the dissection is subcutaneous and at least 2 cm lateral to the oral commissure (Liebman et al, 1982). *(From Larrabee W and Makielski K: Surgical anatomy of the face, Philadelphia, 1993, Raven.)*

above the inferior border of the mandible in 81% of dissections. Anterior to the facial artery, all of the mandibular nerve branches, which innervated the mouth depressors, passed above the lower border of the mandible. The only nerve branches that passed below the mandible anterior to the facial artery innervated the platysma. The nerve was superficial to the posterior facial vein in 98% of the cases and superficial to the anterior facial vein in 100% of the cases (Figure 1.25).

The same study showed that the mandibular nerve may have one (21%), two (67%), three (9%), or four (3%) major branches. In 5% of the cases, there was anastomosis between the buccal and mandibular rami.

Baker and Conley (1979) wrote that in their clinical experience the mandibular branch of the facial nerve is usually 1 to 2 cm below the lower border of the mandible and can be as much as 3 or 4 cm below it. The mandibular branch is deep to the platysma muscle and therefore fairly well protected throughout its course. Liebman and colleagues (1982) performed serial sections of cadavers and described the depth of the marginal nerve around the mouth (Figure 1.25).

SENSORY NERVES

The sensory innervation of the face is from the trigeminal nerve (cranial nerve V). Each division of the trigeminal nerve supplies all tissues from skin to mucosa and corresponds approximately to the three embryological divisions of the face: the frontonasal process (V1), the maxillary process (V2), and the mandibular process (V3). The sensation of the posterior scalp, lower border of the mandible, and neck is supplied by branches of the cervical nerves and plexus.

The ophthalmic division of the trigeminal nerve (V1) supplies sensation to the forehead, anterior scalp, and nasal dorsum via the supratrochlear and supraorbital nerves (Figure 1.26). The infratrochlear and dorsal nasal nerves and terminal branches of the anterior ethmoid nerve provide additional sensation to the nasal dorsum. The upper nasal and septal mucosa are innervated by the anterior ethmoid nerve.

The maxillary division of the trigeminal nerve (V2) innervates the cheek and side of the face, conjunctiva and skin of the lower eyelid, side of the nose and nasal vestibule, and mucosa and skin of the upper lip via three branches: the zygomaticotemporal, the zygomaticofacial, and the infraorbital nerves (Figure 1.27).

The mandibular branch of the trigeminal nerve (V3) has both a sensory and a motor component. There are four clinically important sensory branches to the mandibular nerves: the inferior alveolar nerve, the lingual nerve, the buccal nerve, and the auriculotemporal nerve (Figure 1.28). Areas supplied by the inferior alve-

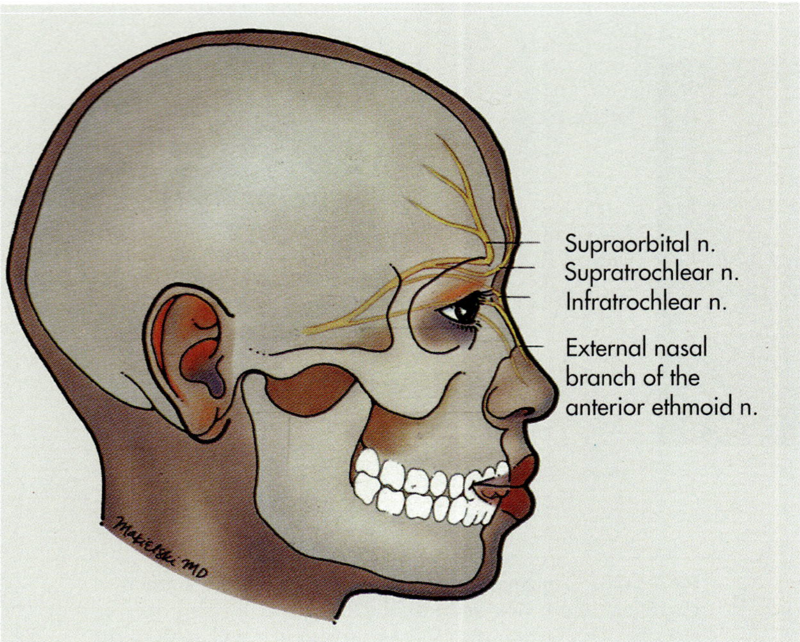

FIG. 1.26. Trigeminal nerve, ophthalmic division. The division provides cutaneous sensation to the forehead, the anterior scalp, and the nasal dorsum through the supraorbital, supratrochlear, infratrochlear, and external nasal branches of the anterior ethmoid nerves. A small lacrimal branch at the lateral canthus also provides sensation to the upper lid. *(From Larrabee W and Makielski K: Surgical anatomy of the face, Philadelphia, 1993, Raven.)*

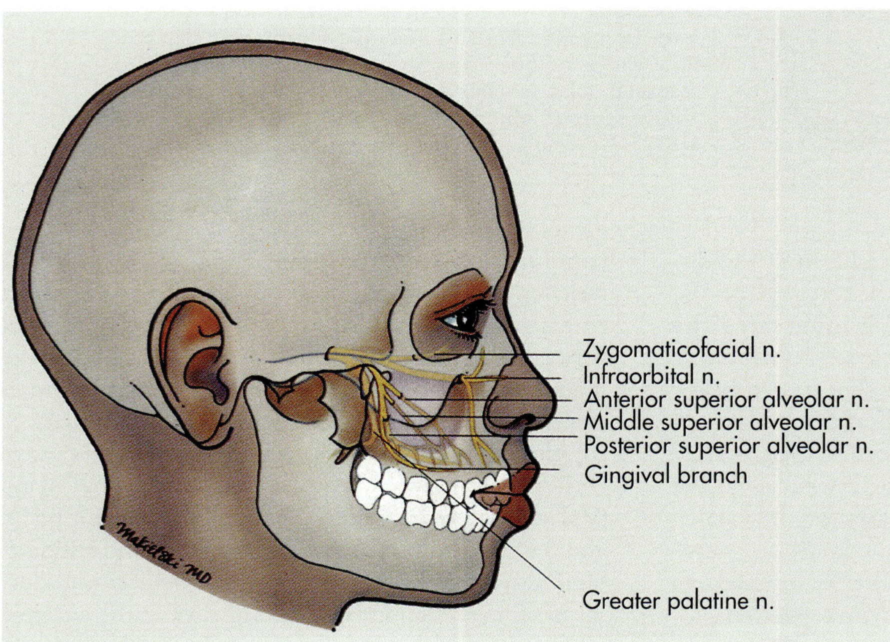

FIG. 1.27. Trigeminal nerve, maxillary division. The division provides cutaneous sensation to the cheek, the side of the face, the lower eyelid, the side of the nose, and the upper lip. There is significant variation in the exact distribution of the anterior superior alveolar, middle superior alveolar, and posterior superior alveolar nerves, which supply sensation to the maxillary dentition. *(From Larrabee W and Makielski K: Surgical anatomy of the face, Philadelphia, 1993, Raven.)*

olar nerve include the lower teeth, gingiva, and mandible. One of its branches, the mental nerve, supplies sensation to the mucosa and skin of the lower lip and chin. Innervation to the anterior two thirds of the tongue, the floor of the mouth, and lingual gingiva is provided by the lingual nerve. The buccal nerve supplies the buccal mucosa and cheek skin. The auriculotemporal nerve provides sensation for temporal skin and portions of the external auditory canal and tympanic membrane. The auriculotemporal nerve also carries some motor fibers to the parotid gland. The motor branch of the mandibular nerve supplies the four muscles of mastication: the temporalis, masseter, and medial and lateral pterygoids.

The supraorbital and supratrochlear nerves are most commonly encountered when performing an endoscopic forehead lift. The supraorbital nerves generally exit from a notch approximately 60% of the time and from a foramen approximately 40% of the time. If they exit from a notch, the supratrochlear nerves also exit from the same notch. If the supraorbital nerves exit from the foramen, the supratrochlear nerves exit

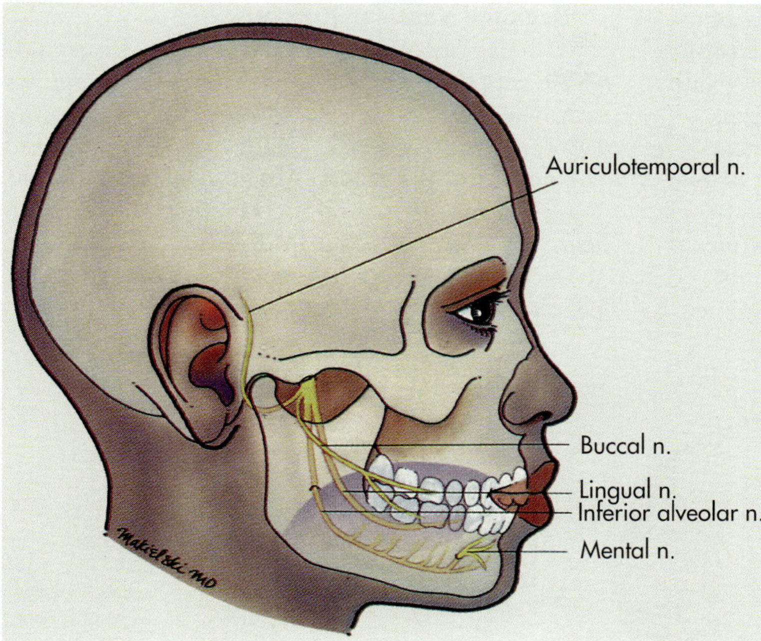

FIG. 1.28. Trigeminal nerve, mandibular division. This division supplies sensation to the lower lip, cheek, temple, anterior two-thirds of the tongue, floor of mouth, and the mandibular dentition. *(From Larrabee W and Makielski K: Surgical anatomy of the face, Philadelphia, 1993, Raven.)*

from a separate foramen. There are multiple branches of the supraorbital and supratrochlear nerves. The medial segments of the supraorbital nerves penetrate the corrugator muscles. One of the largest branches of the supratrochlear nerve goes laterally toward the lacrimal gland.

VASCULAR PATTERNS OF THE FACE

The vascular system is a three-dimensional linkage of neighboring vascular territories. Major distributing vessels travel close to the underlying bony skeleton, emerging from the deep tissues at fixed points, either from bony foramina or where the deep fascia approximates the underlying bone (Figure 1.29). For instance, several branches of the external carotid artery (the occipital, posterior auricular, and superficial temporal arteries) emerge near the skull base, whereas the facial artery emerges along the lower border of the mandible. Other important facial vessels arise at the bony foramina of the mandible and maxilla (the infraorbital and mental arteries) and at the orbital margins (the supraorbital, supratrochlear, dorsal nasal, and medial palpebral arteries).

The distributing arteries then branch into smaller perforator vessels, which form the basis for the muscular and cutaneous vascular systems. Typically, perforator branches enter their respective muscle groups on the deep surface, closely following the connective tissue architecture of the muscle as they divide and subdivide into smaller nutrient vessels before extending to the cutaneous surface.

Arteries

Branches of the perforator arteries extend to the cutaneous surface as either septocutaneous or musculocutaneous arteries. Septocutaneous vessels travel generally within the fascia (septa) of the muscle. In contrast, musculocutaneous vessels pass directly through the muscle tissue, providing multiple nutrient branches to the surrounding muscle as they travel vertically to the cutaneous tissues.

Veins

Venous outflow from the skin occurs by way of a subdermal venous plexus, which generally enters the deep venous system through valves in the venae communicantes. Venous drainage may also occur by way of the paired vena comitantes, which accompany the small cutaneous arteries.

Cutaneous Vascular Plexus

The cutaneous tissues and their nutrient vessels form a stack of interconnected vascular tissue planes called the vascular plexus, consisting of the fascial plexus, the subcutaneous plexus, and the subdermal plexus (Figure 1.30). The deepest structure in the cutaneous vascular plexus is the fascial plexus, at the level of the deep muscle fascia. The fascial plexus derives its blood supply from small vessels that branch off septocutaneous and musculocutaneous arteries as they penetrate the muscular fascia, and from retrograde flow from the overlying subcutaneous plexus. Overlying the fascial plexus is the subcutaneous plexus, a significant network of vessels corresponding to the level of the superficial fascia or SMAS. The vascular density of the subcutaneous plexus demonstrates tremendous regional variation and has a reciprocal relationship with the density of the overlying subdermal plexus.

The subdermal, or cutaneous, plexus is the most significant of the horizontal vascular layers and plays a primary role in the distribution of blood to other regions of the cutaneous system. The subdermal plexus lies at the junction between the reticular dermis and the underlying subcutaneous fat.

Regional Vascular Anatomy

The majority of skin and subcutaneous tissue in the face is supplied by branches of the external carotid system. The exception is a masklike region of the central face that encompasses the eyes, the upper two thirds of the nose, and the central forehead. The ophthalmic branch of the internal carotid system provides the primary blood supply to this region, with anastomoses to the facial and superficial temporal branches of the external carotid artery providing additional blood supply.

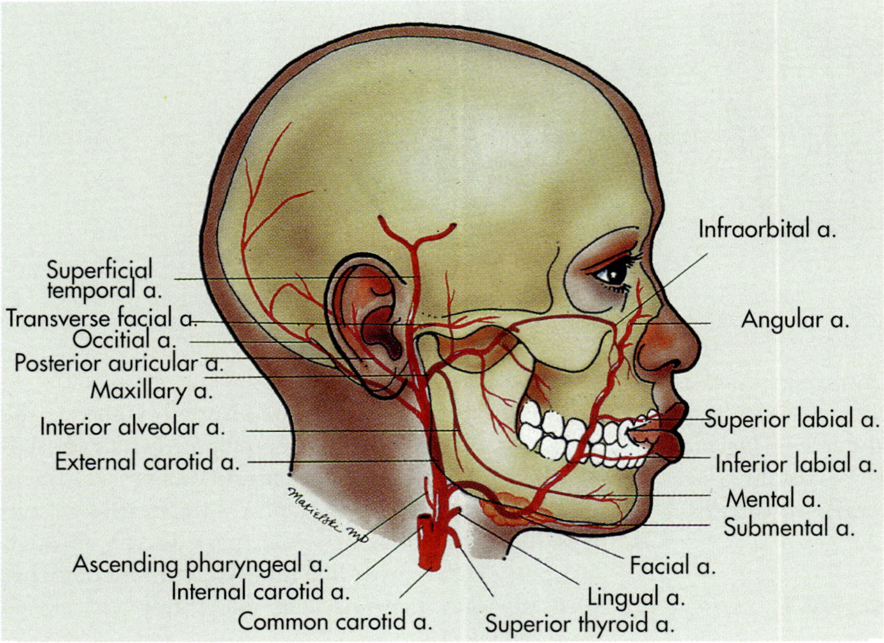

FIG. 1.29. External carotid artery distribution to the face. The external carotid artery separates in the neck from the common carotid artery, and, after giving off the superior thyroid, the lingual, and the ascending palatine arteries, divides into the facial artery and a posterior division that terminates in the superficial temporal artery. *(From Larrabee W and Makielski K: Surgical anatomy of the face, Philadelphia, 1993, Raven.)*

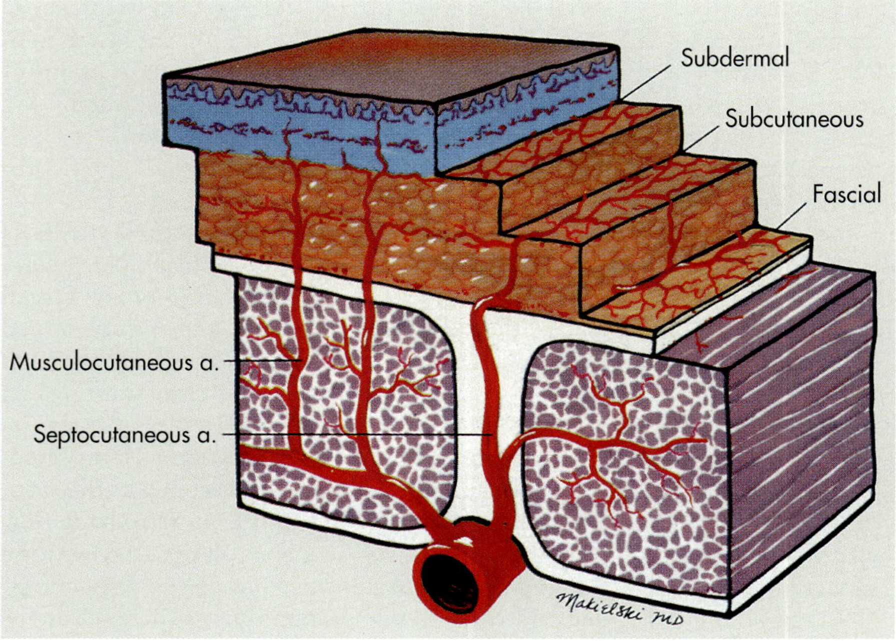

FIG. 1.30. Cutaneous vascular plexus. The cutaneous vascular plexus forms a stacked series of interconnected vascular tissue planes that derive their blood supply from septocutaneous and musculocutaneous arteries. The fascial, the subcutaneous, and the subdermal (cutaneous) layers are shown. Illustrated after Scharnack. (From Daniel and Kerrigan, 1990.) *(From Larrabee W and Makielski K: Surgical anatomy of the face, Philadelphia, 1993, Raven.)*

The blood supply to the temporal area is particularly important for endoscopic surgery. The superficial temporal artery is the terminal branch of the external carotid system, arising deep within the parotid gland and emerging between the condyle of the mandible and the external auditory meatus (Figure 1.31). As the artery nears the zygomatic arch, it lies just deep to the dermis within the substance of the temporoparietal fascia, or SMAS; this fascia also transports the temporal branch of the facial nerve.

Before crossing the zygomatic arch, the superficial temporal artery generates a small horizontal branch known as the transverse facial artery. The transverse facial vessel runs parallel and inferior to the zygomatic arch to supply the lateral orbital area. At the superior border of the zygomatic arch, the superficial temporal artery gives off a second branch, the middle temporal artery. This artery immediately penetrates the superficial layer of the deep temporalis fascia to supply the superficial temporal fat pad and the deep temporalis fascia. It also contributes to perfusion of the temporalis muscle.

Within 2 cm of crossing the zygomatic arch, the superficial temporal artery divides into two or three terminal branches. If there are two branches (more common), the anterior branch supplies the forehead, forming anastomotic connections with the ipsilateral supraorbital and supratrochlear vessels and the contralateral anterior branch of the superficial temporal artery. The posterior branch supplies a wide territory over the parietal skull and has rich anastomotic connections with adjacent and contralateral arteries.

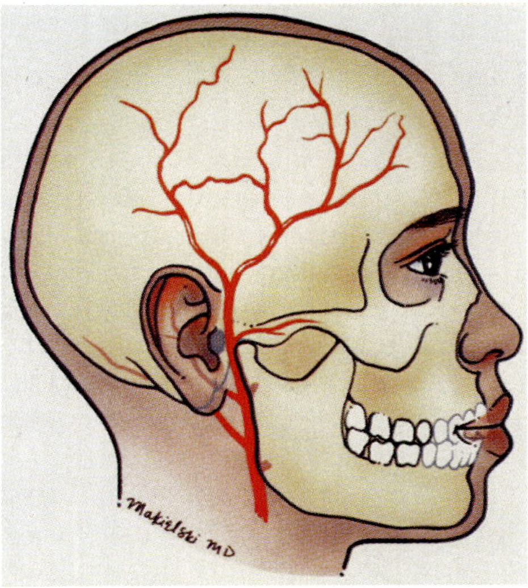

FIG. 1.31. Superficial temporal artery distribution. The most common branching pattern is demonstrated with a bifurcation into the anterior and posterior branches. Inferior to the zygomatic arch, the transverse facial artery is seen. *(From Larrabee W and Makielski K: Surgical anatomy of the face, Philadelphia, 1993, Raven.)*

When a third branch exists, it runs just superior to the supraorbital ridge and is called the horizontal branch. The size of this additional artery varies inversely with the ipsilateral supraorbital and supratrochlear vessels; its physiological importance varies considerably.

FOREHEAD

The forehead is the area of the face most commonly addressed endoscopically. Its anatomy is fairly straightforward, and key relationships have been described previously. This section briefly reviews the functional relationships of the fascial, muscular, and neurological structures and describes them from a superior endoscopic approach.

The overall appearance of the upper face is determined by: (1) the shape and position of the bones of the orbit, (2) the quality and position of the eyelid skin, and (3) the action of the forehead and brow musculature. In order to precisely evaluate and treat the aging forehead and brow, an understanding of the three-dimensional anatomy is essential.

The youthful brow is positioned above the orbital rim; it is slightly higher laterally than medially. The male brow is usually more horizontal and positioned more inferiorly than is the female eyebrow. The female brow is usually more arched, with the peak of the eyebrow located between the lateral limbus and the lateral canthal angle.

The central forehead and scalp consist of five characteristic layers previously described (Figure 1.32, see mnemonic in legend). The skin (S) is thick, averaging 2381 μm in thickness, and is densely adherent to the abundant underlying subcutaneous tissue (C). The galea aponeurotica (A), or epicranial aponeurosis, is a thin tendinous sheet of connective tissue that envelops the entire skull. It is a mobile structure located just superficial to the loose areolar tissue. The galea aponeurotica splits anteriorly to surround the frontalis muscle and posteriorly to encircle the occipitalis muscle (Figure 1.33). Below the superior temporal line, the galea becomes confluent with the temporoparietal fascia. It is within and just deep to this layer that the superficial temporal vessels and the temporal branch of the facial nerve lie. This layer is also continuous with the SMAS below the zygomatic arch.

The loose areolar tissue or subaponeurotic plane (L) of the forehead and scalp is located between the galea aponeurosis and the pericranium (P). Below the superior temporal line, the areolar tissue is continuous with a similar loose connective tissue, which separates the temporoparietal fascia from the deep temporal fascia. The loose areolar layer is relatively avascular and is the dissection plane for traditional coronal brow and forehead lifts and for coronal approaches to the zygomatic arch and midface. It is this layer upon which the super-

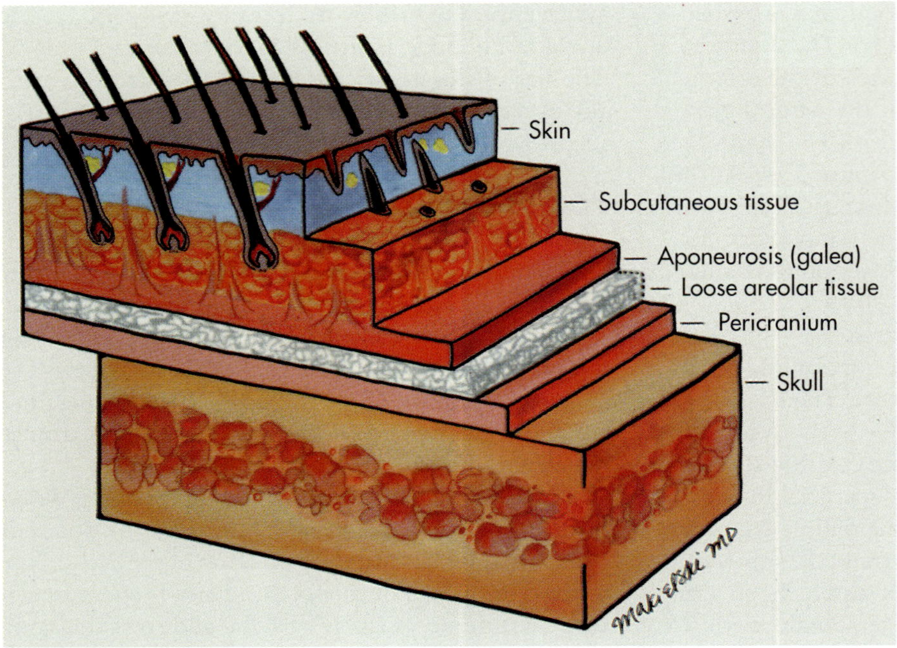

FIG. 1.32. Layers of the scalp. The conventional understanding of the five layers of the scalp is reflected in the time-honored mnemonic; SCALP: *S*kin, Sub*c*utaneous tissue, *A*poneurosis and muscle (galea), *L*oose areolar tissue, *P*ericranium. *(From Larrabee W and Makielski K: Surgical anatomy of the face, Philadelphia, 1993, Raven.)*

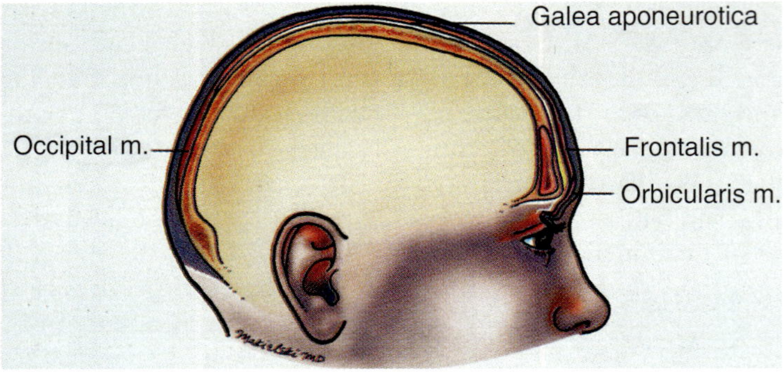

FIG. 1.33. Section through the epicranium. A sagittal section through the epicranium demonstrates the tendinous galea aponeurotica between the frontalis and the occipital muscles.

ficial brow and forehead structures slide over the thickened periosteal layer. The areolar tissue contains a few small arteries and emissary veins. Those veins are valveless and connect the superficial scalp veins with the diploic veins of the skull and the intracranial venous sinuses. The pericranium (periosteum) is a thickened layer of connective tissue, densely adherent to the outer surface of the skull. The pericranium becomes continuous with the periosteum on the inner surface of the skull (endosteum) at the interosseous suture lines of the skull bones. The periosteum covering the outer surface of the skull also becomes continuous with the periorbita (the inner lining of the orbital bones) at the level of the supraorbital rims.

The complex movements of the forehead and eyebrows are a product of the actions of four striated muscles: the frontalis, procerus, corrugator supercilii, and orbital portion of the orbicularis oculi muscles (Table 1.2). The frontalis is connected to the occipitalis muscle through its galeal attachments, and these two muscles act together to tighten the scalp and allow movement of the mobile scalp over the immobile pericranial layer. Contraction of the frontalis muscle elevates the brows. In patients with significant ptosis of the brows, frontalis contracture causes brow elevation, which relieves visual field obstruction. It is the overactivity of the frontalis muscle (in patients with brow ptosis) that causes transverse forehead wrinkles. The nerve supply to the frontalis muscle is the temporal branch of the facial nerve, which travels with the temporoparietal fascia to enter the frontalis on its undersurface.

The procerus muscle interdigitates with the inferior medial extent of the frontalis muscles. Contraction of the procerus muscle causes the medial aspect of the brows to descend and produces horizontal wrinkling over the skin of the root of the nose.

TABLE 1.2
MUSCLES OF THE FOREHEAD

Muscle	Origin	Insertion	Action
Frontalis	Skin and superficial fascia of the orbicularis muscle	Galea aponeurosis	Elevates the brow (produces transverse wrinkles)
Procerus	Fascia of nasal bones and upper lateral cartilages	Skin of medial lower forehead	Descent of medial brow (horizontal glabellar wrinkles)
Corrugator	Superomedial orbital rim	Fascia of lower frontalis muscle and skin of brow	Pulls brow inferiorly and medially (vertical glabellar wrinkles)
Orbicularis oculi (orbital portion) (depressor supercilii)	Medial orbital rim and medial canthal tendon	Medial aspect of bony orbit	Contributes brow descent and motility

The fibers of paired corrugator supercilii muscles interdigitate with the medial fibers of the orbital portion of the orbicularis oculi muscle. Contraction of the slips of the corrugator muscle pulls the brow inferiorly and medially and produces vertical glabellar wrinkling. The supratrochlear and supraorbital neurovascular bundles pierce the corrugator muscle on its deep surface before traveling superiorly on the superficial surface of the frontalis muscle.

With facial aging, there is progressive stretching of the periorbital soft tissues and loss of resting tone of the frontalis muscles. These characteristics cause ptosis of the brows, which is usually more noticeable laterally than it is medially. Ptosis of the brows can be associated with diminution in the upper half of the visual fields. In response to the decreased visual field, involuntary contraction of the frontalis muscle occurs. This overactivity is usually associated with restoration of the brow position and the production of transverse forehead wrinkles.

Temporal Fossa

The temporal fossa is located on the side of the head and is bounded by the superior temporal line (superiorly), the frontal process of the zygomatic bone (anteriorly), and the zygomatic arch (inferiorly). It contains the temporalis muscle and its overlying fascia, the superficial temporal vessels, the temporal branch of the facial nerve, and the auriculotemporal nerve.

The skin of the temporal fossa is thick, a portion of which is hair bearing (posteriorly). The temporal hairline traverses this region in a variable position. The temporoparietal fascia lies just beneath the subcutaneous fat and is a thin, pliable, and richly vascular layer that provides ample tissue for local reconstruction. This layer contains and is supplied by the superficial temporal artery and vein. The superficial temporal artery is narrow in caliber (averaging 1.89 mm) and is one of the terminal branches of the external carotid artery. The superficial temporal artery ascends in a vertical direction anterior to the ear and gives off the middle temporal artery just beneath the zygomatic arch.

The temporoparietal fascia of the temporal fossa is continuous with the epicranial aponeurosis of the forehead and scalp. This layer also contains the temporal branch of the facial nerve, which arises from the upper division of the facial nerve and crosses the midportion of the zygomatic arch on its superficial surface. The temporal branch ramifies into three to five branches, all of which ascend into the forehead no higher than 2 cm above the lateral aspect of the eyebrow. These nerves supply the frontalis, corrugator, procerus, and orbicularis oculi muscles. The temporal branch enters the lateral aspect of the muscles on its surface.

The subaponeurotic plane (loose areolar tissue) of the temporal fossa is located deep to the temporoparietal fascia and superficial to the deep temporal fascia. This loose areolar layer is continuous with the similarly named layer in the forehead and temple. The deep temporal fascia covers the temporalis muscle and contains the deep temporal vessels, which supply the underlying muscle. The deep temporal fascia splits approximately 2 cm above the zygomatic arch to envelop the temporal fat pad and also invests the zygomatic arch on both its superficial and deep surfaces.

The temporalis muscle is fan-shaped and arises from the bony floor of the temporal fossa and the deep surface of the deep temporal fascia. The fibers of the muscle converge and pass deep to the zygomatic arch to insert on the coronoid process of the mandible and the anterior border of the ramus of the mandible. The anterior fibers of the temporalis muscle elevate the mandible, while the posterior fibers retract the mandible. The temporalis is supplied by the deep temporal nerves, which are branches of the anterior division of the mandibular branch of the trigeminal nerve.

In the subaponeurotic plane, the temporal line is the first major landmark. Moving from superior to inferior toward the zygomatic arch, the areolar fascia is encountered, and the superficial layer of the deep temporal fascia is seen. The line of fusion of the superficial and deep layers of the temporalis fascia begins at approximately the level of the supraorbital rim, and inferior to this line the superficial temporal fat pad is visible deep to the superficial layer of the deep temporal fascia.

Branches of the superficial temporal artery and vein can be seen in the temporal parietal fascia. The middle temporal artery arises from the superficial temporal artery at the level of the zygomatic arch or 1 to 2 cm below it. The middle temporal artery always courses superficial to the arch and enters the superficial layer of the deep temporalis fascia just above the arch. The middle temporal artery supplies the fascia and sends a few branches to the temporalis muscle. The sentinel vein is a consistent landmark located approximately 5 mm lateral to the zygomaticofrontal suture line. This generally passes from the subcutaneous layer through the temporal parietal fascia and then into the deeper fascias and muscle. One can occasionally find a second vein somewhat lateral to the first. When one visualizes the sentinel vein endoscopically the temporal branch of the facial nerve is superficial and usually superior to the vein a distance of several millimeters to a centimeter. As elsewhere in the body the venous drainage systems are not extremely consistent in terms of their drainage patterns. There can also be a small vein running with the zygomatical temporal nerve into the orbital system. The zygomatic temporal nerve within the orbit provides parasympathetic fibers to the lacrimal gland and if injured can lead to a dry eye. Once it exits the orbit, however, it is strictly a sensory nerve.

Just above the zygomatic arch lies the temporal parietal fat pad. The temporal branch of the facial nerve runs just superficial to this fat on the undersurface of the temporal parietal fascia. At the lateral orbital rim beginning at the zygomaticofrontal suture line is the area of fascial fusion. Descending from the midline in the subaponeurotic plane one encounters the supraorbital and supratrochlear vessels and nerves. There is considerable clinical variation in the relative size and initial tracking pattern of these nerves. They pierce the frontalis muscle at various levels, with the more medial branches becoming superficial sooner.

The corrugator, procerus, and medial branches of the orbicularis oris (depressor supercilii) muscles are seen clearly from this dissection plane but may blend with each other.

Extending over the orbital rim, the arcus marginalis is encountered. After releasing the attachments of the enveloping fascia of the frontalis muscle (SMAS) from the periosteum, the ROOF is encountered. Medially, it is adherent to the periosteum and extends as a more tenuous layer inferiorly between the orbicularis oculi and the orbital septum.

EYE

The eye is both an intrinsic area of interest for endoscopic surgery and a point of access for procedures, particularly those of the midface. The relationships of the orbicularis oculi muscle have been previously described. In addition to its bony attachments to the orbit rim medially and laterally, the orbicularis oculi is confluent with the frontalis muscles superiorly and is superficial to the zygomatic major and other lip elevators inferiorly.

The relationship of the eyebrow to the surrounding muscular and fascial layers is especially important for endoscopic surgery (Figure 1.34). The galea aponeurotica splits into a deep and superficial layer to surround the frontalis muscle; the deep layer is considerably stronger and more significant. The superficial layer continues on the surface of the orbicularis oculi muscle. The frontalis muscle inserts into the eyebrow as well as interdigitating with the orbicularis oculi muscle. Deep to these muscles and adjacent

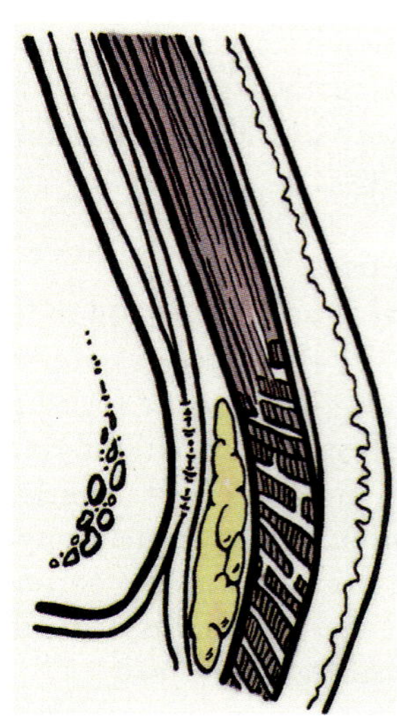

FIG. 1.34. The retro-orbicularis oculi fat (ROOF).

to the periosteum of the supraorbital rim lies the eyebrow fat pad, the ROOF. This fat pad becomes more diffuse and extends into the plane between the septum and the orbicularis muscle as a filmy areolar tissue. The deeper layer of the frontalis muscle fascia attaches to the supraorbital rim periosteum over the medial one half to two thirds of the orbit. Lateral to these attachments, less dense connections exist and these may become quite attenuated in older individuals. The supraorbital ridge represents reactive frontal bone hypertrophy, where the brow fat pad attaches to its undersurface. Laterally, there is no supraorbital ridge and no firm attachments between the brow fat and the bone. In this lateral area, brow ptosis is more rapid in patients with involutional ptosis or paralysis of the seventh nerve. Skin and muscle are attached to the zygomatic bone near the lateral orbicularis. This is the medial extension of the zygomatic cutaneous ligament. There are also vertical orbicularis fibers laterally, and they play a role in creating rhytids in the lateral canthal area.

Deep to the orbicularis oculi over the infraorbital rim lies the SOOF pad. The SOOF is contiguous to the subcutaneous malar fat pad, and elevation of the SOOF will raise the malar pad and help diminish the depth of the melolabial fold. The SOOF is analogous to the eyebrow fat pad (ROOF). There are no branches of the facial nerve over the infraorbital rim or anterior zygomatic prominence. The only nerve at risk over the zygomatic prominence is a sensory branch of the trigeminal nerve, the zygomatical facial nerve, which provides sensation to the lateral orbital area. With aging, the SOOF descends inferiorly and, over the medial orbital rim, somewhat laterally. The origins of the zygomatic major and minor, levator labii superioris, levator labii superioris alaeque nasi, and levator anguli oris can be detached from the zygoma and orbital rim area, either through the periorbital area or through a gingival buccal sulcus incision. The zygomatic major attaches laterally to the lateral canthus. The zygomatic minor, levator labii superioris, and levator labii superioris alaeque nasi attach below the orbital rim and above the infraorbital foramen, and the levator anguli oris attaches below the infraorbital rim.

The orbital septum closely approximates the orbital rim, except in the medial and lateral canthal areas. This fibrous structure originates from the periosteum of the

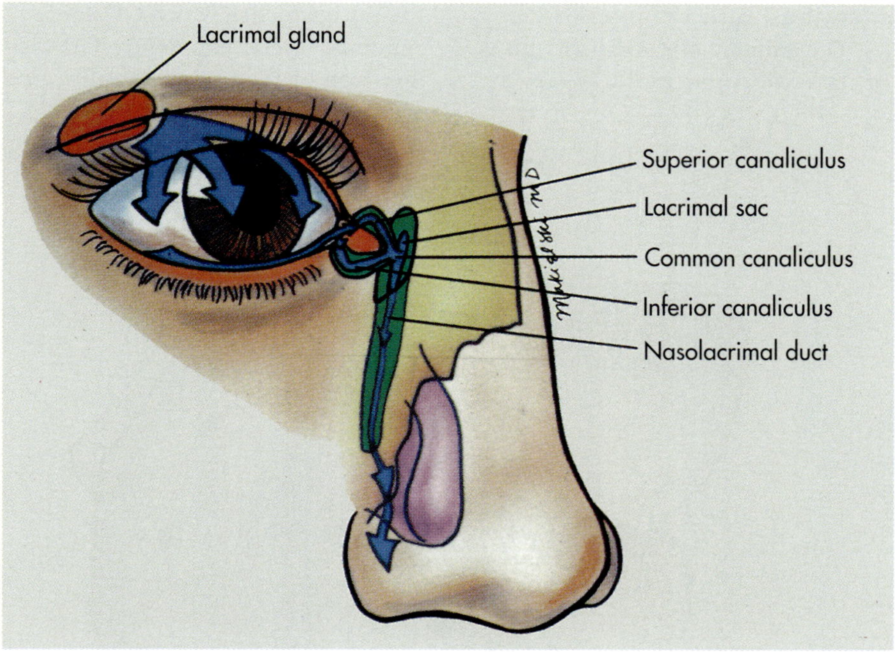

FIG. 1.35. Schematic diagram of lacrimal system. The tear film produced by the lacrimal gland and the multiple accessory gland reaches the upper and lower puncta located 5 to 7 cm from the medial canthus. The lower puncta is usually slightly more lateral than the medial canthus and is the more important of the two. The puncta opening is approximately 0.3 mm in diameter but can be easily dilated to probe the ducts. Immediately beneath the puncta lies the ampulla, an enlargement of the canaliculi before they turn horizontally. The two canaliculi join to form a common duct before draining into the lacrimal sac. The lacrimal sac is approximately 15 mm in height and empties into the nasolacrimal duct, which is approximately 10 to 12 mm in length. It drains into the inferior meatus approximately 15 mm from the nasal floor. Intranasally, the lacrimal sac is located at the level of the middle meatus. *(From Larrabee W and Makielski K: Surgical anatomy of the face, Philadelphia, 1993, Raven.)*

orbital margins, including the tough arcus marginalis of the frontal periosteum. It lies deep to the orbicularis muscle; in the upper lid it fuses with the levator aponeurosis approximately 2 or 3 mm above the tarsus (in the non-Asian lid). In the lower lid, the septum fuses with the capsulopalpebral fascia, which is analogous to the levator aponeurosis of the upper lid, approximately 5 mm beneath the tarsus. Medially, the septum attaches to the posterior lacrimal crest; in the lower lid, it also has some attachment to the anterior lacrimal crest. In the lateral canthal area, the septum follows and fuses with the lateral canthal tendon.

The septum is thinner medially, and the entire septum weakens with age, which allows pseudoherniation of the underlying fat, to occur. The tarsal plates of the upper and lower lids are composed of dense connective tissue (not cartilage). They extend from approximately the punctum medially to 4 to 5 mm from the lateral canthus, and they become less well defined medially and laterally. The upper tarsus is approximately 10 mm in width at the midline; the lower tarsus is considerably smaller. The conjunctiva is firmly attached to the posterior tarsus in both upper and lower lids.

The lacrimal drainage system begins with the upper and lower puncta (Figure 1.35). They are located 5 to 7 mm lateral to the canthus, with the inferior being slightly more lateral. The ampulla of the canaliculus is a slight dilation of its vertical portion just past the puncta before it runs horizontally into the sac. The two canaliculi usually join to form a common canaliculus, which then enters the lacrimal sac superiorly and somewhat posteriorly; they may, however, enter separately. The lacrimal sac is approximately 15 mm in height and rests in the bony lacrimal fossa. The superior few millimeters of the sac are covered by the inferior fibers of the anterior limb of the medial canthal tendon. The lacrimal sac empties into the nasolacrimal duct, which traverses somewhat over a centimeter of the bony canal to enter the inferior meatus in the nasal cavity. The lacrimal system is particularly amenable to endoscopic repairs.

CHEEKS AND NECK

As one approaches the cheek posteriorly, the skin and subcutaneous tissue can be easily lifted over the parotid, with the subdermal plexus easily visualized through the flap. The next layer includes the SMAS, which probably is one layer with the parotid fascia. As the skin flap is elevated anteriorly, the zygomatic cutaneous ligament (McGregor's patch) is encountered superiorly (Figure 1.36). Also at the anterior border of the masseter one encounters a weaker area of cutaneous ligaments, which Owsley (1992) has termed the midface fascial ligaments. The facial nerve branches are seen coursing over the thin masseteric fascia and

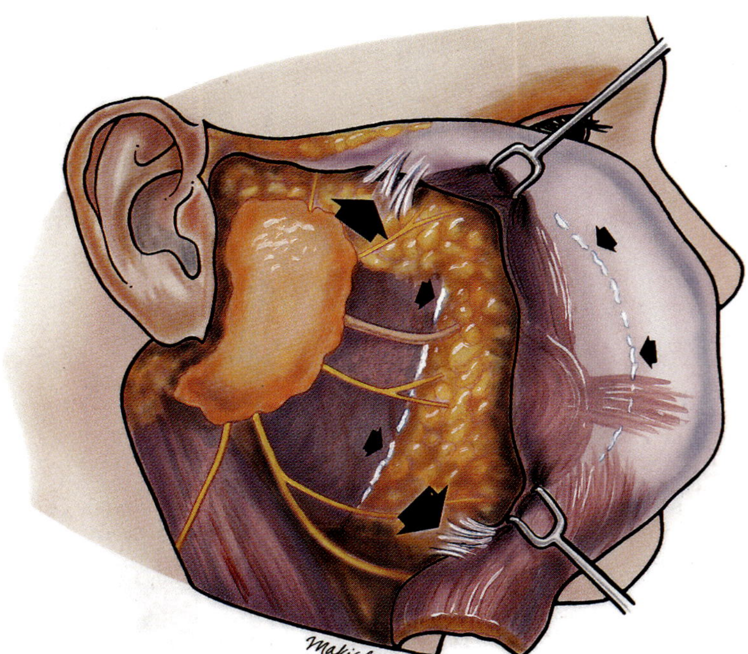

FIG. 1.36. Major retaining ligaments of the face. The SMAS is elevated to demonstrate the retaining ligaments of the face. They are strong ligaments with periosteal attachments termed the zygomatic ligament (McGregor's patch) superiorly and the mandibular ligament inferiorly. Weaker fascial ligaments are seen at the anterior border at the masseteric muscle.

then over the buccal fat pad (Figure 1.37). At the zygomatic major muscle, the SMAS becomes attached to this muscle with its bony insertions (Figure 1.38). The SMAS thus envelops the other muscles of facial expression. Inferiorly, the platysma is continuous with both the midface SMAS and the depressor muscles of the lower lip.

Superficial to this SMAS layer in the cheek lies the malar fat pad, which becomes more ptotic with age. A plane can be developed between the fibromuscular SMAS and this fibrofatty layer or malar cheek pad. This malar fat pad can be repositioned separately from the SMAS. The fibromuscular SMAS, if followed anteriorly, merges with the superficial layer of the orbicularis oris muscle. The fibrofatty malar cheek pad, if advanced posteriorly, flattens the melolabial fold. The orbicularis oris muscle when elevated exposes the SOOF, which is contiguous with the malar fat pad below. Deep to this fatty layer along the orbital rim lie the insertions of the elevator muscles of the lip. There is a perforating branch of the transverse facial artery, which is encountered inferior to the malar eminence and before reaching the zygomatic major muscle. There are no branches of the facial nerve along the zygomatic prominence and infraorbital rim; therefore, this area can be used safely for suturing the malar fat pad. Because of the bony insertions and more discrete nature of the zygomatic major and other lip elevator muscles, it is safer to begin elevation above these muscles and elevate inferiorly toward the platysma. If one attempts the same elevation inferiorly to superiorly, it is more likely that a branch of facial nerve will be damaged as one slips into a deeper plane in the more tenuous SMAS of the midcheek. In the neck area, elevations superficial to the platysma muscle are free of risk to the facial nerve. The paths of the cervical and marginal mandibular branches have been described previously, and both are at risk if subplatysma dissection is performed.

The Buccal Fat Pad

The aesthetically important part of the buccal fat pad lies lateral to the buccinator and provides fullness to the cheek inferior to the malar prominence (Figures 1.39 and 1.40). The fat pad as a whole is a complex three-dimensional structure.

The main body of the buccal fat pad sits on the posterolateral surface of the maxilla overlying the superior portion of the buccinator muscle under the anterior portion of the masseter. It has three main extensions: buccal, pterygoid, and temporal, although some authors have divided it into as many as nine portions.

The buccal extension is the most important from an aesthetic standpoint. It extends anterioinferiorly from the main body in a globular mass with a convex lateral face, covering most of the buccinator. Two surgically vulnerable structures, the facial nerve and the parotid duct, lie in close proximity to the buccal extension. The buccal rami of the facial nerve, which exit the anterior border of the parotid gland, lie on the surface of the masseter, tightly bound by the thin sheet of parotid-masseteric fascia. An extension of this fascia envelops the buccal fat pad; thus, the buccal extension has facial nerve fibers immediately lateral to it. The parotid duct runs immediately superior to the buccal extension before diving through the fibers of the buccinator to enter the oral cavity.

The pterygoid extension continues posteriorly from the main body on the lateral surface of the

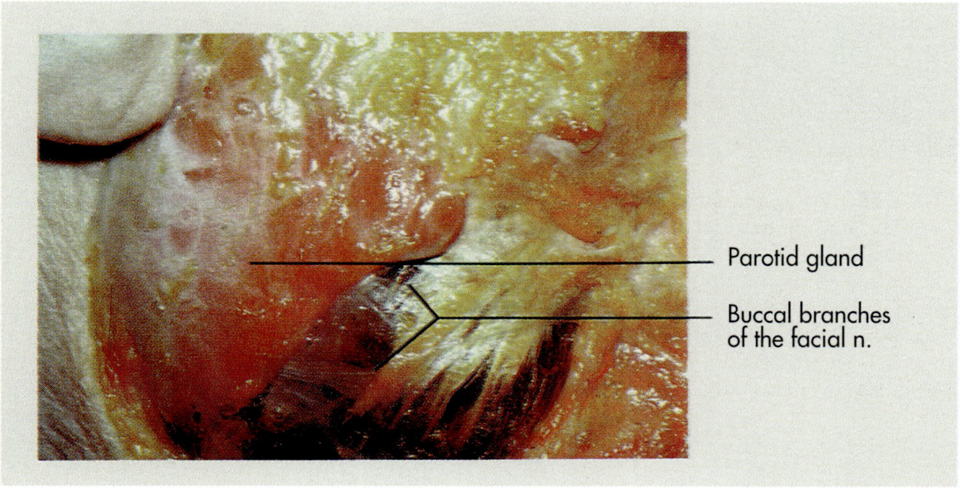

FIG. 1.37. Buccal branches of the facial nerve. The buccal branch of the facial nerve is seen exiting the parotid gland and coursing over the masseter muscle. *(From Larrabee W and Makielski K: Surgical anatomy of the face, Philadelphia, 1993, Raven.)*

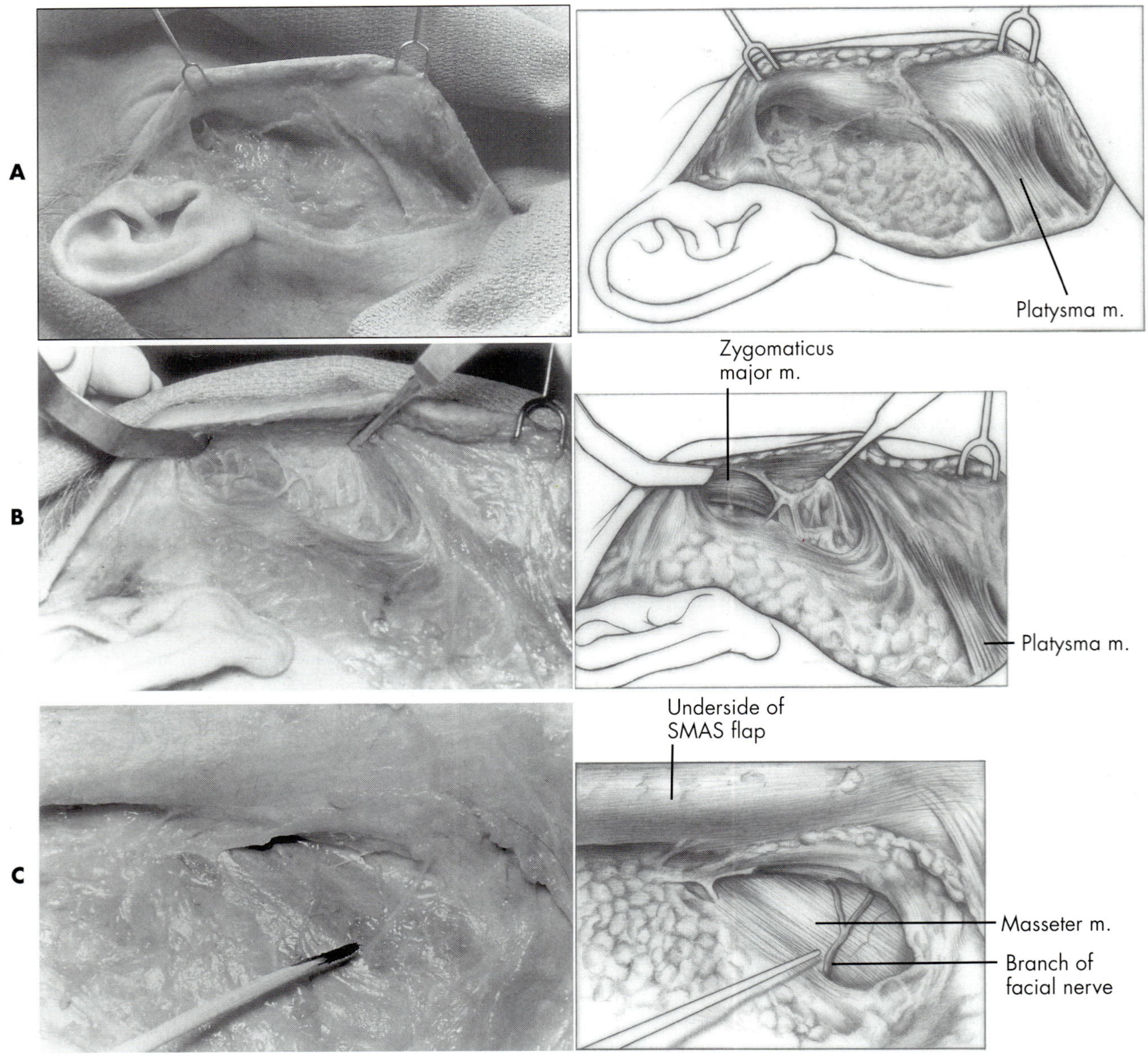

FIG. 1.38. Posterior dissection of the SMAS. **A,** Superficial musculoaponeurotic system (SMAS) flap. The incision has been carried down into the neck to improve exposure. The flap is dissected immediately below the SMAS layer and thus incorporates the SMAS. Platysma runs superiorly and anteriorly to join the SMAS. **B,** The SMAS flap extends anteriorly to the zygomaticus major muscles. The upper half of the fusion of the SMAS with fascia investing zygomaticus major has been incised to give a clear view of muscle. **C,** Close-up of immediate undersurface of SMAS flap in midcheek area. Buccal branches of facial nerve lie in loose connective tissue just deep to the SMAS and overlying masseter muscle.

Continued.

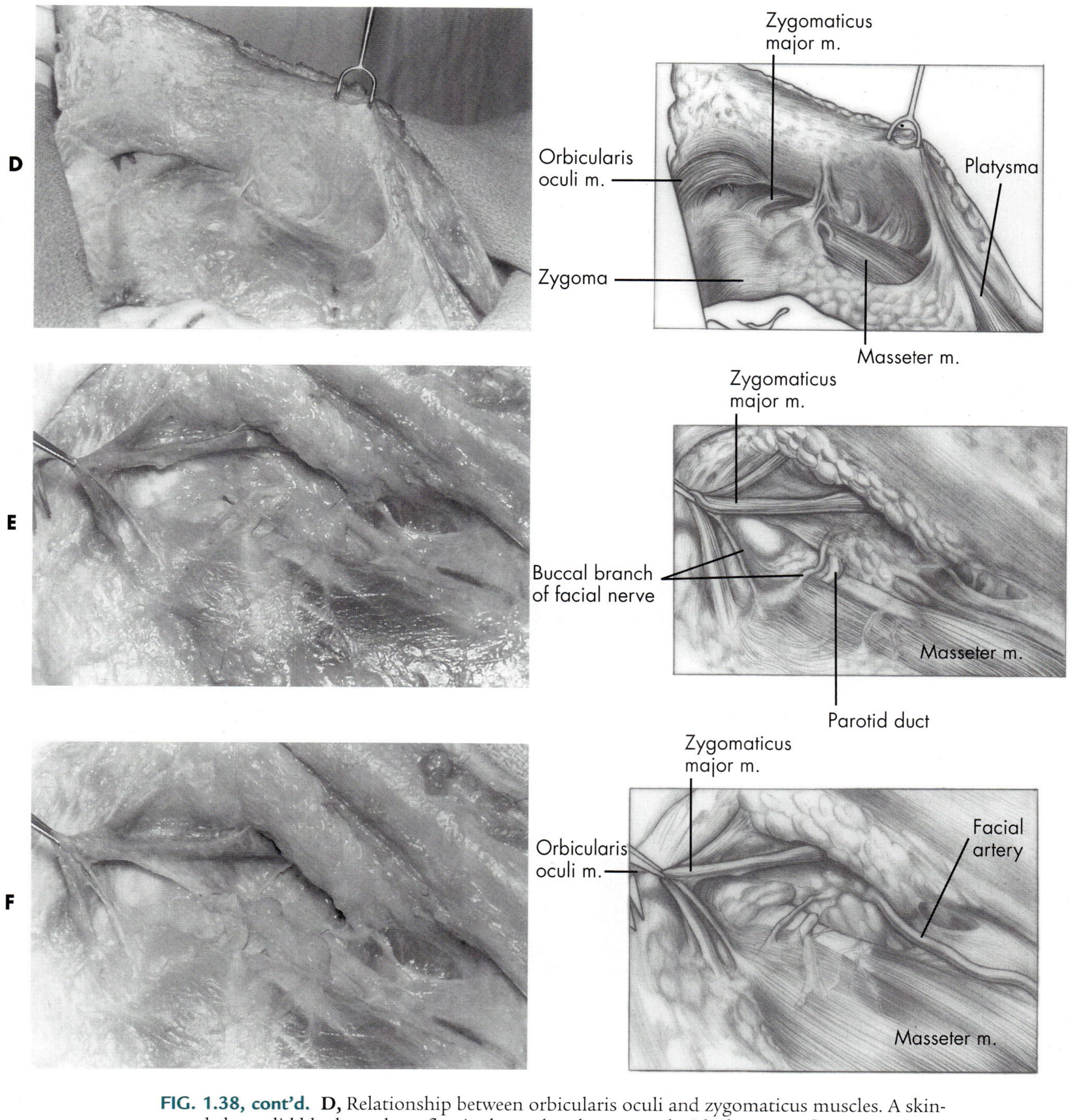

FIG. 1.38, cont'd. D, Relationship between orbicularis oculi and zygomaticus muscles. A skin-muscle lower lid blepharoplasty flap is elevated and connected with the SMAS flap. Tips of scissors are under the orbicularis muscle (partially reflected upward with the SMAS flap). Note attachment of zygomaticus to malar bone. **E,** Close-up of zygomaticus major muscles I. A large buccal branch of the facial nerve enters the upper third of the muscle. The parotid duct runs anteriorly into the buccal fat pad, with a buccal branch of the nerve paralleling 1 cm superiorly. **F,** Close-up of zygomaticus major muscle II. Additional dissection reveals the ascending course of the facial artery. Scissor tips lift the orbicularis muscle superiorly. *(From Larrabee W: Facelift anatomy, Facial Plastic Surgery Clinics of North America, Nov. 1993.)*

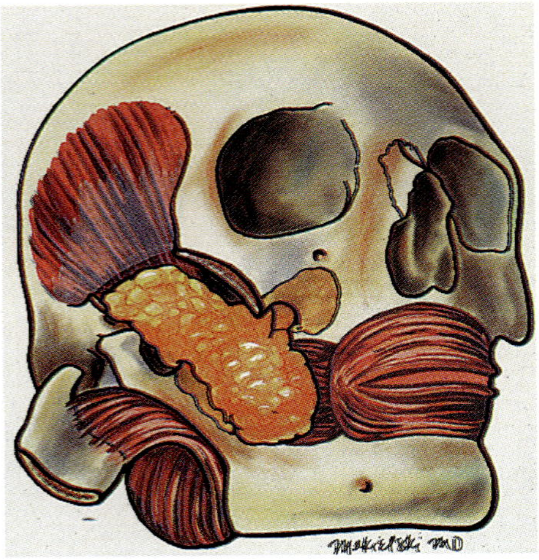

FIG. 1.39. Buccal fat pocket. The zygoma and the masseter are reflected to demonstrate the buccal fat pad and its relationship to the muscles of mastication. In addition to the primary buccal extension, the pterygoid and temporal extensions are seen. The buccal branches of the facial nerve and the parotid duct lie on the superficial surface of the buccal extension. The buccinator muscle is deep to it and must be pierced to approach the buccal fat from an intraoral approach. *(From Larrabee W and Makielski K: Surgical anatomy of the face, Philadelphia, 1993, Raven.)*

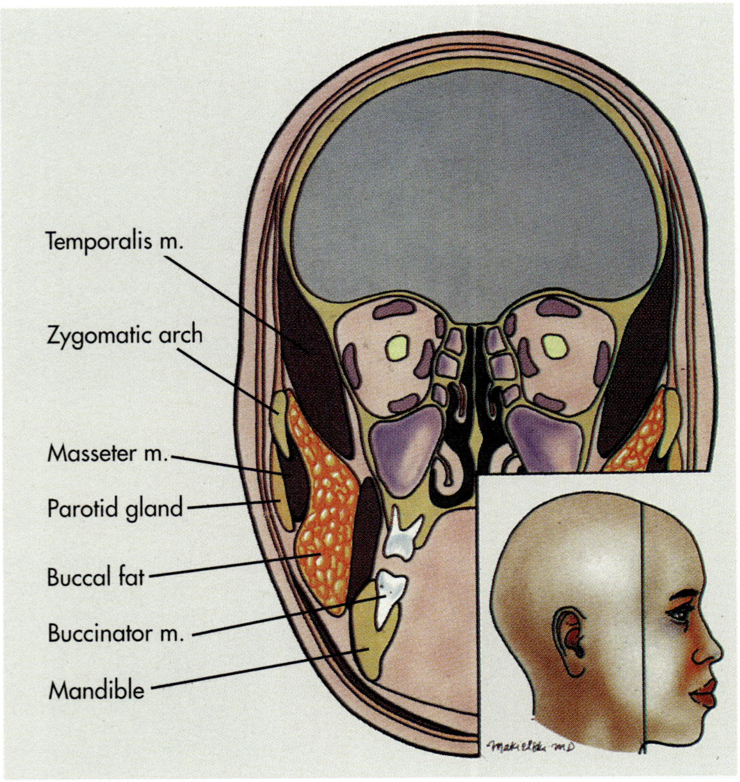

FIG. 1.40. Cross-section of buccal fat pocket. A coronal section through the anterior parotid gland demonstrates the important skeletal and muscular relationships of the buccal fat. Its primary function is to provide a gliding surface for the muscles of mastication. It lies between the temporalis and the masseter muscles in this plane. Its pterygoid extension surrounds the pterygoid muscles. The temporal extension of the buccal fat is separated from the superior temporal fat pad by the deep layer of the deep temporalis fascia. *(From Larrabee W and Makielski K: Surgical anatomy of the face, Philadelphia, 1993, Raven.)*

medial and lateral pterygoid muscles and proceeds medially around the posterior wall of the maxilla and through the pterygomaxillary fissure. It is closely associated with the maxillary artery and maxillary division of the trigeminal nerve and can be encountered during the transmaxillary sinus approach to the maxillary artery. The temporal extension passes posteriosuperiorly from the buccinator muscle under the zygomatic arch and lateral to the coronoid process of the mandible, separating the temporalis muscle from the arch. The superficial temporal fat pad is a separate structure, separated from the buccal fat pad's temporal extension by the deep layer of the deep temporalis fascia.

The blood supply of the buccal fat pad is from the branches of the facial artery, which lies along the most anterior portion, and the transverse facial artery, which has anastomoses with the facial artery in the region of the buccal extension. There are also contributions from the internal maxillary to the deeper portions, principally via the buccal artery. The nerve supply is from the buccal branch of the mandibular nerve before its distribution to the skin and mucosa of the cheek.

SELECTED READINGS

Abul-Hassan HS, Ascher G, Acland RD: Surgical anatomy and blood supply of the fascial layers of the temporal region, Plast Reconstr Surg 77:17-24, 1986.

Baker DC and Conley J: Avoiding facial nerve injuries in rhytidectomy, Plast Reconstr Surg 64:781-795, 1979.

Barton FE: The SMAS and the nasolabial fold, Plast Reconstr Surg 89:1054-1059, 1992.

Barton Jr FE: Rhytidectomy and the nasolabial fold, Plast Reconstr Surg 90:601-607, 1992.

Beard C and Quickert MN: Anatomy of the orbit, ed 2, Birmingham, Ala, 1977, Aesculapius.

Bernstein L and Nelson RH: Surgical anatomy of the extraparotid distribution of the facial nerve, Arch Otolaryngol 110:177-183, 1984.

Cardosa C: The anatomy of the platysma muscle, Plast Reconstr Surg 66:680-683, 1980.

Castro CP and Zani R: Masseter muscle rotation in the treatment of inferior facial paralysis, Plast Reconstr Surg 52:370-373, 1973.

Conley JJ: Salivary glands and the facial nerve, New York, 1975, Grune and Stratton.

Correia PC and Zani R: Surgical anatomy of the facial nerve as related to ancillary operations in rhytidoplasty, Plast Reconstr Surg 52:549-552, 1973.

Davis BA, Anson BJ, Budinger JM, et al: Surgical anatomy of the facial nerve and the parotid gland based upon a study of 350 cervico-facial halves, Surg Gynecol Obstet 102:385-412, 1956.

Dingman RO and Grabb WC: Surgical anatomy of the mandibular ramus of the facial nerve based on the dissection of 100 facial halves, Plast Reconstr Surg 29:266-272, 1962.

Dzubow LM: Facial flaps biomechanics and regional applications, Norwalk, Conn, 1990, Appleton and Lange.

Ellenboger R: Pseudoparalysis of the marginal mandibular nerve of the platysma face lift operation, Plast Reconstr Surg 63:364, 1979.

Faigin G: The artist's complete guide to facial expression, New York, 1990, Watson-Guptill Publications.

Fatah MF: Innervation and functional reconstruction of the forehead, Br J Plast Surg 351-398, 1991.

Freilinger G, Gruber M, Happak W, et al: Surgical anatomy of the mimetic muscle system and facial nerve: importance for reconstruction and aesthetic surgery, Plast Reconstr Surg 16:167, 1992.

Furnes DW: The retaining ligaments of the cheeks, Plast Reconstr Surg 83:11-16, 1989.

Gosain AK, Yousif NJ, et al: Surgical anatomy of the SMAS: a reinvestigation, Plast Reconstr Surg 92:1254, 1993.

Grant JCB: An atlas of anatomy, ed 6, Baltimore, 1972, Williams & Wilkins.

Griesman B: Muscles and cartilages of the nose from the standpoint of a typical rhinoplasty, Arch Otolaryngol 39:334-341, 1944.

Hamra ST: Composite rhytidectomy, Plast Reconstr Surg 90:1, 1992.

Hussein S, Ascher G, Acland R: Surgical anatomy and blood supply of the fascial layer of the temporal region, Plast Reconstr Surg 77:17-24, 1986.

Jost G and Levet Y: Parotid fascia and face lifting: a critical evaluation of the SMAS concept, Plast Reconstr Surg 74:42-51, 1984.

Larrabee W and Makielski K: Surgical anatomy of the face, Philadelphia, 1993, Raven.

Larrabee W and Sherris S: Principles of facial reconstruction, Philadelphia, 1995, Raven.

Lemke BN and Stasior OG: The anatomy of eyebrow ptosis, Arch Ophthalmol 100:981-986, 1982.

Letourneau A and Daniel R: The superficial musculoaponeurotic system of the nose, Plast Reconstr Surg 82:48-55, 1988.

Liebman EP, Webster RC, Berger AS, et al: The frontalis nerve in the temporal brow lift, Arch Otolaryngol 108:232-235, 1982.

Liebman EP, Webster RC, Gaul JR, et al: The marginal mandibular nerve in rhytidectomy and liposuction surgery, Arch Otolaryngol Head Neck Surg 104:179-181, 1988.

Lightoller GHS: Facial muscles, J Anatomy 60:1-85, 1925.

Manchot C: The cutaneous arteries of the human body, New York, 1983, Springer-Verlag.

McKinney P and Gottlieb J: The relationship of the greater auricular nerve to the SMAS, Ann Plast Surg 14:310-314, 1985.

Mitz V and Peyronie M: The superficial musculo-aponeurotic system (SMAS) in the parotid and cheek area, Plast Reconstr Surg 58:80-88, 1976.

Owsley JQ: Aesthetic facial surgery, Philadelphia, 1994, WB Saunders.

Owsley JQ: Lifting the malar fat pad for correction of prominent nasolabial folds, Plast Reconstr Surg 91:463, 1993.

Pensler J, Ward J, Parry S: The superficial musculoaponeurotic system in the upper lip: an anatomic study in cadavers, Plast Reconstr Surg 75:488-492, 1985.

Ramirez OM, Maillard GF, Musolas A: The extended subperiosteal face lift: a definite soft-tissue remodeling for facial rejuvenation, Plast Reconstr Surg 88:227, 1991.

Reeh MJ, Wobig JL, Wirtschaffer S: Ophthalmic Anatomy, American Academy of Otolaryngology-Head and Neck Surgery.

Rubin LR: Anatomy of a smile, Plast Reconstr Surg 53:384-387, 1974.

Rubin LR, Mishriki Y, Lee G: Anatomy of the nasolabial fold: the keystone of the smiling mechanism, Plast Reconstr Surg 83:1, 1989.

Rudolph R: Depth of the facial nerve in face lift dissections, Plast Reconstr Surg 85:537-544, 1990.

Salmon M: Arteries of the skin, New York, 1988, Churchill Livingston.

Stuzin JM, Wegstrom L, Kawamoto HK, et al: Anatomy of the frontal branch of the facial nerve: the significance of the temporal fat pad, Plast Reconstr Surg 83:265-271, 1989.

Tardy ME and Brown RJ: Surgical anatomy of the nose, Philadelphia, 1990, Raven.

Taylor GI, Palmer JH, Mchanamny D: The vascular territories of the body (angiosomes) and their clinical applications. In McCarthy JG, editor: Plastic surgery, vol 1, Philadelphia, 1990, WB Saunders.

Tolhurst DE, Carstens MH, Greco MJ, Hurwitz DJ: The surgical anatomy of the scalp, Plast Reconstr Surg 87:603-612, 1991.

Tremolada C, Fissette J, Candioni P: Anatomical basis for a safe and easier approach to composite rhytidectomy, Aesth Plast Surg 18:386-391, 1994.

Wasset M: Superficial fascial and muscular layers in the face and neck: a histological study, Aesthetic Plast Surg 11:171-176, 1987.

Yousif NJ, Gosain A, Matloub H, et al: The nasolabial histological reappraisal, Plast Reconstr Surg 93:60-69, 1994.

Yousif NJ and Mendelson BC: Anatomy of the midface, Clin Plast Surg 22(2):227-240, 1995.

Zide BM and Jelks GW: Surgical anatomy of the orbit, New York, 1985, Raven.

chapter two

Endoscopic Cameras, Light Sources, and Optics

Douglas Dedo

Today's endoscopes are based upon modifications to early telescopes used by our predecessors in medicine and surgery. In 1879, the same year in which Thomas Edison invented the incandescent lamp, Nitzi developed the first distally lighted cystoscope.[1] He used a platinum wire filament cooled by circulating water in a telescope that had very large diameter lenses. Because of their large diameter, the early scopes had limited clinical application. Later, after the turn of the century, Chevalier Jackson introduced distally lighted scopes with incandescent bulbs. Today, fiber illumination in hollow or open endoscopes has replaced the incandescent bulb to provide bright, dependable lighting.[2]

In 1950, the British optical physicist, H.H. Hopkins, of Reading University, developed the Hopkins rod lens telescope that is so popular today.[3] In this telescope, the air-containing spaces between the lenses were replaced with glass rods, separated by "air lenses." This improved the illumination, increased the field of vision, and improved image contrast. As a result, these rods allowed a marked decrease in the diameter of the tube or housing of the telescope without a concomitant reduction in the quality of the viewing field.

ENDOSCOPE

An endoscope is actually a combination of two different systems: an optical system consisting of rod lenses and a fiberoptic light system. This latter system transmits light from the attached light guide to the distal end of the endoscope to illuminate the surgical site. The lens (image carrying system) collects the reflective light and relays the image back to the eye or camera on the objective end of the telescope.

The design of the endoscope is a balancing act between the optical and light systems. In a tube of fixed diameter, the amount of light transmitted must be balanced with the image that will be reflected back to the objective lens. As the number of light fibers increase, so does the risk of blooming or whiting out the reflected image. Hence, in the case of a video camera placed on the objective lens, only white light would be perceived. Conversely, if the number of light fibers is inadequate, the image is dim, with poor quality and definition.

As the diameter of the lens is increased, there is a natural decrease in the number of light fibers because of a fixed volume of the two housings. In Figure 2.1, the light fibers travel in the periphery of the housing, while the rod lenses occupy the center section. Usually, these light fibers are in three bundles placed evenly around the lenses.

The field of view of any endoscope is limited by the diameter and angle of the distal lens. As the diameter of the scope increases, the field of vision increases. From a 3-mm to a 4-mm endoscope, the field of vision increases approximately 4 degrees. The angle of view is controlled with the angle of the distal lens. As the distal lens increases from 0 to 130 degrees, the angle of view from the long axis of the scope will vary from straight out to almost looking back at the observer (Figure 2.2). The entire optical system forms a sort of telemicroscope, which allows for viewing magnified images of objects at a short distance.

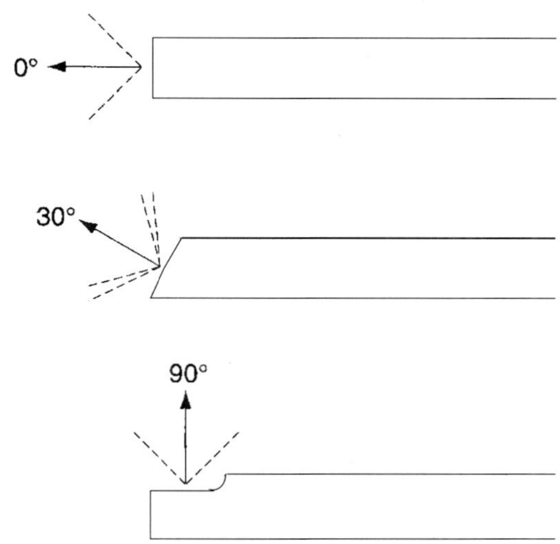

FIG. 2.1. The angle of view is limited by the angle of the objective lens.

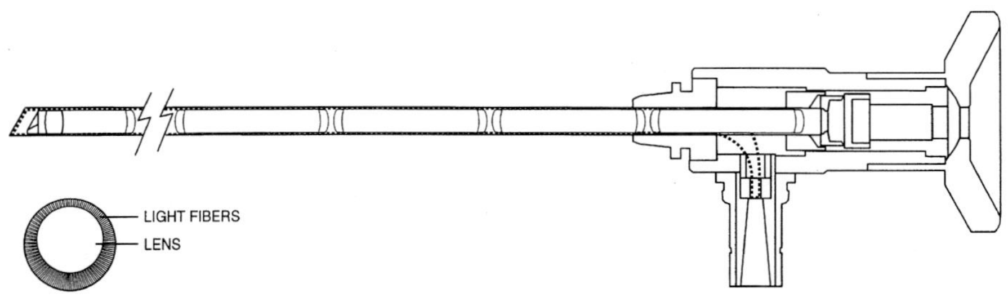

FIG. 2.2. The endoscope is a fine balance between the light fiber system that travels in the periphery around the lens collecting system.

CAMERAS AND CAMERA OPTICS

An optical coupling device on the camera (Figure 2.3) serves two purposes: it mechanically attaches the camera to the endoscope and, more important, it optically transfers the image from the endoscope's optical system to the camera's active pickup device. Often referred to as an endoscopic adapter, this optical coupler is either permanently attached to the camera head or screws into the head by a threaded ring. A permanently attached adapter virtually eliminates the chance for fogging to occur between the lens of the adapter and the camera head. The endoscopic adapter focuses and magnifies the endoscopic image onto the imaging sensor of the camera head for monitor viewing.

The amount of magnification depends upon the focal length of the endoscopic adapter, with the lower focal length corresponding with lower magnification. It is possible to purchase a variety of lenses with different focal lengths (25 mm to 40 mm) for use in various situations. A better solution, however, is to purchase a camera with a variable focal length zoom adapter. The built-in zoom adapter enables the surgeon to vary the magnification of the image at any point throughout the procedure, without the inconvenience of changing lenses.

A poor quality adapter will not allow for a clear image. The adapter and the endoscope optics must work together to produce a good image on the monitor. The endoscope, the endoscopic adapter, the camera head, the camera processor, and the monitor all contribute to image quality, the optics within the endoscopic adapter can degrade the image.

There are two types of cameras. The beam splitter camera allows the surgeon to visualize the field through the endoscope while the image is simultaneously seen on the video monitor. This is the most popular camera for endoscopic sinus surgery. The closed camera, on the other hand, limits the surgeon's operative field to that seen on the monitor. This creates a new dimension for surgery as one operates by remote control. This latter system is most popular with surgeons who perform arthroscopic surgery.

Each camera system has two components: a camera head and a central processing unit. The camera head contains the active device that transforms the optical image delivered by the endoscopic adapter into an electronic signal, which can then be transmitted down the light cable to the camera processor unit. This active device is called a charged coupled device (CCD). A CCD is a semi-conductor that has the property of turning photons into electrons. The optical image is projected onto the CCD surface, which is approximately 20 to 35 mm^2 in area. This surface is subdivided into approximately half a million individual picture elements, called pixels, which are small silicone elements. This has the effect of dividing the continuous optical image into discrete "tiles." To reproduce the continuous optical image as closely as possible, the number of pixels are maximized. The greater the number of pixels on the CCD, the higher the image resolution. From the CCD interface, the electronic image is transmitted down the camera cable to the processor of CCU.

There are two camera configuration options available for video-endoscopy: single-chip cameras that use one CCD and three-chip cameras that use three CCDs. The main difference in images produced by the two types is in horizontal resolution, which translates to detail recognition and color. Most single-chip cameras reproduce color by using a mosaic filter pattern. In this filter pattern, one of four different colored filters is placed over each pixel; this filter array requires an electronic process to reconstruct the colors and detail of the original image. Because not all of the color is available at each pixel, this reconstructive process does not fully recover all of the color and detail information that was present in the original optical image. So, from a theoretical standpoint, single-chip cameras have lower resolution and less accurate color reproduction than three-chip cameras. It should be noted, however, that the current state-of-the-art single-chip camera technology produces images that are very close in performance to three-chip cameras.

Three-chip cameras, on the other hand, use a prism that separates light into the three primary colors of red, green, and blue (RGB). There are three sensors, and each sensor transmits one color to the video monitor. There is no electronic process required for color conversion, and, therefore, the colors are reproduced more accurately. Because all of the information on each pixel is available for resolution, the number of lines increase from approximately 470 to 750. Unfortunately, the size of the three-chip camera makes it larger and potentially more difficult to handle. Expect an additional cost of $3000 to $4000 per camera.

An exception to the independent camera head is the video-endoscope. Variations of a one-piece camera/scope are: chip on a stick configuration, which places a sensor at the distal end of an endoscope, or connects the endoscope permanently to the camera head in order to optimize ergonomics. Video-endoscopes seem to be smaller and less expensive than the traditional combination of camera and scope because of the reduced optical requirements of the design. However, the reduced optical channels may also have reduced capabilities for drawing information from the scene. Drawbacks of many of the current video-endoscope configurations include system malfunctions and compatibility. If the system does not work, then neither the scope nor the camera can be used. This is in contrast to the independent camera and universal endoscope, where one can fail and the other will still function when using a one-piece camera and scope. Compatibility with other medical and surgical specialities may require additional purchases within the hospital because the endoscope measurement requirements may differ from specialty to specialty.

CAMERA CONTROL UNIT

The second part of any camera system is a camera control unit (CCU) that houses the power supply and electronics to process the information from the image sensors in the camera head and convert it to a standard video signal (Figure 2.4). White balancing to adjust for

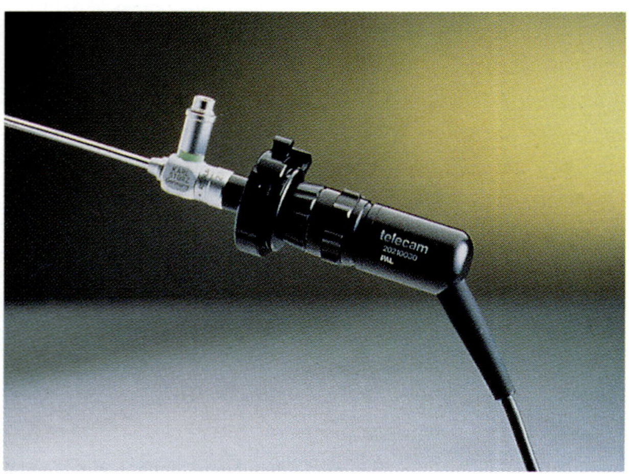

FIG. 2.3. Telecamera integral zoom/focus head attached to endoscope.

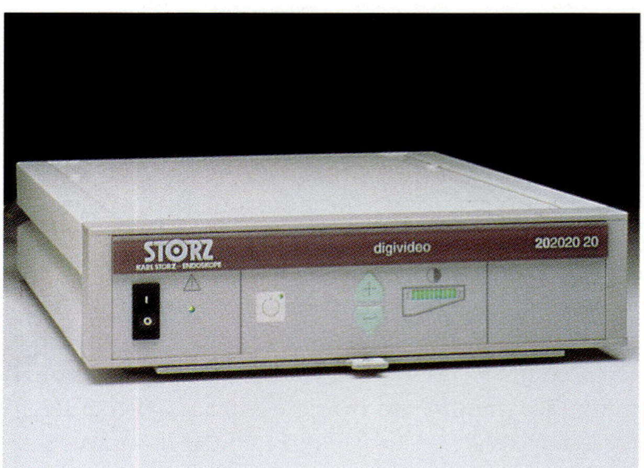

FIG. 2.4. Digivideo camera control unit.

different color temperatures of light sources is done either automatically through the camera head or in some units manually on the CCU. Automatic exposure and color bar by the CCU further refine the video output.

MONITOR

The television monitor for endoscopic surgery is a high-resolution monitor with upwards of 450 to 600 lines (Figure 2.5). This is in comparison to the home television unit that has only 250 lines of resolution. The limiting factor for the resolution of any video system is the lowest number of lines of resolution for any electrical component. If the camera has 600 lines of resolution and the video monitor has 400 lines of resolution, the maximum lines of resolution would be 400. In the future, we may expect to see high-density, high-resolution monitors with 1000 to 1200 lines of resolution.

On the back of the monitor are up to three types of inputs and outputs that relate to the three common standards by which video signals are sent to a monitor: composite, Y/C or S-video, and RGB. Generally, the best image is provided in the following order of desirability: RGB, Y/C, and composite. The differences lie in the way portions of the video signal—chrominance or color, luminescence or brightness, and synchronizing signals—are transmitted to the monitor. Composite video combines the elements of brightness, color, and synchronization into one signal. The combined signal reduces the amount of band width available to the components of luminescence, chrominance and synchronization. It also requires that the monitor (or other receiving device) separate these components. The translation often produces artifacts that are due entirely to the decoding process. The result is a sort of herringbone fuzziness at the boundaries between different colors. Y/C or S-video separates the brightness and color information into two distinct signals. It is capable of higher resolution than composite video because of the wide band width available on each channel. It also means that there is no requirement to separate these two signals at the monitor, thereby avoiding the decoding artifacts, which results in better color. The synchronizing signals are encoded with a luminescence signal, thus providing greater band width for chroma. RGB separates the synchronization, luminescence, and color information into four channels: red, green, blue, and synchronization, so the outcome is true color and high resolution. RGB is usually recommended when using a three-chip camera to get the full advantage of the true picture information.

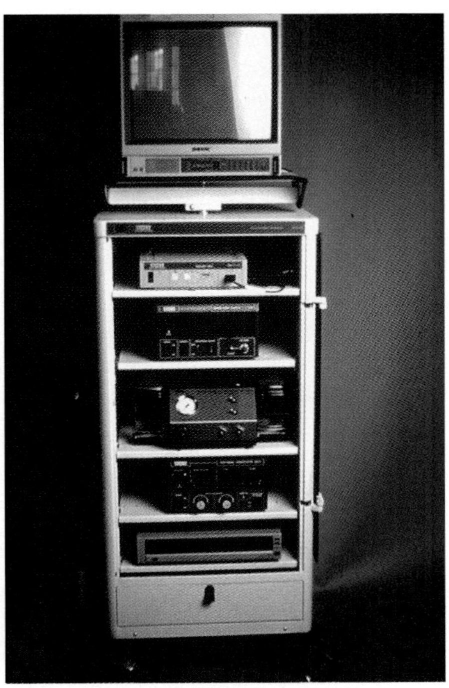

FIG. 2.5. Video setup with monitor on top for endoscopic surgery.

It is necessary to consider each component in the imaging chain when selecting the best output. The choices may be limited by the camera, monitor, or documentation accessories. Not all cameras, monitors, videocassette recorders, video printers, or image capture devices have RGB outputs. In these instances, Y/C is a recommended video output.

LIGHT SOURCES

The light sources that provide the illumination for the endoscopes differ in terms of illumination technology type, and the power of the source (usually expressed in watts). The power of a light source is a rough measure of its brightness, and as the wattage is increased, so is the illumination. This is always true when comparing sources of the same type. However, when different sources use similar wattage of power, they may produce different levels of brightness.

Endoscopic light sources come in different technology types that include halogen-tungsten, metal halide, and xenon, with power ratings from 150 to 500 W. The halogen-tungsten incandescent light source produces light in a yellow-green spectrum and is quite versatile. It is inexpensive, costing between $500 and $6000. The problem with this light source is that, as the wattage is increased, the lamp burns out quicker. Over time, the actual output decreases as the bulb gradually burns out. As a result, at the end of a bulb's life (approximately 100 hours), the output of the light source, and possibly the color as seen on the monitor will be altered.

The metal halide light units are sealed with a filament impregnated with one of the halogen metals. A

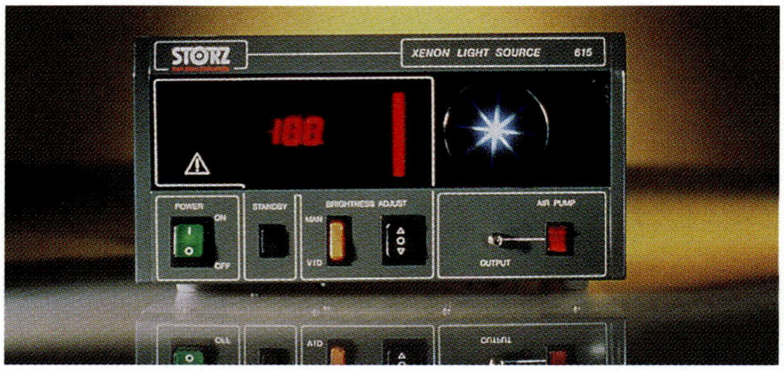

FIG. 2.6. Xenon light source.

particular metal will determine whether it is under the red or blue spectrum. These units cost between $3000 to $7000. The problem with the metal halide lamp is the visible spectrum or output is not constant. When the bulb is turned on, it takes time for it to reach its intended color temperature. These lamps usually burn for 200 to 250 hours.

The xenon light source (Figure 2.6) is a standard to which most light sources are compared. It is pure white light and most closely approaches the color of sunlight. The light source is actually a metal ceramic vessel filled with xenon gas under pressure. It always outputs the same color temperature throughout the life of the bulb. The cost is between $4000 to $21,000, and these lamps last from 400 to 1000 hours.

LIGHT-GUIDE CABLES

The problem with the early illuminated telescopes was that the light bulbs barely produced adequate light and they also produced heat that was highly undesirable. After the discovery of the way to "pipe" light from one location to another using fiberoptics, the light source became remote, thus keeping heat outside of the body while providing sufficient illumination.

Fiberoptics have the interesting property of containing the flow of light. Light that enters one end of an optical fiber will come out the other end with almost no loss. This happens through a mechanism of internal reflections. Fibers range in size from 30 to several hundred microns (a micron is one one-thousandth of a millimeter, or approximately 40 millionths of an inch). Thousands of these fibers are bundled together, surrounded with a protective jacket and fitted with metal end fittings in order to make an endoscopic light-guide cable. The cable is typically inserted into a light source at one end and attached to the light-guide post of the endoscope at the other.

Fluid-filled light cables transmit light through a fluid-filled medium. Although fluid cables are capable of carrying a greater amount of light, the cables themselves are less flexible and much more expensive. Due to recent innovations in fiber-optic technology, fiber-

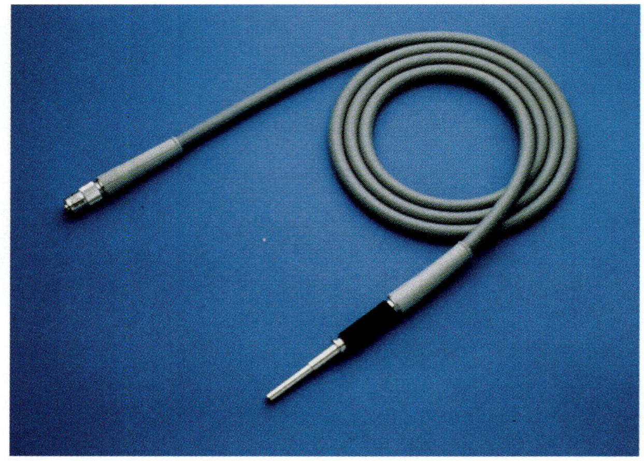

FIG. 2.7. Fiber-optic light cable.

optic cables are now capable of carrying almost as much light as do fluid cables, but at a much lower cost (Figure 2.7).

Light-guide cables are available in different diameters. The correct diameter depends upon the size of the endoscope being used. Matching the right cable to the right scope will prevent overheating and underillumination. Generally speaking, a smaller scope requires a smaller light guide.

ACCESSORIES

The previously described equipment forms the basic components required for any endoscopic procedure. Video documentation with video recorders or video printers is also available.

A key advantage of using the endoscopic video system is the ability to document surgical findings.

VCRs and printers must be selected carefully to match the same resolution as the video camera system. The resolution of the VCR or printer will determine the resolution of the image on the monitor.

Digital image enhancement systems can in real time enhance contrast and detail recognition and provide edge corrections of the endoscopic image. These enhancements provide the surgeon with improved detail recognition and increased information for diagnostic evaluation.

TROUBLESHOOTING

If the viewed video image does not appear accurate, start at the beginning of the imaging chain with the light source and check every device along the way. Light bulbs and fiberoptic bundles lose their intensity over time and need to be replaced. It is recommended to regularly check the number of hours on the light bulb of your light source, and replace the bulb when needed.

The light guide or cable will degrade over time in two different ways: discoloration and breakage. Discoloration will change the color appearance of the light that comes out of the light guide. By holding one end of the light guide to a light bulb or fluorescent lamp, any discoloration can be appreciated, and it will look considerably more yellow than the light source. Breakage occurs when individual fibers break within the protective housing. Using the same viewing arrangement, small black dots will appear in the projected light cone as fibers that are broken. A few broken fibers will not necessarily affect the transmission of light, but when one third of the fibers are missing, it is time to replace the light cable. Every black dot presents a small amount of light that is not getting from the light source to the endoscope.

Check the monitors frequently. Cameras provide color bars for checking the color, hue, and brightness of the monitor. When the monitor is improperly set, a clear vivid video image will be lost in a poor picture on the monitor.

REFERENCES

1. Lesserson JA, Schaeter SD: Instrumentation for endoscopic sinus surgery, Ears Nose Throat J 73:522-531, 1994.
2. Snow JB: Introduction to peroral endoscopy. In JJ Ballanger, editor: Diseases of the nose, throat, ear, head and neck, ed 14, Philadelphia, 1991, Lea and Febiger, p 1247.
3. Krause DE, Grybauskos VT, Friedman M: Instruments and equipment for endoscopic sinus surgery, Otolaryngol Clin North Am 22:4703-4711, 1989.

chapter three

The Nursing and Surgical Assistant Perspective in Endoscopic Forehead Surgery

Julene E. Cray, Nancy Jurek, and Ashley Shobe

With the rapid advancement of laser and endoscope technology, the surgeon and staff must be acutely aware of all safety parameters associated with both of these tools. The safety aspect of endoscopic laser cosmetic surgery is vital to the success of each procedure. Lack of communication and inadequate education are the major causes of laser accidents during endoscopy procedures.[1] The surgical staff (surgeon, circulating nurse, surgical assistant, and anesthesiologist) must function as a team to ensure proper and efficient use of the laser and endoscopic instrumentation.

The nursing care and setup require the nurse and surgical assistant to be technically oriented while maintaining the overall patient safety as their top priority.

PREOPERATIVE NURSING CARE AND SETUP

On the morning of surgery, before the patient arrives, the chart is prepared and reviewed for completeness: signatures, age, weight, past and current medical conditions, surgeries, allergies, medications, laboratory work-up values, postoperative instructions given, postoperative medications ordered, and preoperative pictures taken. The physician's orders are noted and the consent to operate is prepared.

The patient is scheduled to arrive 45 minutes before the procedure. During this time, the nurse greets the patient and his or her companion. The nurse answers any questions the patient or companion may have and informs them of the estimated time of completion, including recovery time. They are assured that the recovery nurse will review all postoperative instructions and appointments at time of discharge.

The patient is then directed to the changing room to remove clothing and jewelry before donning the gown, surgical hat, and foot covers. The patient is given a warm blanket in the preoperative chair while the nurse gives him or her the opportunity to express any fears or apprehensions. The nurse gently reassures the patient of his or her decision to have endoscopic cosmetic surgery. The vital signs are taken and the nursing checklist is completed, which reviews with the patient any controlled preexisting conditions, allergies, current medications, and when the patient last ate or drank and voided. The caregiver's telephone number is confirmed, and the location where the patient will be spending the first night after surgery is also confirmed. The consent is reviewed and then signed, the surgical routine is explained, the written postoperative instructions are discussed, and the patient is encouraged once again to raise any questions or fears at this time. The nurse explains that swelling and bruising in the forehead, brow, and eye area are not uncommon. The patient is also told to expect some blurry vision upon awakening in the recovery room as a result of the protective eye ointment used during the procedure.

The surgical assistant will introduce him or herself to the patient. The anesthesiologist will review all of the anesthesia protocol and the patient will then be walked to the operating room. The patient is positioned supine, and the gown is untied to prevent binding and provide more comfort for the patient. A warm blanket is placed next to the patient, a pillow is placed under the knees, and the elbows and heels are padded. The nurse communicates to the patient what he or she is doing and the reasons why. The intravenous line is started, and all appropriate monitors are placed on the patient for the induction of monitored anesthesia care.

PREOPERATIVE SETUP

The preoperative setup is prepared 1 hour before the surgery is scheduled to begin. The surgical assistant will select all of the instrumentation needed and sterilize or disinfect it, if necessary. The circulating nurse will help set up the room by placing the equipment in the correct position (Figure 3.1). The endoscopic video monitor (Karl Storz Imaging, Inc, Culver City, Calif.) can be placed on a swing arm and positioned over the patient's right side. The nurse will also test the function of the laser, the smoke evacuator, the electrocautery, the suction and video cart power source, light source, and monitor.

As the surgical assistant opens the sterile supplies and instrumentation on the sterile back table, the circulating nurse prepares the preoperative tray with a marking pen, examination gloves, 4×4 gauze, alcohol swabs, and a 20-cc syringe with local anesthetic. Also placed on the tray for the circulating nurse are examination gloves, comb, and small rubber bands. The surgical preparation solution is prepared on a sterile field with sterile 4×4 gauze. Tumescent solution (500 cc lactated Ringer's with 25 cc lidocaine 1% and 1 cc Adrenalin) is prepared and attached to a venoset, which is threaded through the Kline pump and connected to a 22-gauge, 3.5-inch spinal needle ready for injection by the physician.

The circulating nurse ensures at this time that all laser safety controls are in place according to the laser safety checklist. The laser should be positioned over the surgeon's dominant shoulder for ease of maneuverability. This also prevents the arm from crossing over the sterile field and making it awkward for the assistant to retract and assist.

The smoke evacuator is essential to ensure adequate plume evacuation. The filters in the smoke evacuator need to be changed according to the manufacturer's instructions. Wall suction is not sufficient, and if used for plume evacuation, the carbon particles may clog the entire wall suction system.

The key to the laser must be retrieved from its secure location. The key should not be left in the laser when unattended to prevent unauthorized operations, in accordance with the requirements of the Occupational

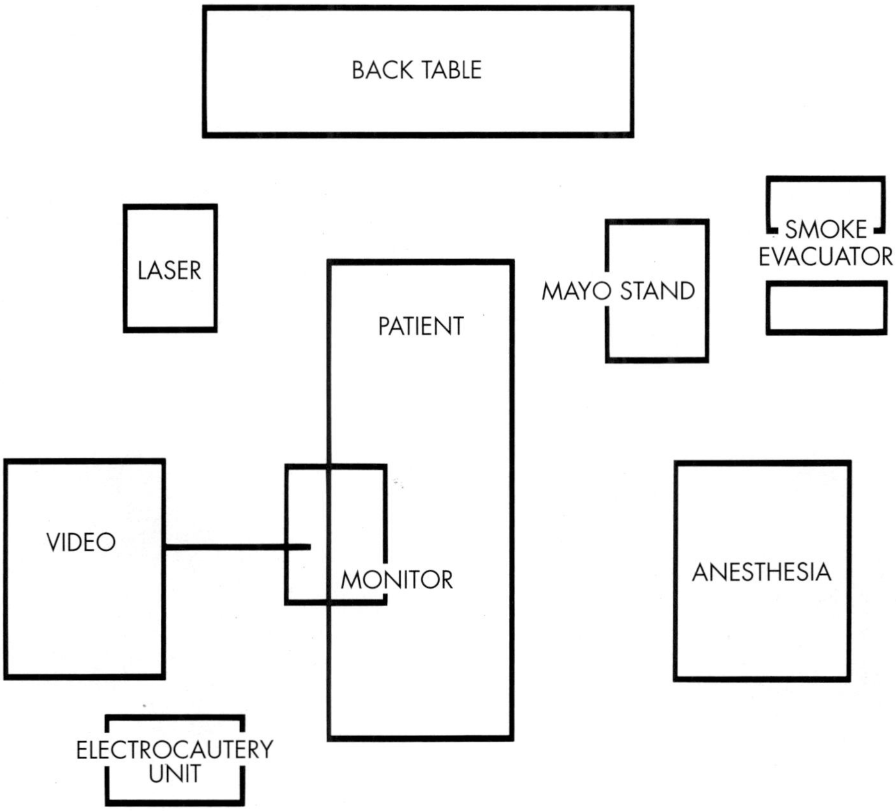

FIG. 3.1. Diagram of placement of equipment: laser, video cart and monitor, anesthesia, smoke evacuator, and electrocautery unit.

Safety and Health Administration (OSHA).[2] The laser is then test fired for beam alignment and function. To minimize the possibility of a fire hazard, a basin of water or normal saline should be on the back table, and the location of the nearest industry standard fire extinguisher should be noted.

Danger signs should be placed on all doors leading into the operating suite to clearly warn anyone wishing to enter. An appropriate pair of safety glasses can also be attached to the sign for use by the person entering. All staff in the room should have safety eyewear available for use during the laser activation. The patient's eyes are usually covered with moist 2×2 gauze and tape.

The physician then marks the scalp incisions and the guide lines he or she will use for asymmetry. He or she then injects the local and the tumescent solution to the forehead, temple, and adjacent scalp areas. The circulating nurse binds the hair away from the incision sites by placing small rubber bands around each section (Figure 3.2). Next, the nurse performs the surgical preparation of the neck, face, and hair with Betadine solution (never alcohol or Hibiclens if the laser is to be used), making sure to soak the banded areas of hair as well as wiping the oral airway and oxygen tubing.

The surgical assistant has draped the patient from the neck to the feet with sterile drapes and puts the following equipment on the sterile field (Figure 3.3):

1. Thirty-degree endoscope inserted into sheath, with sterile light source cable and a three-chip camera attached to the eyepiece of the scope
2. Endoscopic bipolar cautery, with sterile power cord and suction tubing
3. Flexible insulated suction cautery
4. Infusion tubing for the tumescent solution
5. Argon tubing for the cooling of the CO_2 laser fiber
6. External bipolar cautery
7. Laser smoke evacuator tubing with cone

The ends of each of the above are handed off the field to the circulating nurse to be connected to the proper equipment.

The articulating arm of the CO_2 laser is draped with a sterile plastic cover, and the 3.0- by 450-mm fiber (Sharplan Lasers, Inc, Allendale, N.J.) is attached to the Fiberlase 3.0 handpiece with a coupler device. The articulated arm is counterbalanced and is left hanging over the back table until it is used (Figure 3.4).

After the skin is prepped, the surgical assistant will complete the sterile draping by securing a sterile towel around the hair with staples (3m Precise DS-25, 3M Medical, St. Paul, Minn.).

The circulating nurse then connects all of the previously described instrumentation to the appropriate equipment and aids the assistant in whiting out the camera on the video monitor.

The Mayo stand is set up with the following instrumentation (Figure 3.5):

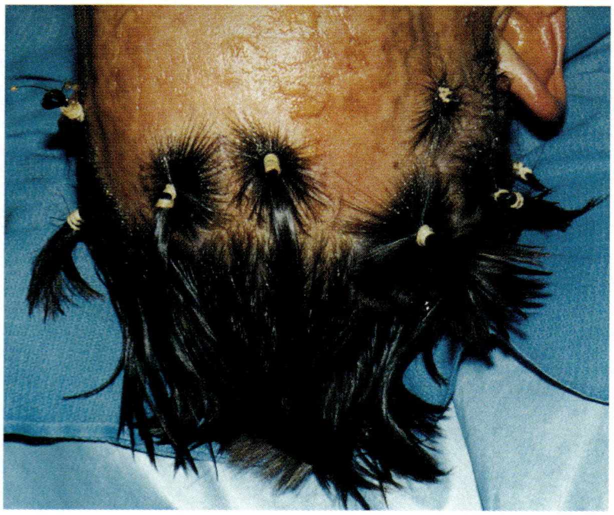

FIG. 3.2. Rubber bands are used to bind the hair away from the incisions.

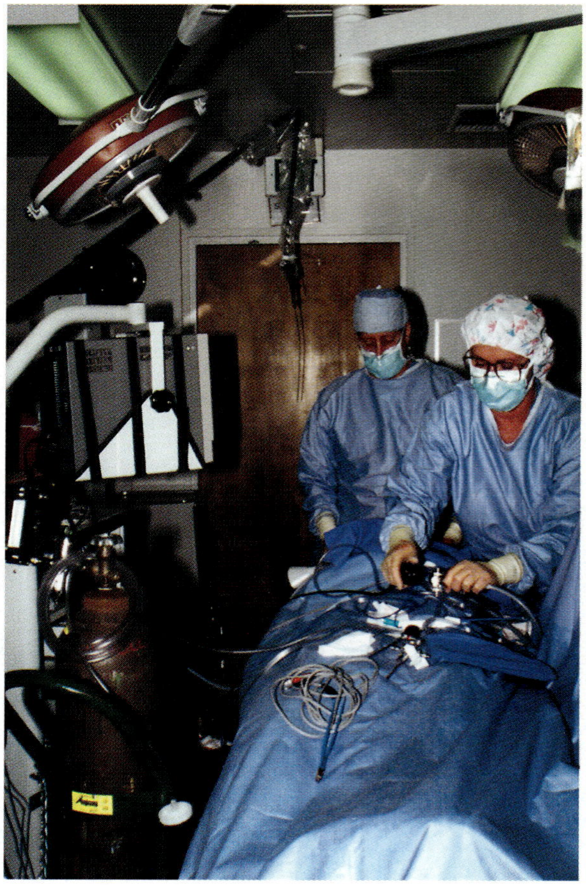

FIG. 3.3. The sterile field with instrumentation shown.

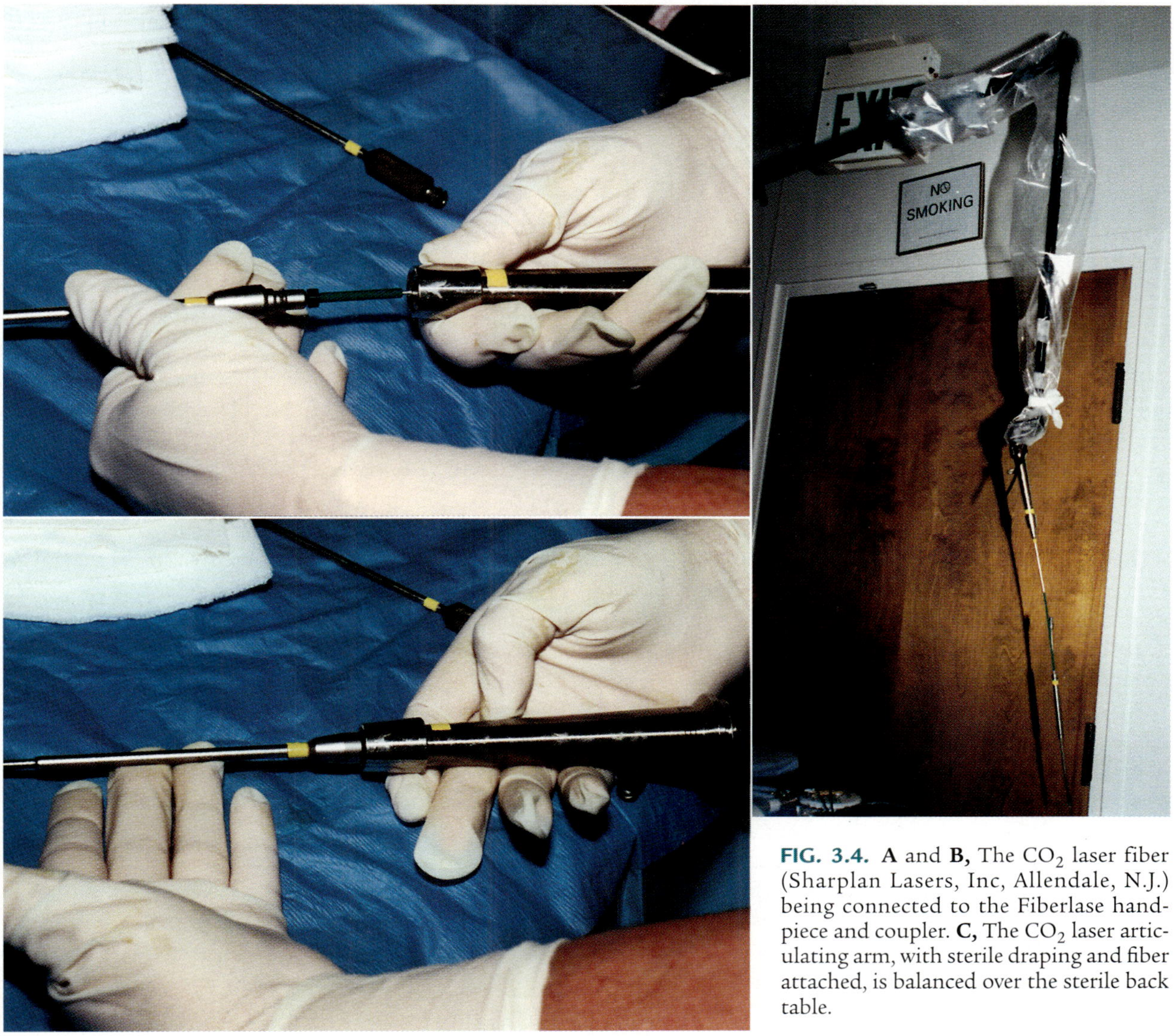

FIG. 3.4. **A** and **B,** The CO_2 laser fiber (Sharplan Lasers, Inc, Allendale, N.J.) being connected to the Fiberlase handpiece and coupler. **C,** The CO_2 laser articulating arm, with sterile draping and fiber attached, is balanced over the sterile back table.

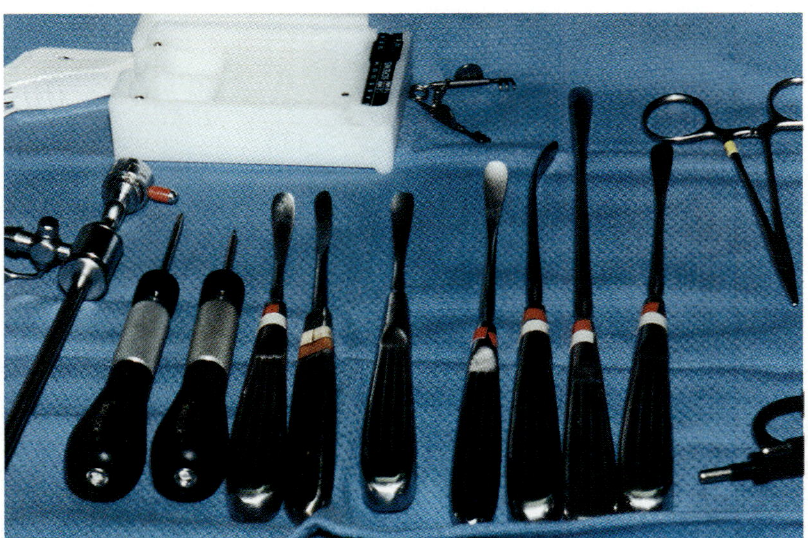

FIG. 3.5. Mayo stand instrumentation. (Karl Storz Imaging, Inc, Culver City, Calif.)

1. Additional endoscopic sheath
2. Self-tapping screwdrivers and bone screws, Osteomed 1.6- by 12-mm screws, No. 208612 or (Anspach 2- by 12-mm screws, Part No. 912-112 if Anspach is used, a microdrill and power source is required.)
3. Small incision skin retractor
4. Six to seven various elevators (Karl Storz Imaging, Inc, Culver City, Calif.)
5. Needle holder with 310 Prolene or Polysorb (P-12)
6. Three endoscopic dissectors: horizontal, vertical and straight

"Trouble-shooting for equipment malfunctions (and failures) should be in place and back-up systems should be available to ensure successful completions of a closed endoscopic procedure without conversion to an open salvage technique."[3]

INTRAOPERATIVE NURSING

As the surgical team begins the procedure, it is like a well-choreographed dance, with each member responding to the movements of the other.

The endoscopic incisions are very small and often require the surgical assistant to guide the distal end of the endoscope into the incision, then lifting the incisions with two small skin hooks to allow passage of the endoscope. The assistant positions and stabilizes the head while providing traction of tissue. The surgical assistant is sometimes required to hold the videoscope so the physician is free to use both hands for manipulating the instrumentation. The assistant is often kept busy securing all the tubing and cords on the sterile field in a neat and orderly manner. Most important, the fiber-optic light cord must be prevented from becoming kinked in order to protect the delicate fibers inside. The surgical assistant must also be available to assist the anesthesiologist in maintaining a patent airway by lifting the chin or adjusting the oral airway tube.

The circulating nurse, besides being responsible for all of the documentation associated with a surgical case, will assist in adjusting the overhead lights in and out of the surgical field and turning room lights off and on at the request of the physician. The video monitor and xenon light source need to be put on standby when the scope is not in use to prevent the light source from igniting the dry drapes. It is also the responsibility of the nurse to assume the role of the laser safety advocate. The nurse needs to be attentive to the communication from the surgeon as to what settings are preferred, and then he or she must input them correctly. Once the laser is turned on, the laser is the nurse's number one responsibility along with the patient. The laser needs to be put on standby whenever there is a pause in its use. This is extremely important because most of the accidents that occur with lasers are from misdirected beams that produce flammability hazards.[4]

POSTOPERATIVE NURSING AND INSTRUMENTATION

When the procedure is complete, all instrumentation is disconnected, and surgical drapes are removed. The rubber bands are removed from the hair. Antibiotic ointment is placed on all stapled incisions lines. A sterile Hydrosorb pressure dressing (Calgon Vestal, No. 1694-NX, Avitar Inc, distributed by Merck & Co, Inc, St. Louis, Mo.) is placed over the forehead and covering the brows; Surgipad is used over the scalp, which is covered with Sof-Kling (Johnson & Johnson, Arlington, Tex.) and an Ace wrap to help prevent swelling and bruising. When the patient is stable, he or she is transferred to the recovery room via gurney. The head is elevated 30 degrees and ice bags are placed on the forehead and scalp. Usually, the patient is in the postanesthesia room for approximately an hour until all discharge criteria are met and the caregiver arrives to transport the patient.

POSTOPERATIVE CLEANING AND STERILIZATION OF THE ENDOSCOPE

Endoscopic instruments require specific processing procedures to ensure patient safety and comply with the Bloodborne Pathogen Standard of OSHA.[5]

Endoscopes for cosmetic surgery are designed to minimize trauma, and are therefore made as small as practical. (For more detailed information about the endoscope, please see Chapter 2 on endoscopes.) These endoscopes can be delicate and must be handled with care. This care not only includes the proper cleaning and sterilization process but also the inspection before and after use for any sign of damage. Dents along the shaft and scratches on the lenses are the most noticeable signs of damage. Look through and rotate the telescope to check the clarity of the view. Scratches, fingerprints, or residual debris will be obvious and will cause an impaired view. Additionally, debris may act as an abrasive and scratch the lens.

The impairment of the fibers can also cause darkened areas in the field of view. The fiberoptics are intact when the light is evenly distributed at the distal tip. Foggy images may result from moisture entering a damaged seal around the lens. A partially or completely obstructed view may be the result of damaged lenses within the endoscope shaft or eyepiece.

Failure to properly maintain and use these instruments may result in trauma to delicate tissues, perforation, infection, or breakage of the instruments, which can produce foreign bodies.[6]

Cleaning

Cleaning is the first and most important step in reprocessing the endoscopic instrumentation. To prevent blood, protein material, and other contaminants from drying on the endoscope, it should be placed immediately after use in a cleaning enzyme/disinfectant solution that dissolves sugars and proteins. The instrumentation should be disassembled into the component parts before cleaning. Manual cleaning is the safest and most effective method. Do not put other instruments on top of the scopes. The external and internal surfaces of the endoscope must be cleaned. If an instrument is not properly cleaned, it cannot be sterilized or disinfected.[5] Always refer to the manufacturer's guidelines for appropriate cleaning instructions.

Sterilization

Routine ethylene oxide (ETO) gas sterilization is recommended for all endoscopes. However, the cost and restrictive policies surrounding ETO prohibit most surgery centers and offices from using this method. Therefore, high-level disinfection is commonly used in these settings.

Some endoscopes are marked "autoclavable," which means that they can be steam-autoclaved only and not flashed-autoclaved. However, the life of these scopes will be longer if ETO or chemical disinfection is used.

Disinfection

Glutaraldehyde (14-day, 2% concentration without surfactants, eg, Cidex [Johnson & Johnson, Arlington, Tex.]) is the most commonly used disinfectant for endoscopic equipment. Only Environmental Protection Agency–registered disinfectant solutions capable of high-level disinfection should be used. It is important to follow solution manufacturers' instructions and pay close attention to proper dilution and recommended minimum exposure times for the endoscopes. Prolonged exposure may result in tarnishing or corrosion.[6]

After removal from the disinfectant, glutaraldehyde manufacturers are now recommending three separate, copious rinses of at least 1 minute each.[5] The disinfectant can be caustic to skin and mucous membranes, so it is imperative that the endoscopes be rinsed properly with sterile water. The endoscope should be dried with a sterile soft cloth, and alcohol can be applied to the fiber surfaces to complete the drying process.

The endoscopic equipment (telescope, fiber-optic light cable, and sheaths) should be stored safely and properly.

CONCLUSION

In summary, the operative assistance by the nurse and surgical technician are critical to the innovative methods being employed by the surgeon in endoscopic forehead surgery. In this rapidly advancing field of high technology, we must maintain our standard of care for the patient. The challenge of increasingly sophisticated equipment and new procedures will continue to take us into the 21st century. We as health care professionals must continue to cooperate as a team and learn together for the benefit of our patients.

REFERENCES

1. Zickefoose, S: Nasal surgery using laser with endoscopy surgery. AORN J 50(5):979-988, 1989.
2. American National Standards Institute. Safe Use of Lasers in Health Care Facilities. Laser Institute of America Publishers, Orlando, Fla., February 1996, p 8.
3. Muschenheim R: Nursing care for endoscopically treated patients. In Sasaki G, editor: Endoscopic aesthetic reconstructive surgery, Philadelphia, 1996, Lippincott-Raven, pp 3-12.
4. Anonymous. Laser use and safety. Health Devices, 21:306-310, 1992.
5. Young E: Disinfecting and sterilizing endoscopic instrumentation: what are your choices? Min Invas Surg Nurs 10(1):27-29, 1996.
6. Karl Storz Imaging, Inc. Hopkins rigid telescopes, instructions for use, Karl Storz Imaging, Inc, Culver City, Calif., 1994.

4

chapter four

Aesthetic Considerations for the Upper Third of the Face

William H. Beeson and Gregory S. Keller

The upper third of the face is a very dynamic and expressive area of the face, and it, including the periorbital area, is a focal point not only for the expression of our emotions and personality, but also in an aesthetic sense. It is important to have an aesthetic concept of beauty with regard to this area of the face. Because beauty is the harmony, symmetry, and proportion of one's face, it is crucial to look at the cephalometrics of the upper third of the face. DaVinci described the basic tenets of the face as being divided into thirds (Figure 4.1, *A*) and being five widths of an eyelid (Figure 4.1, *B*). The eyebrows should lie at the approximate level of the superior orbital rim, with the highest point of the brow being the lateral one third (a point tangent to the lateral limbic margin).

Some surgeons have found anthropometric and cephalometric parameters to be helpful when considering foreheadplasty. Farkas and Kolar1 noted that the most attractive women had a forehead that was smaller in proportion (as well as being shorter in height) when compared to the middle and lower third of the face. McKinney2 has suggested that the normal distance from the midpupil to the upper brow is 2.5 cm. A lesser distance could be an indication for foreheadplasty or browlift. Farkas and Kolar have noted that the acceptable distance from the trichion to the glabellar area should be approximately 61.9 mm and from the brow to the anterior hairline, approximately 5 cm. When measurements are less than these, foreheadplasty may well be indicated.

EYEBROW

Ideally, the eyebrow is a gracefully arching structure, located at the level of the superior orbital rim in men and slightly above that plane in women. In women, the medial aspect of the eyebrow is tangent to a vertical line drawn through the lateral nasal ala margin. The lateral brow terminates on an oblique line crossing through the nasal ala and lateral canthus. The medial and lateral extents should be in a horizontal plane. The superior point of the brow is the lateral third (approximately the margin of the later limbus). The medial extent of the brow has a "clubbed-head" configuration, whereas laterally the brow gradually tapers (Figure 4.2).

There are characteristic sexual features of the forehead and eyebrows. The superior orbital ridges from the upper border of the orbit, separating the midface from the forehead. The protrusion of the supraorbital rim is more prominent in its lateral third in men. Pneumatization of the frontal sinus accounts for prominent frontal bossing—an overlying protrusion of the frontal bone. Women have a smoother, gentler, continuous curve from the supraorbital rim to the upper forehead as a result of the lack of frontal bossing and a less prominent superior orbital rim.

PHYSIOLOGY AND FUNCTION

Physiologically, the function of the brow is limited: it serves primarily to protect the eye. Brow hairs not only shade the eye, but also function to prevent perspiration, dust, and other irritants from coursing down the forehead area and into the eye. Although the eyebrows may have a somewhat limited function physiologically, they do play a significant role in projecting one's mood through action of the frontalis, corrugator supercilia, orbicularis oculi, and procerus muscles, all of which have an effect on eyebrow motility. Inferior displacement of the medial portion of the eyebrows project malice. A similar displacement laterally gives the appearance of sadness, and a fatigued appearance is portrayed when the overall area becomes ptotic.

Ptosis of the upper brow can contribute significantly to superior and lateral visual field defects. There may also be interference with the motility of the upper eyelid. Ptosis of the upper brow is often associated with "gravitational" aging syndrome, but not all cases of ptosis are associated with aging. Some cases may be the result of congenitally low set brows or an acquired form of dermatochalasis. It goes without saying that effective management of the ptotic brow is essential in obtaining the desired aesthetic improvement in the periorbital area.

As we age, a number of things happen. Skin loses its moisture and elasticity, fat redistributes itself, muscles atrophy, and the skeleton gradually resorbs. These changes have significant influence on the upper one third of the face. In fact, the periorbital and forehead are often the first areas to exhibit changes, which many people seek to surgically rectify. Although the normal aging process significantly affects the aesthetics of the upper third of the face, facial animation and muscle dynamics dramatically influence aesthetics in this area of the face, even at a very early age.

Ellis and Masai[3] have pointed out that three basic patterns of behavior can be identified regarding the animation of the upper half of the face: eyebrow raising, frowning, and squinting. These patterns are usually established in the individual by the age of 6 and will influence greatly the aging process of the upper one third of the face (Table 4.1).

1. Brow lifting is a result of frontalis muscle activity.

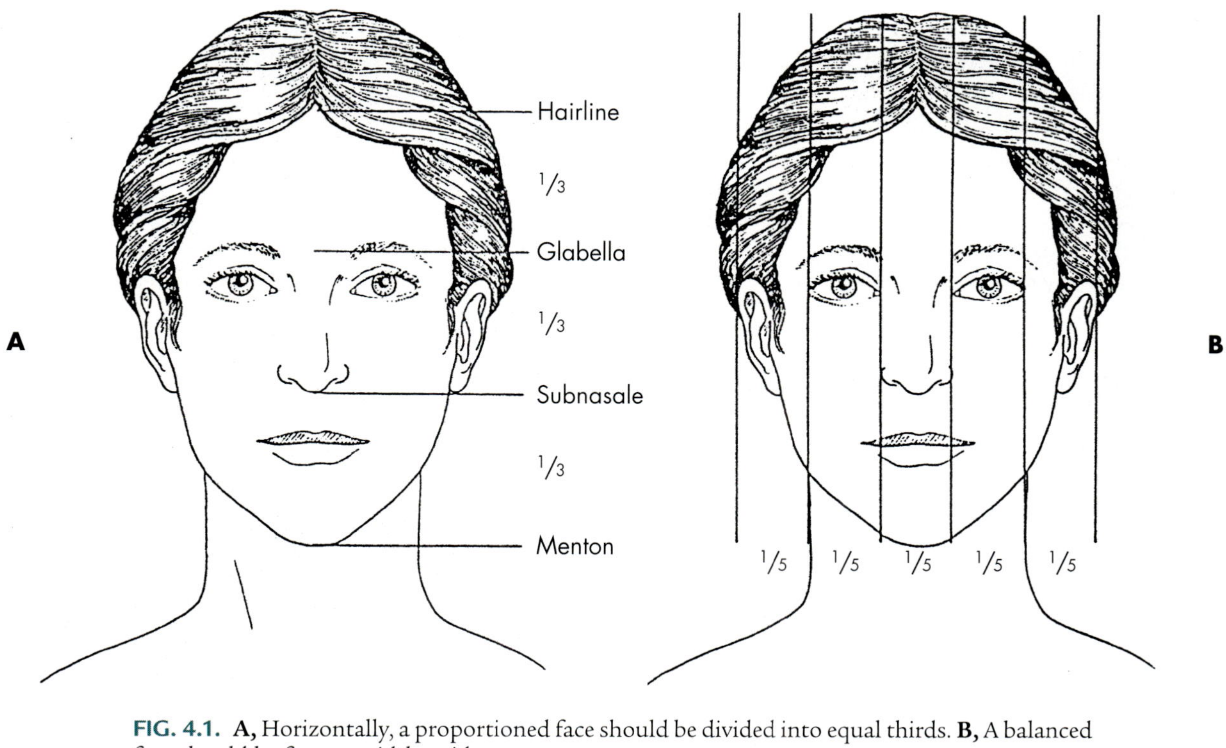

FIG. 4.1. **A,** Horizontally, a proportioned face should be divided into equal thirds. **B,** A balanced face should be five eye widths wide.

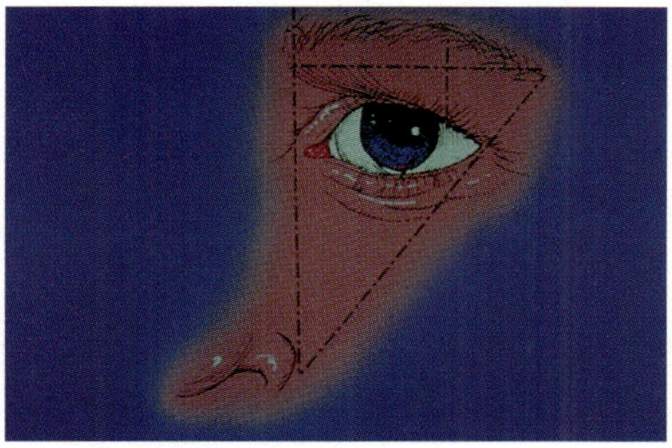

FIG. 4.2. Ideal eyebrow symmetry and proportion.

TABLE 4.1
UPPER FACIAL ANIMATION

Action	Muscles Involved	Results
Brow lift	Frontalis	Brow ptosis
Frowning	Corrugator supercilia	Glabellar rhytids
Squinting	Orbicularis oculi	Crow's-feet/laugh lines

Contraction results in brow ptosis, which usually promotes further horizontal wrinkling.

2. Frowning is a natural expression of anger or puzzlement. It pulls the medial end of the eyebrows together by action of the corrugator supercilia muscles in the medial part of the orbicularis ocular. It develops very deep, vertical glabellar lines.
3. Squinting is a dominant pattern in individuals with uncorrected errors of refraction, long-term stress, or prolonged exposure to light. It is the orbicularis oculi muscle acting unopposed by the frontalis muscle laterally that causes the common "crow's-feet" or "laugh lines."

Thus, it appears that adults animate the upper third of the face according to a pattern that is well established in late childhood, although environmental factors may play an important role in establishing this pattern early in life.

Proportion, Balance, and Symmetry vs. Aesthetic Trends in Fashion

Although it is true that proportion and balance play an important part in our concept of beauty, it is important to note aesthetic trends and cultural differences. For example, in the 1960s the style for the upper third of the face was a "wide-eyed" look, with high-arched, sharply manicured eyebrows. This stands in contrast to today's "natural" trend, with a narrower eyelid and a lower set, more dense eyebrow (the "Brooke Shields" look).

Indications for aesthetic foreheadplasty are ptosis of the lateral one third of the eyebrow, glabellar ptosis, and vertical glabellar rhytids. Physicians should have a thorough understanding of the anatomy of the region and be aware of the various surgical approaches that can be used to correct this problem, as well as the complications that can be associated with each of the procedures.

PATIENT SELECTION

In evaluating candidates for management of the ptotic eyebrow, and when considering which surgical approach to employ, it is imperative to assess: frontal hairline and general hair density, the presence of redundancy in the glabellar area, the presence or absence of forehead rhytids, and general skin pigmentation. It is also important to inquire about a history of hyperpigmentation or history of hypertrophic scarring.

Traditionally, there have been three approaches to management of the ptotic brow: direct approach, mid-forehead, coronal approach, and pretrichial approach. As with any surgical procedure, there can be complications and undesired results. Artz et al[4] reported their series of 40 patients who underwent foreheadplasty by traditional surgical techniques: 18 coronal, 19 anterior hairline approach, 2 mid-forehead, 1 supraorbital (or direct brow lift). Approximately 15% of patients had a complication or a condition that required additional surgical treatment. It should be noted that management of the upper third of the face is not a "benign" process and that close attention to basic tenets of patient selection, a thorough knowledge of the anatomy, and adherence to meticulous surgical technique is of critical importance. Today, endoscopic foreheadplasty opens a new vista for surgical management of the upper third of the face. However, the aesthetic parameters and indications for patient selection remain the same, regardless of treatment modality.

REFERENCES

1. Farkas LG, Kolar JC: Anthropometrics and art in the aesthetics of women's faces. Clin Plast Surg 14(4):599-616, 1987.
2. McKinney P, Mossie RD, Zubowsi ML: Criteria for the forehead lift. Aesthetic Plast Surg 15:141, 1991.
3. Ellis DA, Masai H: The effect of facial animation on the aging upper half of the face. Arch Otolaryngol Head Neck Surg 115:710-713, 1989.
4. Artz JS, Dinner MI, Foflietti MA: Planning the aesthetic foreheadplasty. Ann Plast Surg 25(1):1-6, 1990.

chapter five

Endoscopic Forehead and Brow Lift

Gregory S. Keller and Robert Hucherson

Endoscopic forehead and brow lifting techniques have become the most popular of endoscopic facial plastic surgery techniques over the past several years. The forehead, with its unusual combination of readily accessible dissection planes and muscular slings, appears to be ideally suited for endoscopic manipulations.

Although endoscopic techniques have been used for bronchoscopy, sinusoscopy, esophagoscopy, and cystoscopy since the turn of the century, the use of endoscopes to visualize and incise the corrugator, procerus, and depressor musculature and to perform temple lifts was not reported until 1991.[1,2] Since then, a myriad of techniques have emerged for surgery on the forehead and brow.[3-26]

In order to place these techniques into context and to present a balanced view of forehead endoscopy, this chapter is divided into three parts: first, a principles and concepts section; then, an atlas section presenting a basic technique; and finally, a patient evaluation section that allows the surgeon to classify common patient problems that require variations of the basic technique.

PRINCIPLES AND CONCEPTS OF ENDOSCOPIC FOREHEAD AND BROW SURGERY

The Three Basic Methods Used to Alter the Forehead

Basically, there are three ways to effect a change in the forehead: (1) myotomy of the small facial expressive muscles that depress the brow (corrugator, procerus, orbicularis oculi, depressor supercilii) or elevate it (frontalis), (2) denervation of these facial expressive muscles, and (3) shifting of the forehead backward to elevate the brow (Box 5.1). Forehead lifting procedures use these manuevers to achieve the goals of brow elevation, reduction of horizontal forehead rhytids, reduction of vertical glabellar rhytids, elevation of lateral canthal hooding produced by a downward sagging of the forehead tissues in the region of the brow tail, and reduction of infrabrow skin overhang produced by downward sagging of the forehead tissues in the region of the brow body.

In most forehead procedures, myotomy of the brow depressor muscles, with a subsequent backward elevation of the forehead and brow, is used to modify rhytids, to elevate the brow, to diminish infrabrow overhang, and to diminish lateral hooding. In some procedures, however, myotomy alone is performed for the purpose of diminishing rhytids by interrupting the muscle's rhytid-producing action. Other procedures use a combination of myotomy to release some of the depressor muscles that lower the brow (orbicularis) and denervation of various temporal nerve branches to release others (corrugator, procerus, orbicularis).

Either myotomy alone or in combination with denervation can weaken the depressor muscles of the brow. If the weakening of the depressor muscles is sufficient, the elevator muscles (occipitalis-galeal-frontalis sling) work with less opposition from these depressor muscles and, in some instances, can elevate the brow without posterior fixation of the scalp.[9,27]

BOX 5.1. THREE BASIC METHODS USED TO ALTER THE FOREHEAD

1. Myotomies of corrugator, procerus, orbicularis oculi, depressor supercilii, and frontalis muscles
2. Denervation of these muscles
3. Shifting of the forehead backward to elevate the brow

BOX 5.2. UNIQUE CONCEPTS OF ENDOSCOPIC FOREHEAD LIFTING

1. Small incisions rather than a single large incision
2. Creation of an optical cavity
3. Release of the brow with myotomy and/or denervation
4. Elevation of the brow through posterior fixation of the scalp

Four Technique Concepts Common to Endoscopic Forehead Rhytidectomy Methods

Despite the multiplicity of methods for endoscopic forehead and brow lifting, all of them accomplish their goals in one or more of the manners previously enumerated. In reviewing different methods for forehead and brow lifting, four concepts are unique and shared by most methods of endoscopic aesthetic forehead surgery: (1) the use of several small incisions rather than a large coronal or pretrichial incision, (2) the creation of an optical cavity, (3) release of the brow via myotomy, and (4) elevation of the brow via posterior shifting of the forehead and scalp. In a sense, these unique concepts represent procedure steps that are accomplished in sequential order (Box 5.2).

Use of several small incisions rather than a coronal or pretrichial incision. By the use of a series of small incisions, access is gained to the forehead and brow for both the endoscope (for visualization) and instruments or laser (for manipulation, incision, modification). The use of small incisions allows the surgeon to minimize damage to the sensory nerves (supraorbital) that normally are interrupted with larger (coronal or pretrichial) incisions and to diminish the hair loss that accompanies large incisions that resect hair-bearing scalp. There are many variations of small incision placement that are tailored for hair loss patterns, size of forehead, surgical access, and other considerations.

As these incisions have evolved, they have become smaller and oriented in the scalp over the frontal bone in a vertical direction. Most of these small vertical incisions become undetectable and have a cosmetic advantage over a single larger incision or a horizontal incision, which can alter hair direction.

Figure 5.1 illustrates typical incisions that we use for most female patients. Other authors' incisions are illustrated in subsequent chapters.

We use four vertical incisions in the frontal area. The lateral frontal fixation incisions are 1 cm in length and are placed at or lateral to the lateral canthus over the frontal bone. This lateral placement keeps the incisions closest to the region of the brow tail to gain maximal upward pull on this region, the area most likely to fail in both endoscopic and coronal forehead lifting techniques.

These laterally placed incisions have an outward vector of pull to relieve infrabrow crowding. This outward vector of pull brings the "fallen in" glabellar area upward and outward. Postoperative outward "splaying" of the interbrow distance is minimized by using a lateral incision placed at the level of the lateral canthus when compared to an incision placed at the level of the lateral limbus. The lateral limbus incision, placed closer to the medial edge of the brow, exerts a more powerful pull on the medial brow edge than does the incision placed at the level of the lateral canthus. The lateral limbus incision splays the brows to a greater degree and elevates both the medial forehead and the medial brow more (usually a less preferable result).

Two central incisions that are placed behind the hairline in the vertical plane of the medial brow are used. With the movement of the lateral (fixation) incisions so far outward, the ability to use them for visualization or instrumentation when modifying the medial musculature becomes difficult. With two central incisions, the endoscope can be placed through one, and instrumentation can be placed in the other while the small midline muscles are released.

The temple incisions are 2 cm long and are placed diagonally (in a similiar direction as the temple portion of a face-lift incision) rather than vertically. The bottom portion of the incision is at approximately the superior orbital rim. This placement allows for a maximal outward and upward force on the brow tail, which usually needs to be "unrolled" from a position that has fallen over the vertical portion of the orbital rim.

For patients with male pattern baldness, it is often necessary to vary these incisions. For males, 1-cm vertical incisions are usually placed along the male fringe. If a small vertical incision can be hidden in a frontal tuft, or if a frontal tuft is going to be created with hair transplantation techniques, a single 1-cm incision can also be placed in the midline (Figure 5.2).

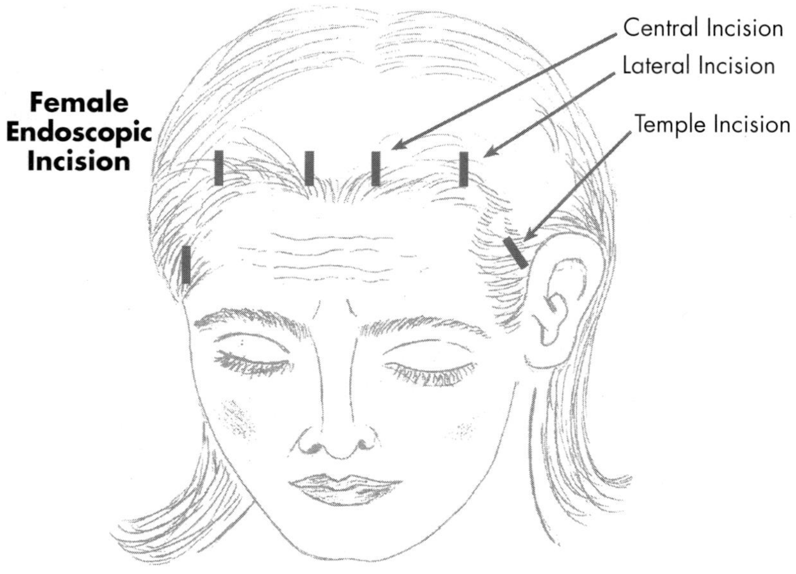

FIG. 5.1. Endoforehead incisions: women.

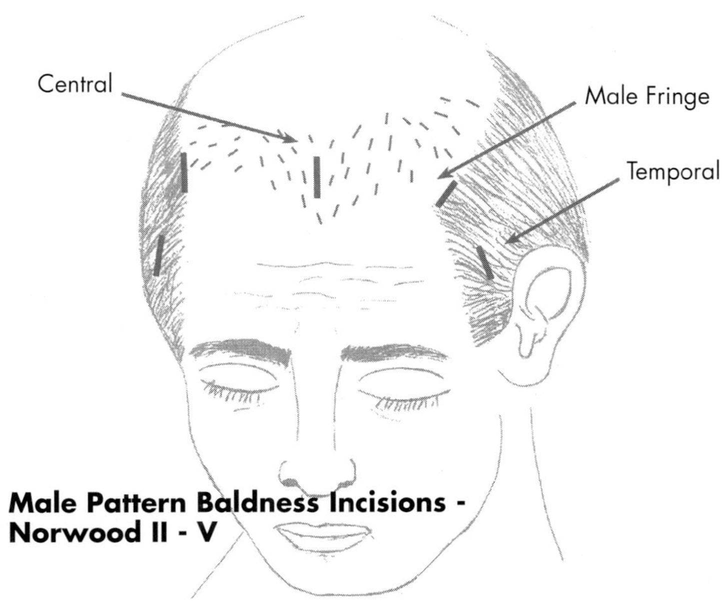

FIG. 5.2. Endoforehead incisions: male pattern baldness (Norwood types II–V).

If a frontal tuft is missing, and one is not going to be created, the frontal area may be accessed in retrograde fashion through a blepharoplasty incision (Figure 5.3). Alternatively, the frontal area medial to the supraorbital nerve may be left alone, and a segmental endoscopic temple lift is performed through the temple and fringe incisions. Other authors, as described in subsequent chapters, use horizontal incisions placed high on the forehead for patients with baldness.

In women who have a high forehead and want to lower the hairline, a pretrichial or trichophytic incision is constructed (Figure 5.4). In women with a receding (male pattern) hairline, a single vertical central incision (rather than two midcentral incisions) is used to access the mid-forehead, similar to Norwood types II–V male pattern baldness patients.

The trend in endoscopic forehead lift surgery has been to tailor the position of various portions of the brow; therefore, many exceptions to this incision plan are possible. For instance, when the midbrow needs significant elevation, the lateral fixation incisions are placed at the lateral limbus to achieve a greater vector of pull at the midbrow. When the medial brow needs

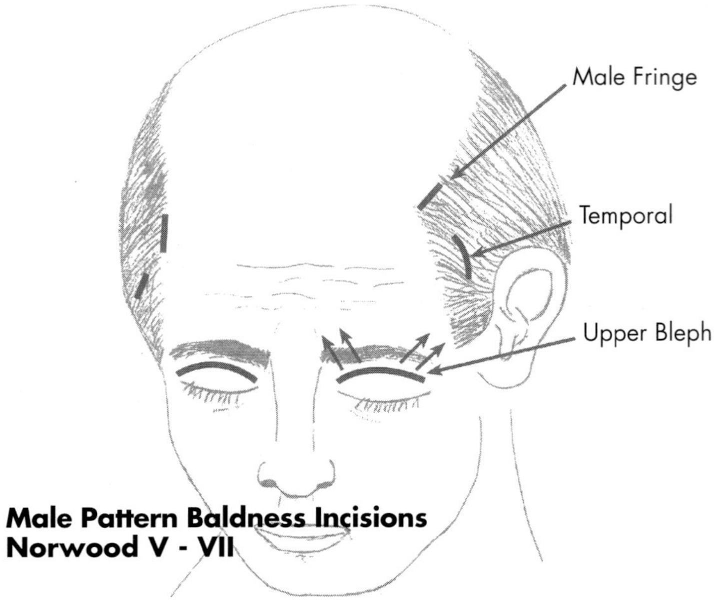

FIG. 5.3. Endoforehead incisions: male pattern baldness (Norwood types V–VIII).

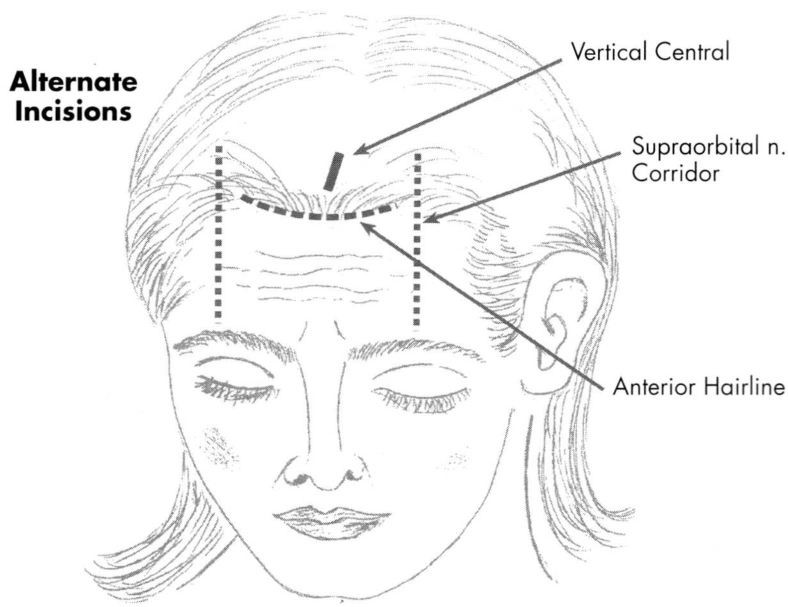

FIG. 5.4. Alternate frontal incisions for female patients with high hairlines.

elevation, backward fixation can be performed from the central incisions.

It is, however, the tail of the brow that, because of its lack of suspension by the frontal musculature, normally requires the most elevation. For this reason, the standard incision plan is the one most frequently used.

The creation of an optical cavity. Because there is no natural cavity in the forehead into which an endoscope may be placed (such as the bronchus in bronchoscopy and the bladder in cystoscopy), the surgeon must create his or her own cavity and hold it open with instrumentation. These optical cavities are created in the naturally occurring planes that exist in the forehead and temple (Box 5.3). In the forehead over the area of frontal bone, optical cavities may be created in the subcutaneous, subgaleal, subperiosteal, or (most commonly) in a composite of several of these planes.

The subperiosteal plane is stiffer than the subgaleal or subcutaneous planes, and a retraction backward of the rigid periosteum for brow elevation "stretches" or

BOX 5.3. OPTIONS FOR CREATION OF AN OPTICAL CAVITY OVER THE FRONTAL BONE

1. Subperiosteal
2. Subgaleal
3. Subcutaneous
4. Composite of these three planes

"unfolds" the forehead less than subcutaneous or subgaleal elevation. This lack of forehead stretch produces less elevation of the forehead for any given degree of brow elevation than dissection in either the subcutaneous or subgaleal planes. One centimeter of brow elevation is often achieved for every 1.2 cm of backward pull on a subperiosteal flap, giving a ratio of 1.2:1. Another advantage of the subperiosteal plane is that it is easy to dissect it quickly and blindly from the superior incisions.

The musculature of the forehead, however, lies in the subgaleal plane. A transition must be made to the subgaleal plane in order to access this musculature. A transition to the subgaleal plane must also be made over the descending process of the frontal bone at approximately the level of the brow, if the surgeon wishes to continue over the malar eminence in the supraperiosteal plane. If he or she wishes to pass over the malar eminence in the subperiosteal plane, this transition does not have to be made.

The subgaleal plane dissection causes less edema and ecchymosis than does the subperiosteal plane dissections. For this reason, procedures that are geared primarily to deactivate muscle and require minimal brow and forehead elevation are often performed in the subgaleal plane. If a greater amount of brow elevation is required, the dissection is performed in the subperiosteal plane to minimize forehead elevations. In patients with a short forehead, where a greater degree of forehead lengthening is desired, the subgaleal plane is advantageous, especially where prominent horizontal forehead rhytids are present. Use of the subgaleal plane produces a greater amount of forehead lengthening than the subperiosteal plane.

The subcutaneous plane is often used when the forehead requires lowering. Often, a limited subcutaneous dissection is performed through a horizontal pretrichial or trichophytic incision, and the dissection is transitioned to a subgaleal plane for muscle modification. As the forehead is pulled backward, the pretrichial skin may be excised as underlying frontalis muscle is advanced.

In the temple, the optical cavity is usually created in the plane immediately above the superficial layer of deep temporal fascia. This layer may be followed medially over the malar eminence and medial one third of the zygoma. On occasion, the temple cavity may be created in the subcutaneous plane. This is usually performed in order to perform myotomies on the orbicularis muscle for crow's-feet. The orbicularis muscle may also be sutured upward to elevate the brow tail.

If a dissection in the subperiosteal plane over the zygoma and malar eminence is required, a transection of the superficial layer of deep temporal fascia is performed approximately 1 to 2 cm above the zygomatic arch, and the optical cavity is created over the superficial fat pad (the fat pad between the superficial and deep layers of deep temporal fascia).

Figure 5.5 illustrates the common planes of optical cavity creation that we use. A subperiosteal dissection is created over the frontal bone to the level of the brow. At the level of the brow, in the midline, a transition is made to a supraperiosteal plane over the nose between the insertions of the corrugator muscle, preserving these insertions. The periosteum is either pushed away from the musculature, and/or the periosteum is incised to gain access to the corrugator, procerus, depressor, and orbicularis musculature in the subgaleal plane. A transition to the supraperiosteal plane is also made over the orbital rim and the descending (zygomatic process) portion of the frontal bone and onto the malar eminence. In the temple, the optical cavity is created over the superficial layer of deep temporal fascia. The two cavities are usually joined over the temporal line. Note that dissection is extended posteriorly to allow redraping of the skin after backward fixation.

Release of the brow. In order to elevate the brow, the muscles, periosteum, and fascial connections that depress the brow or bind it down to the bone in the proximity of the orbital rim must be released. This release can be divided into a medial frontal portion (medial to the supraorbital nerve), a midfrontal portion (lateral to the supraorbital nerve and medial to the lateral orbital rim), and a lateral frontal/temporal (or brow tail) portion (fascial and orbicularis oculi attachments to the lateral orbital rim, temporal line, and malar eminence).

In its medial frontal aspect, the brow is held downward to bone by the periosteum and small muscles of facial expression, namely the corrugator, the orbicularis oculi, the depressor supercilii, and the procerus. The corrugator, procerus, and portions of the orbicularis oculi are innervated by a branch of the temporal branch of the facial nerve that travels along the superior brow. The remainder of the muscles are innervated by branches of the zygomaticus branch or the buccal branch of the facial nerve that travels to these muscles via a pathway inferior to the orbit.

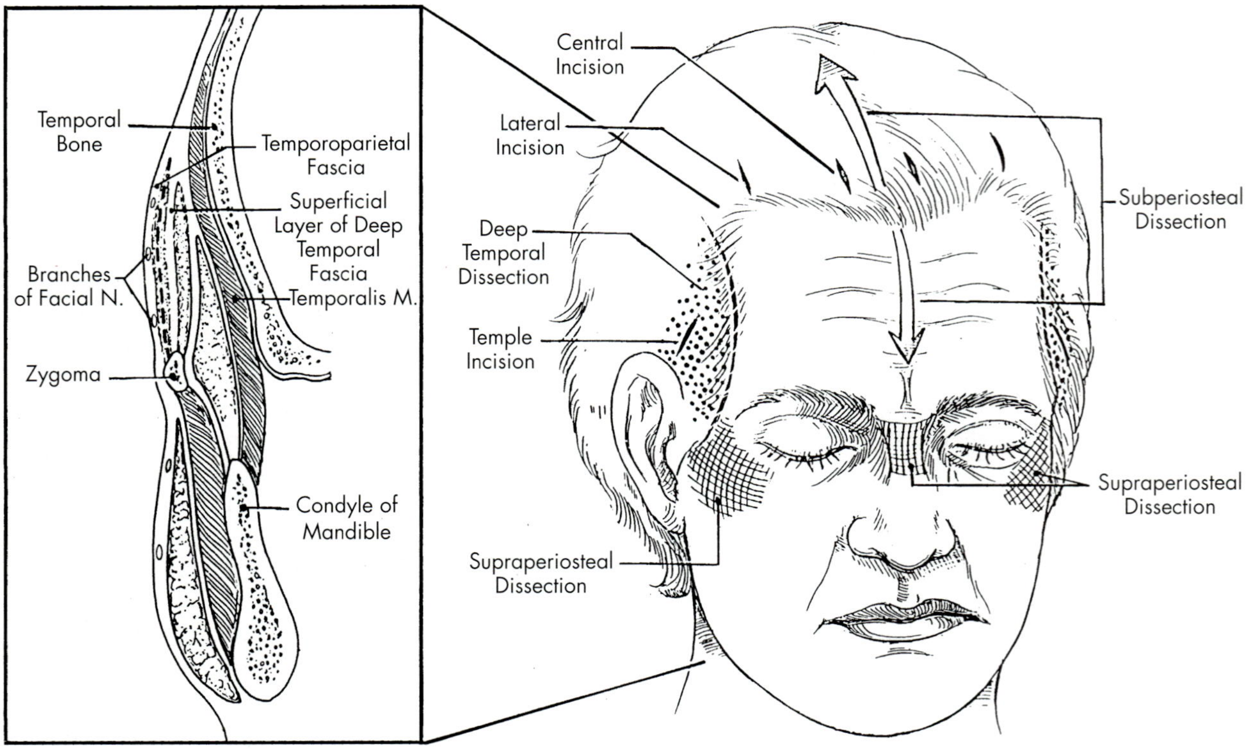

FIG. 5.5. Usual composite of surgical planes used in endoforehead lift.

Incision of these muscles near their bony attachments is considered by most surgeons (including ourselves) to be required to release the medial aspect of the brow. Isse,[9,38] however, argues that simple denervation of portions of the corrugator (along with myotomies of the procerus, depressor supercilii, and portions of the orbicularis oculi muscle) by incising the frontalis nerve branches along the brow, medial to the supraorbital nerve and lateral to the supratrochlear nerve, can, at times, be enough to elevate the medial brow.

Isse[9,38] bases his argument on the "agonist-antagonist" concept of the action of the depressor muscles (corrugator, orbicularis oculi, depressor supercilii, procerus) and the elevator muscles of the brow (occipitalis-galea-frontalis sling). When denervation of the depressor muscles occur, Isse reasons, the pull of the elevator muscles becomes relatively stronger than that before denervation, which causes the position of the brow to move upward. As evidence of this, Isse cites a patient of his who had a laceration that interrupted the nerve unilaterally. One year after the accident, the patient had an elevation of the brow on the side of the interruption.[28, 29]

In the lateral frontal portion of the brow (the area between the supraorbital nerve and the lateral orbital rim), the periosteum is first released below the bony rim. The orbicularis oculi is then incised horizontally after the retro-orbicularis oculi fat pad is penetrated (Figure 5.6).

In the lateral frontal/temporal portion of the brow, the conjoint tendon (fusion of the galea and periosteum and superficial and deep temporal fascia) is incised at the level of the brow, and the frontal and temporal cavities are connected. The orbicularis is then elevated and incised vertically along the vertical orbital rim. A horizontal release of the soft tissues is then performed over the malar eminence. These manuevers allow the brow tail to be elevated.

Elevation of the brow via posterior shifting and fixation of the scalp. After the optical cavity is created and the release of the brows' attachments to the orbit are performed, the surgeon is able to shift the scalp and underlying periosteum posteriorly. In shifting the scalp posteriorly, the brows are elevated without excision of the scalp.

Fixation of the scalp's new position to a point on the bone is accomplished through the use of screws, sutures, plates, skin and scalp excision, and soft-tissue rolls, as discussed in subsequent chapters. Fixation in the temple area is usually accomplished with sutures.

After the scalp is shifted posteriorly, a redundancy in the scalp soft tissue posterior to the fixation point is created. This is quickly taken up by contraction of the occipitalis-galea-frontalis sling posterior to the

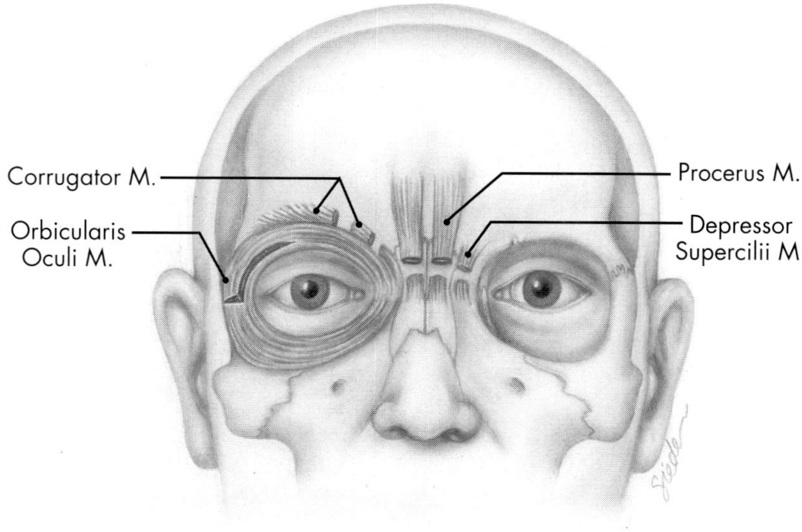

FIG. 5.6. Myotomies of the depressor muscles (corrugator, orbicularis oculi, depressor supercilii, and procerus) performed to "release" the brow.

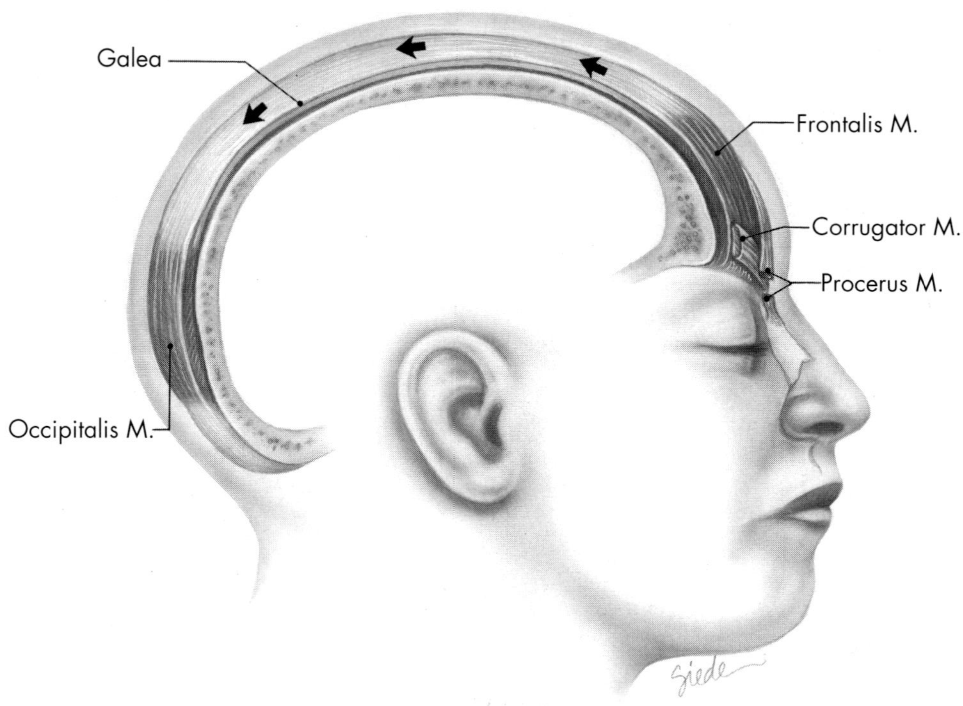

FIG. 5.7. With release of the depressor muscles, the occipitalis-galea-frontalis sling pulls the scalp backward.

point(s) of fixation. Usually, the redundancy disappears within several minutes (Figure 5.7).

Endoscopic Forehead Lifting: A Basic Technique Atlas

As we have noted previously, a wide variety of endoscopic techniques are used in practice today. Most of these are probably effective in forehead rejuvenation to varying degrees.[30]

As we have evolved as endoscopic surgeons, during 6 years of experience with more than 700 patients, our technique has evolved also. Some of this has been the result of sharing experience with other surgeons. Some has been the result of refining our own results.

Although we do not use a single technique for all patients, we do use a basic technique for most of them. The advanced digital images that are presented in this chapter enable us to express our methods in pictorial form, rather than through a series of drawings.*

Endoscopic forehead rejuvenation surgery, like most other operations, can be divided into a series of steps, with options occurring in each step. The five steps in our technique of endoscopic forehead lifting are: (1) marking, anesthesia, and incisions, (2) blind creation of the optical cavity, (3) temple dissection, (4) frontal dissection with muscle release and myotomy, and (5) fixation (Box 5.4).

BOX 5.4. BASIC ENDOSCOPIC FOREHEAD LIFTING: FIVE STEPS

1. Markings, anesthesia, and incisions
2. Blind creation of the optical cavity
3. Temple dissection
4. Frontal dissection with muscle release and myotomy
5. Fixation

Marking, anesthesia, and incisions. We first mark the midline from the glabella to the scalp. The position of the notch of the supraorbital nerve and/or supratrochlear nerve are also marked, if palpable. A semicircular area is inscribed 2 cm above the brow. This delineates an area where blind undermining is not performed, in case the supraorbital nerve emerges from a foramen above the orbital rim.

A variety of anesthesia techniques are used. These range from local anesthesia to conscious sedation to monitored anesthesia coverage (MAC) to a general anesthesia. MAC or a general anesthesia is most often used with a subperiosteal plane approach over the frontal bone, because the sound of the scraping dissection is usually disturbing to the patient.

The six incision locations are then marked. Before the incisions are made, 1% lidocaine with epinephrine, diluted with an equal amount of .25% bupivacaine (50/50 mixture), is used for the supraorbital blocks, the occipital nerve blocks, infiltration of the incisions, infiltration of the forehead and temple as necessary, and a "ring" block. Tumescent solution is then injected over the entire surface to be undermined and dissected.[32]

Two central incisions are placed at the level of the medial brows, equidistant from the midline and approximately 1 cm behind the hairline. These are vertical and 1 to 1.5 cm in length. These incisions are used for the access of both the endoscope and instruments and are usually not used for fixation.

Two lateral incisions are placed at the level of the lateral canthus. These incisions are used for both access of the endoscope and instruments and for fixation. They are basically vertical in orientation, but are canted laterally so that the vector of the incision is diagonal in a posterior and lateral direction. This angle can usually be tailored to fit the line of transition between temporal thinning hair and full frontal hair, thereby fitting into the patients natural hair pattern.

The lateral incisions are placed 1 cm behind the hairline and are 1 to 1.5 cm in length. When a lateral incision is constructed, its anteriormost position is noted on the underlying bone by either placing a drill mark at the anterior level of the incision or by using a laser to place a mark directly on the bone. When making both the lateral and the central incisions, it is helpful to place a small retractor into the incision to hold it apart[33] (Figure 5.8).

Two diagonal temple incisions are then made. The incisions are approximately 2 cm behind the hairline and 2 cm in length. The midpoint of these incisions is approximately at a horizontal line connecting the two superior orbital rims. The path of these incisions can be connected to the temple portion of a face-lift incision.

Blind creation of the optical cavity. Blind dissection is initially required to create a pocket in which to place the endoscope. Although the plane and extent of the posterior dissection can vary, we currently use a slightly curved elevator (Karl Storz, No. 479408) (Figure 5.9) through the right lateral incision to create a subperiosteal pocket. The dissection is performed anteriorly and posteriorly, sweeping the elevator in a counterclockwise circular pattern. This same pattern is repeated through each of the other lateral and central incisions so that all of these incisions are connected by the subperiosteal dissection. Usually, the elevator will reach downward to a point approximately 2 cm above the brow (see Figure 5.9).

In the glabella, the medium straight dissector (a longer elevator—Karl Storz No. KST 664-1) (Figure 5.10, *A*) is used to continue the subperiosteal dissection downward until resistance is felt. In the midline, this point represents the insertion of the corrugator muscles. By pushing through this point, a supraperiosteal plane may be followed downward over the dorsum of the nose (Figure 5.10, *B*).

Laterally, the subperiosteal dissection is carried to the level of the brow, using a medium-length curved dissector (Karl Storz, No. KST 664-3). If the shorter dissec-

* For our ability to obtain these digital images, we are indebted to Karl Storz GMB for the use of their 4-mm optical chain and Imagemanager technology to produce the superb pictures that appear here. The ability to capture high-quality endoscopic pictures has, since the days of Brubaker and Brubaker's camera,[31] been a problem.

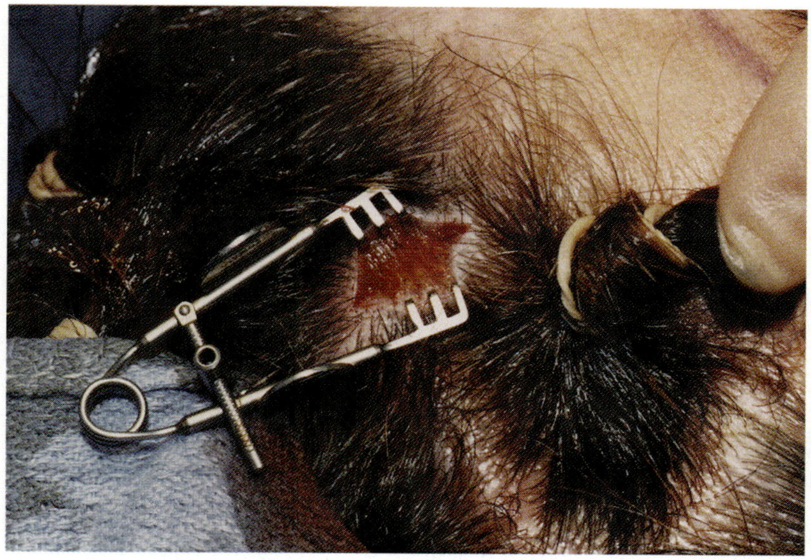

FIG. 5.8. Small retractor holding right lateral incision apart.

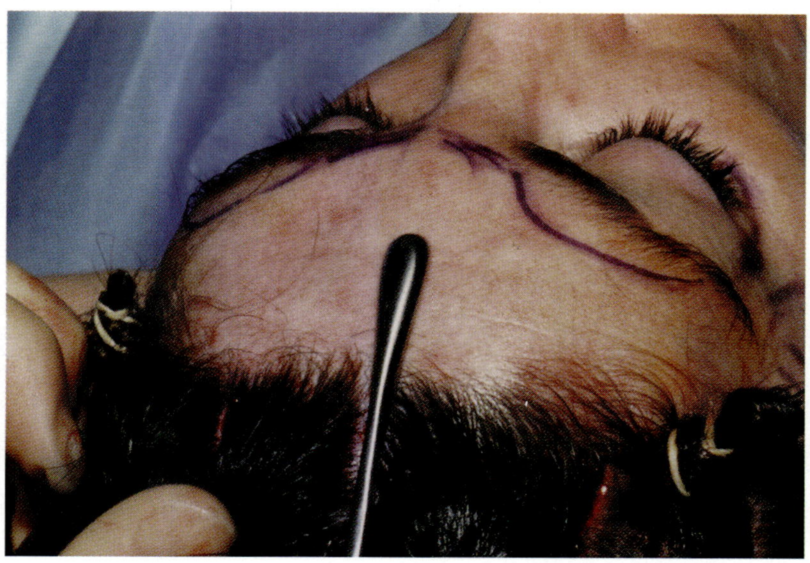

FIG. 5.9. Elevator used to blindly undermine in the subperiosteal plane over the frontal bone. A semicircular area above the supraorbital nerve is not elevated.

tor (Karl Storz No. 479408) is not long enough, a spoon elevator (Karl Storz No. 502505DB) may also be used. The undermining is carried to the level of the brow.

Following this, the same spoon elevator or medium length curved dissector (Karl Storz No. KST 664) is used to undermine posteriorly in a subperiosteal plane. Dissection is carried to the occiput or nuchal ridge (Figure 5.11).

Attention is then turned to the right temple incisions. The incision is carried downward through the temporoparietal fascia, which moves with the scalp when it is moved forward and back, to the deep temporal fascia. The deep temporal fascia is a glistening white layer immediately overlying the temporal muscle. It does not move when the scalp is retracted upward (Figure 5.12).

Retracting the scalp upward, loose fibrous areolar tissue is seen between the temperoparietal fascia and the deep temporal fascia. This loose areolar tissue, the "innominate fascia," is a landmark. By sweeping it upward with the temporoparietal fascia (using Karl Storz No. 479408), the facial nerve is safe (Figure 5.13). Posteriorly, this layer is dissected backward over the extent of the temporalis muscle. Posterior to the muscle, the same dissector is used to dissect in a subperiosteal plane, sweeping in a clockwise fashion until

A

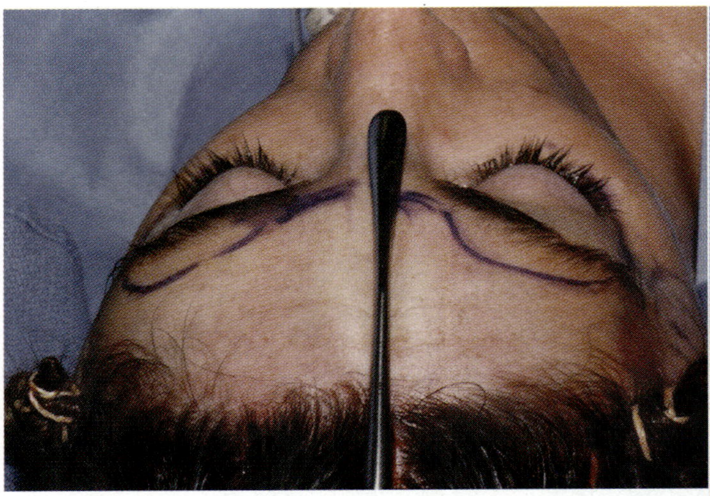

B

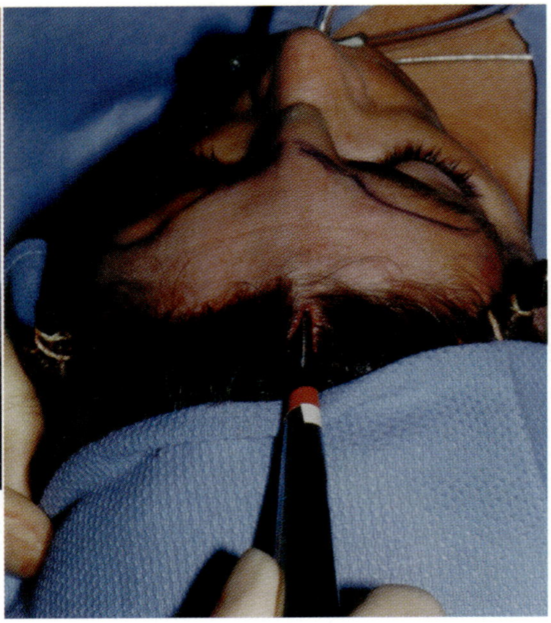

FIG. 5.10. **A,** Position of elevator between corrugators. **B,** Elevator as used to undermine between the corrugator muscles and transition to a supraperiosteal plane.

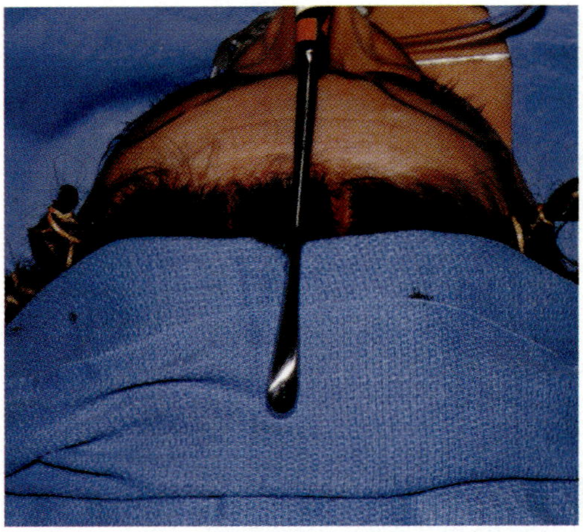

FIG. 5.11. Elevator extends the subperiosteal dissection toward the occiput.

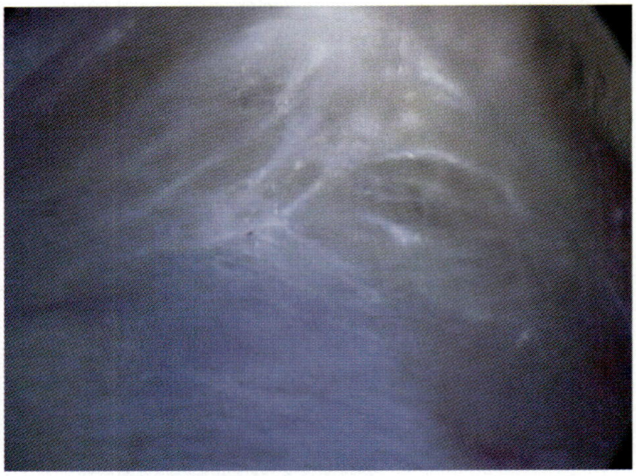

FIG. 5.13. Loose areolar tissue of the innominate fascia is swept upward.

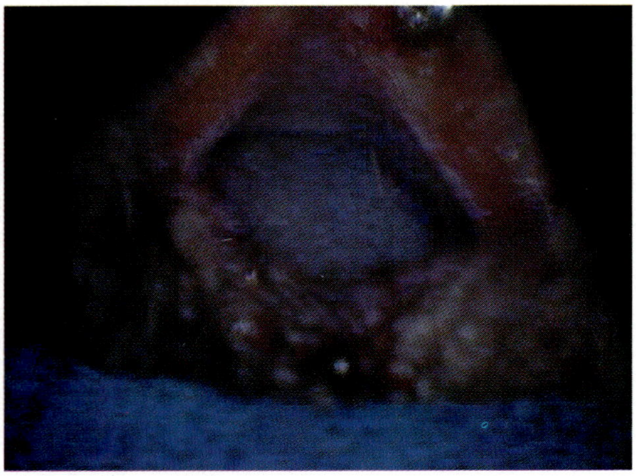

FIG. 5.12. Retracted temporal incision shows the temporoparietal fascia adherent to the skin. Deep temporal fascia is seen as a glistening white layer.

the lateral incision is reached, which connects the two temporal and lateral incisions in the subperiosteal plane. Dissection is continued inferiorly until the temporal line is reached.

The innominate fascia is then elevated anteriorly to the hairline. It is important to not undermine blindly anterior to the hairline, because it is here that the fascial layers become complex. Accurate dissection under direct vision makes the remainder of the case go much smoother. The blind undermining on the left side is then performed in similar fashion.

Temple dissection. Following the blind dissection, the elevator (Karl Storz No. 479408) is used to elevate along the superficial layer of deep temporal fascia, proceeding from the hairline toward the malar eminence. Both the endoscope, encased in the Karl Storz wide visualization sheath (Karl Storz No. 50200EM) (Figure

A

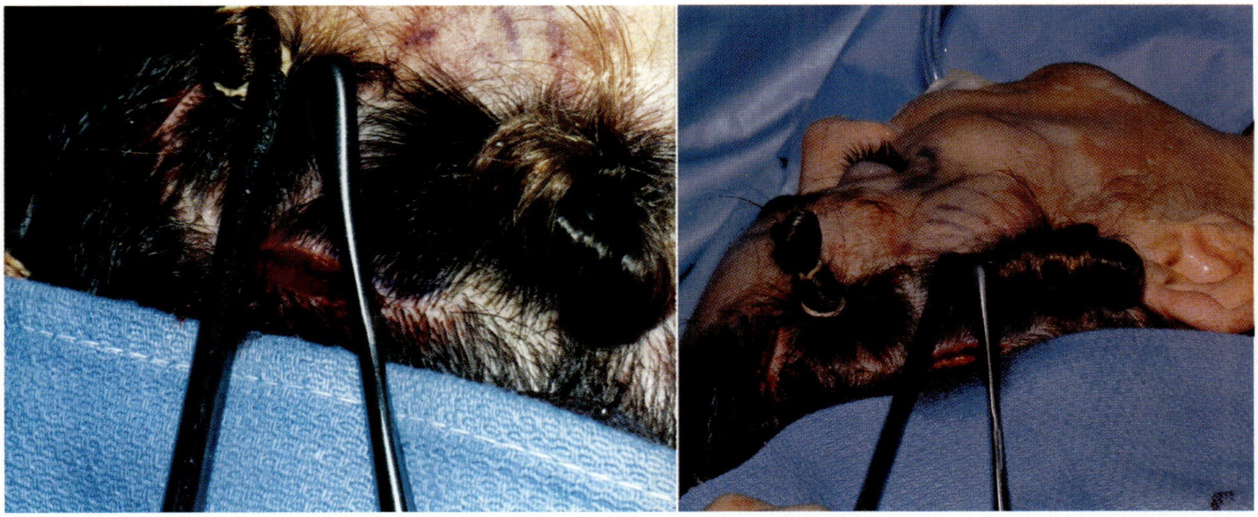

B

FIG. 5.14. **A,** Karl Storz wide sheath is shown in position with instruments. **B,** Elevator and sheath are both placed in the right temporal incision.

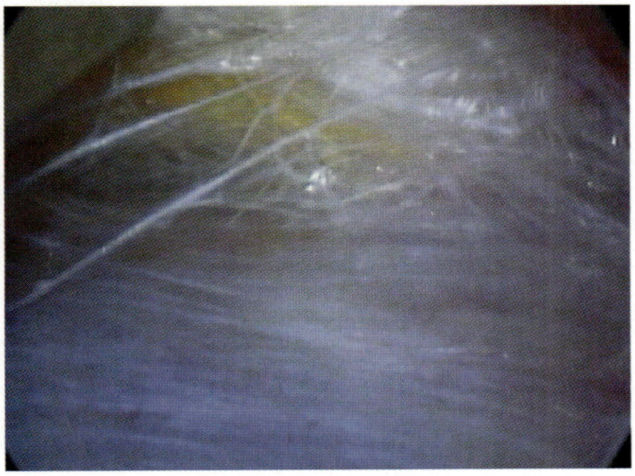

FIG. 5.15. Above the innominate fascia, the temporoparietal fat pad is seen.

5.14, *A*) and the elevator are placed in the right temporal incision (Figure 5.14, *B*). To avoid "digging oneself into a hole," a wide zone of dissection is created. All of the loose areolar tissue (the innominate fascia) is swept upward. The innominate fascia is a landmark, enabling the surgeon to stay clear of the facial nerve, which travels in the lower portions of the temperoparietal fascia (Figure 5.15). Often, the temporoparietal fat pad can be seen and should be swept upward (Figure 5.16, *A*, *B*).

As the dissection progresses, a yellowish tinge can often be seen through the superficial layer of deep temporal fascia (Figure 5.16, *A*). This is the superficial fat pad lying between the superficial and deep layers of the deep temporal fascia. It usually appears at a level consistent with the horizontal plane of the brow. As the dissection proceeds downward and medially, toward the malar eminence, an outline of the zygomaticotemporal vein ("sentinel vein") can be seen at the level of the zygomaticofacial suture (see Figure 5.16, *B*).

When the surgeon wants to dissect over the zygomatic arch in a subperiosteal plane, he or she makes a horizontal incision in the superficial layer of deep temporal fascia, exposing the superficial fat pad (Figure 5.16, *C*). Dissection then proceeds over the fat pad until the arch is encountered. This is not a part of our basic forehead dissection.

As the basic dissection is carried downward and medially toward the malar eminence, a layer of fat will be seen immediately superior to the zygomatic arch, the prezygomatic fat pad. Several veins (perforating branches of the zygomaticotemporal) can be seen in the superior portion of this pad. The most medial and superior of these emerges near the zygomaticofrontal suture (sentinel vein). A second branch emerges near the lateral portion of the malar eminence and often is accompanied by a sensory nerve (zygomaticotemporal) (Figure 5.17).

This vein is cauterized at its base with a bipolar cautery (Karl Storz No. 50203BE or No. HP840021) and severed with endoscopic scissors (Karl Storz No. 50203S). The vein immediately lateral to this is often in the vicinity of the facial nerve, where it crosses the zygoma (Figure 5.18).

Dissection is carried medial and inferiorly over the malar eminence in the supraperiosteal plane using either the endoscopic scissors (Karl Storz No. 50203S), the medium-length straight elevator (Karl Storz No. KST664-1), or the "spoon" elevator (Karl Storz No. 502505DB). This dissection plane is superior to the "soof." If desired, the zygomaticus muscle can be identified, and the dissection can be carried into the cheek

A

B

C

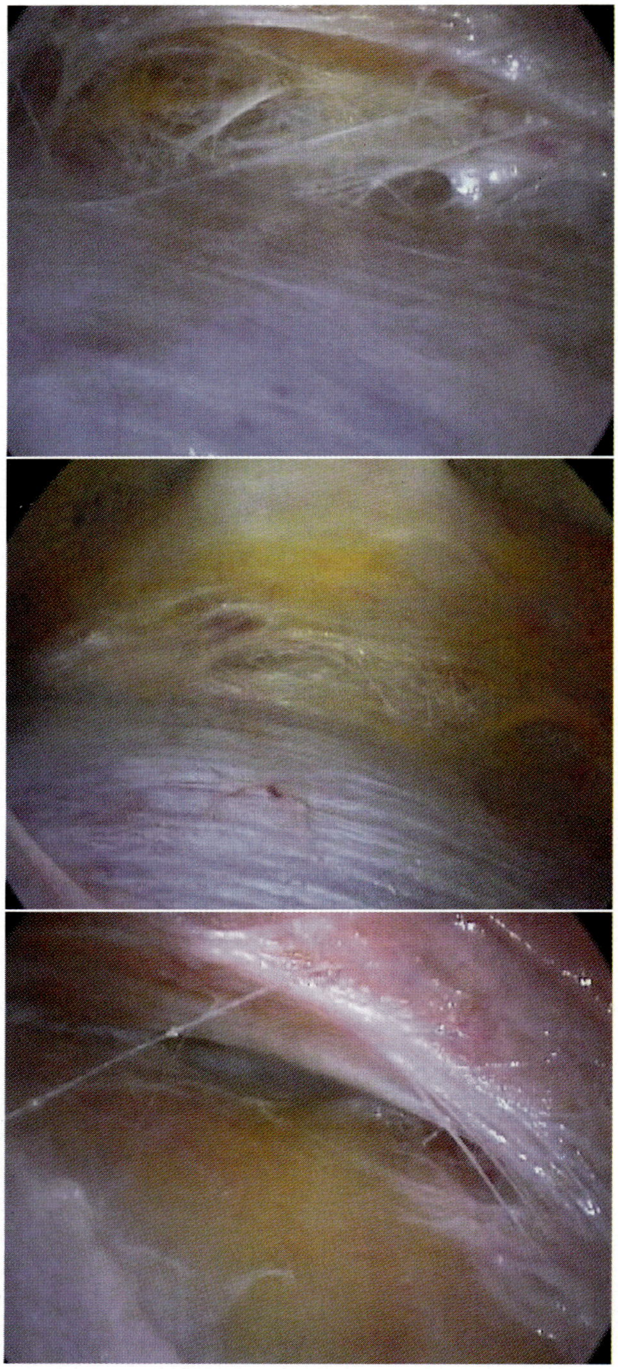

FIG. 5.16. **A,** Temporoparietal fat pad is swept upward with the innominate fascia. Through the superficial layer of deep temporal fascia, the superficial fat pad (between the layers of deep temporal fascia) can be seen. **B,** As the dissection is carried downward and medially, a branch of the zygomaticotemporal vein ("sentinel vein") can be seen as a purple outline in the fascia at the level of the frontozygomatico suture. **C,** When an incision is made in the superficial layer of the deep temporal fascia, the superficial fat pad can be seen. This approach is used when it is desired to carry the dissection over the zygomatic arch in the subperiosteal plane.

in the plane of the superficial fascia (Figures 5.19 and 5.20). Laterally, the dissection is carried over the medial one third of the arch, to the second perforating vein.

The surgeon's attention is then turned medial and superior. From the temporal incision (again with both the endoscope with the wide sheath [No. 50200EM] and the dissector [No. 479408] in the same incision) (Figure 5.21, *A*), the temporoparietal fascia is separated from the superficial layer of deep temporal fascia in the direction of the superior hairline (Figure 5.21, *B*). When the temporal line is encountered, the elevator (No. 479408 or No. KST 664-3) is used to incise and elevate the periosteum over the lateral margin of the frontal bone, thereby connecting the temporal with the frontal optical cavities (Figure 5.22).

The dissection is then carried downward (Figure 5.23), connecting the frontal and temporal optical cav-

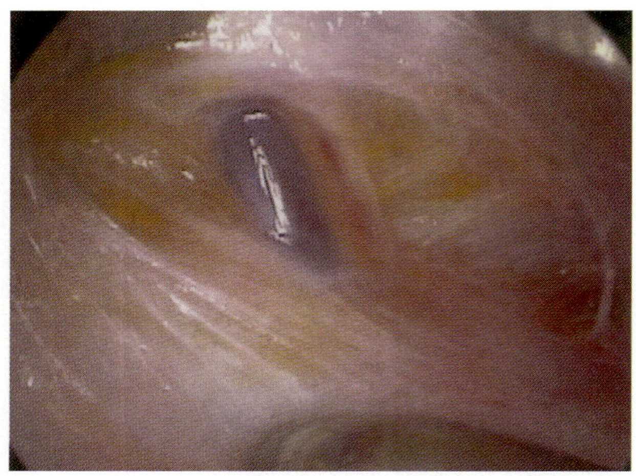

FIG. 5.17. Vein is uncovered.

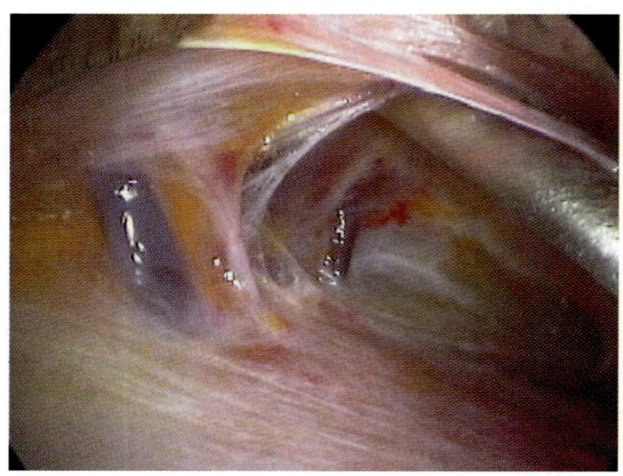

FIG. 5.18. Dissection showing another vein lateral to that shown in Figure 5.17. A nerve passing above this may represent a frontal branch of the facial nerve.

ities in a subperiosteal plane to the level of the brow. At the level of the brow, near the frontozygomatic suture, a branch of the zygomaticotemporal communicating vein can often be identified several millimeters lateral to the brow (Figure 5.24). This vein is often accompanied by one of the temporal branches of the facial nerve. Often, this vein can be seen through the skin preoperatively.[34]

The vein may be cauterized with the bipolar suction cautery (Karl Storz No. HP840021 or No. 50203BE) and severed at its base, close to the bone. Over the zygomatic process of the frontal bone, the dissection is transitioned to a supraperiosteal dissection, which communicates with the dissection over the malar eminence (Figure 5.25).

The same procedure is then completed in the left temporal optical cavity. On the left side, a right-handed surgeon (during parts of the operation) sometimes uses two ports for dissection. The surgeon may place the endoscope in the lateral incision, and the medium curved instrument in the temporal incision to dissect the periosteum from the temporal line. This is easiest if the two incisions are already connected superiorly.

Frontal dissection with muscle release and myotomy. In the frontal area, the endoscopic sheath (No. 50200EM) and instrument (spoon elevator, Karl Storz No. 50205DB) may be used in a two-port dissection. The endoscope is placed in the port to the left of the instrument for a right-handed surgeon, beginning with the instrument in the right lateral incision and the endoscope in the right central incision. The periosteum is elevated to the level of the orbital rim (Figure 5.26, *A-C*).

A

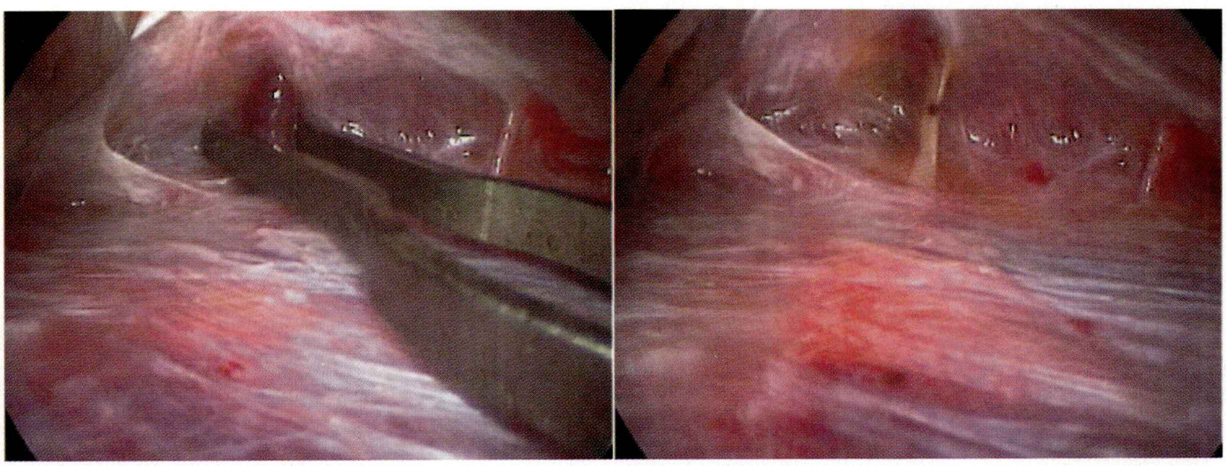

B

FIG. 5.19. **A,** In another patient, the bipolar cautery is placed on the vein. **B,** Vein is cauterized.

A

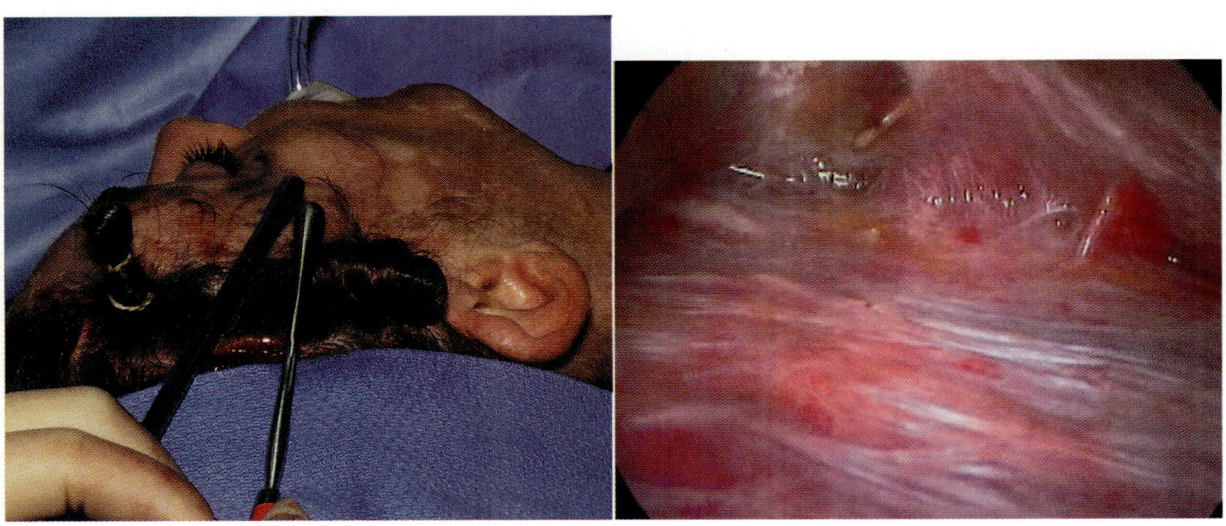

B

FIG. 5.20. **A,** Elevator and endoscope shown externally over the malar area to be dissected. **B,** Dissection is carried over the malar eminence.

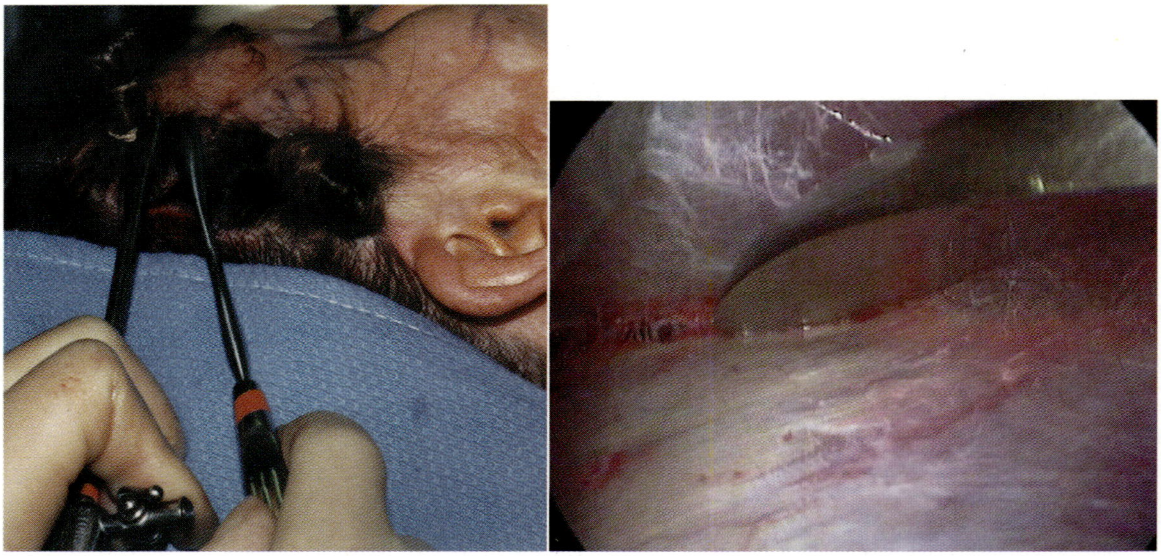

FIG. 5.21. **A,** Position of the endoscope and elevator is shifted superiorly and laterally. **B,** In another patient, dissection on the superficial layer of deep temporal fascia proceeds to the temporal line (conjoint fascia).

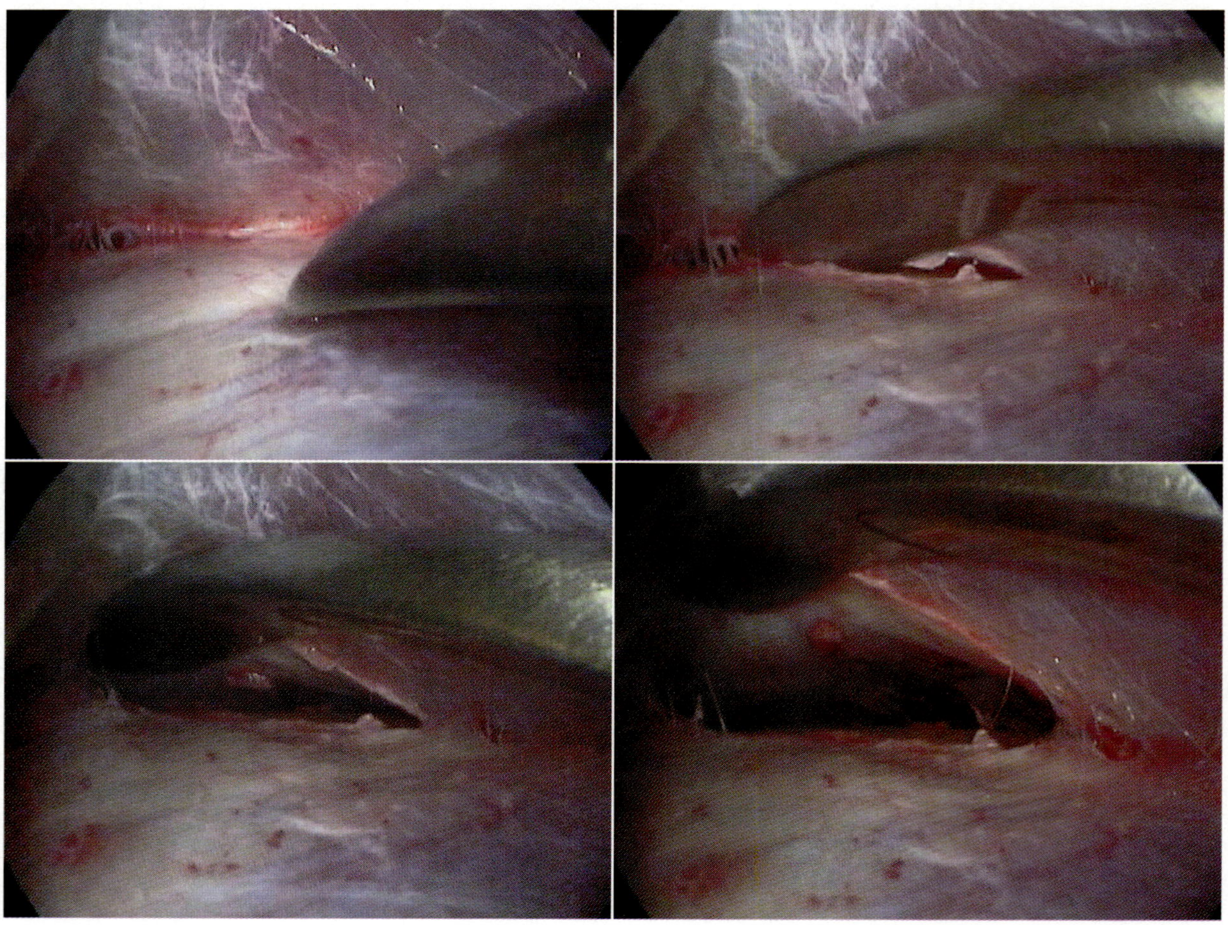

FIG. 5.22. **A,** Elevator is placed on the temporal line. **B,** Incision of the frontal periosteum at the temporal line. **C,** Elevation of the frontal periosteum. **D,** Connection of the temporal and frontal dissections from lateral to medial.

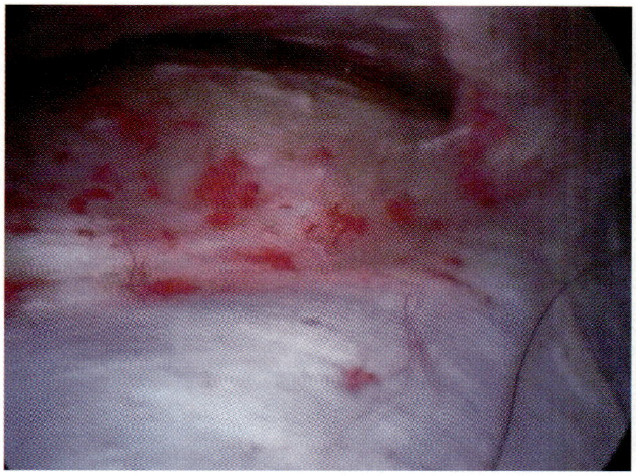

FIG. 5.23. Periosteum is elevated downward toward the brow, which enlarges the connection between the frontal and temporal cavities.

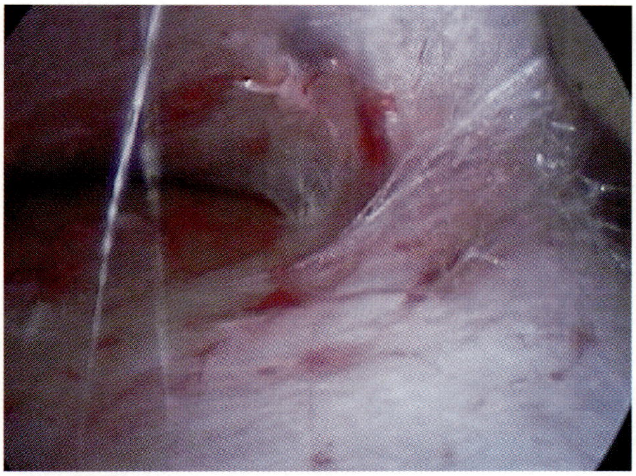

FIG. 5.24. At the level of the brow (at approximately the level of the frontozygomatic suture and slightly lateral to it), a branch of the zygomaticotemporal vein may be encountered.

In the two-port dissection, the endoscope is then placed in the right central incision, and the instrument (knuckle elevator No. 50205CA or shovel elevator No. KST 534) is placed in the right lateral incision. The subperiosteal dissection is then carried over the orbital rim (Figure 5.27), elevating the arcus marginalis and exposing "roof" fat (Figure 5.28). Progressing medially, the arcus marginalis is elevated until the supraorbital bundle is found (Figure 5.29). If the periosteum is thick or adherent, it may be necessary to incise it with a sickle knife below the level of the brow.

The supraorbital nerve usually emerges from a notch that is inferior to the supraorbital rim. Two important variations of this anatomy are noteworthy. The supraorbital nerve may emerge from a foramen (Figure 5.30) above the supraorbital rim. Or a lateral supraorbital nerve branch (innervating the lateral portion of the forehead) may emerge superior to the rim, with the main branch emerging from a notch below the rim (Figure 5.31). Because of these variations in the anatomy of the nerve, it is important for the surgeon not to blindly undermine the periosteum to the supraorbital rim, in order to avoid cutting the nerve. We usually blindly undermine only to a level 2 cm above the rim.

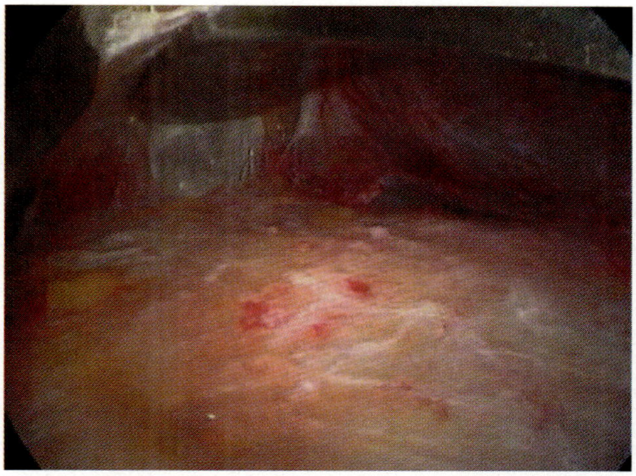

FIG. 5.25. Supraperiosteal elevation over the malar eminence with the medium straight elevator.

The endoscope is then placed in the left central incision, and the elevator is placed in the right central incision to push the periosteum off of the corrugator and procerus muscles (Figure 5.32). Veins in the areas of the medial brow and the supraorbital nerve are isolated and cauterized with the bipolar suction cautery (Karl Storz No. HP840021 or No. 50203BE). The same procedure is performed on the left side.

Recently, new instrumentation has made this procedure easier. The Karl Storz optical dissector sheath (No. KST 521) (Figure 5.33) can be used to perform both the visualization and the subperiosteal undermining through a single incision. Using the optical dissector sheath, the periosteum and arcus marginalis may be quickly elevated through a single port (Figure 5.34). The supraorbital bundle, in this case emerging from a foramen (Figure 5.35), may be identified, and the periosteum is swept off of the corrugator and procerus muscles with this device (Figure 5.36).

The optical dissector sheath is then removed, and the wide angle visualization sheath (No. 50200EM) is then reinstalled. The endoscope is placed through the left central incision, and the high-energy pulsed carbon dioxide laser (placed in the right central incision) (Figure 5.37) is used to incise the procerus muscle with 250 mj of energy (8 W) through a thin flexible waveguide (Sharplan Lasers). The use of the high-energy laser allows relatively charless cutting with hemostatsis. If the laser is unavailable, the straight endoscopic scissors (No. 50203S) or horizontal curved scissors

A

B

C

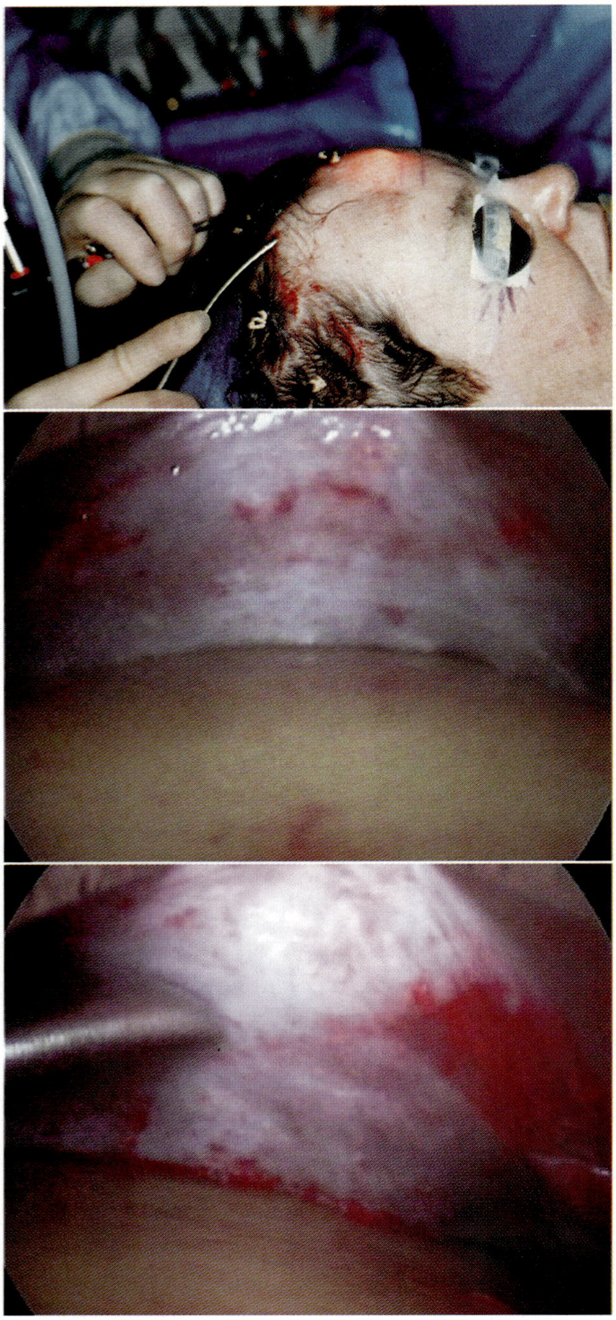

FIG. 5.26. **A,** Endoscope is placed in the right central incision, and the spoon elevator is placed in the right lateral incision. **B,** Endoscope is used to suspend the subperiosteal cavity created by blind dissection. **C,** Spoon elevator is used to elevate the periosteum toward the orbital rim. (In this instance, the endoscope is in the left central incision, and the elevator is in the left lateral incision.)

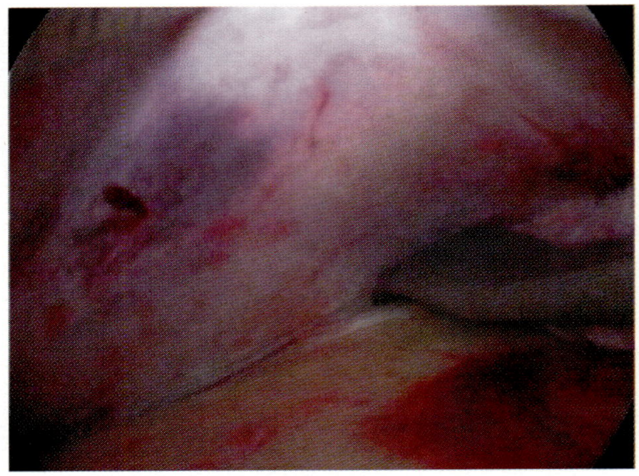

FIG. 5.27. Knuckle elevator is shown elevating the periosteum over the orbital rim. Currently, we use the "shovel" elevator for this purpose.

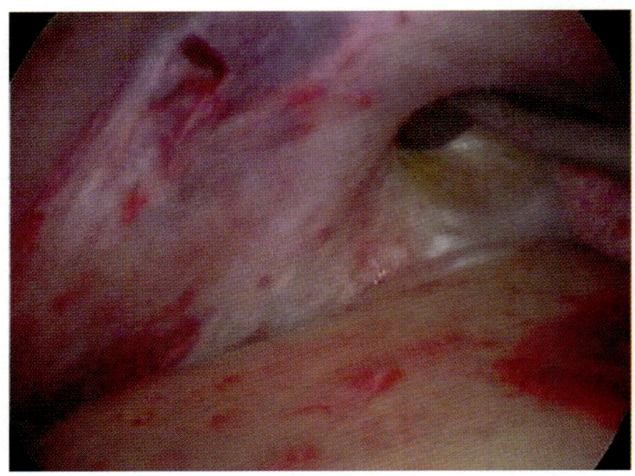

FIG. 5.28. "Knuckle" is pushed upward to elevate the arcus marginalis below the brow. "Roof" fat is exposed.

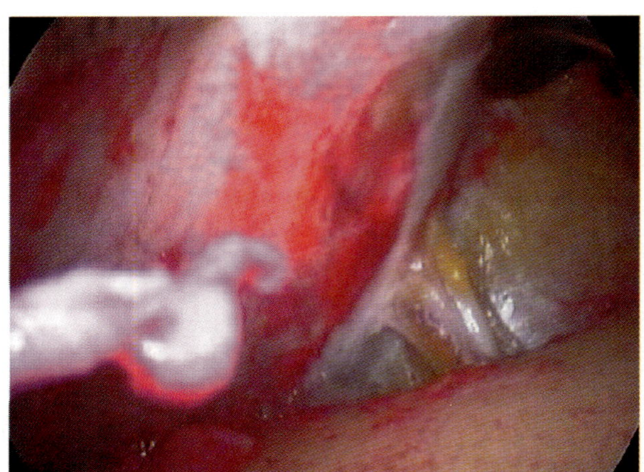

FIG. 5.29. Elevation of the arcus marginalis proceeds medially until the supraorbital bundle is encountered.

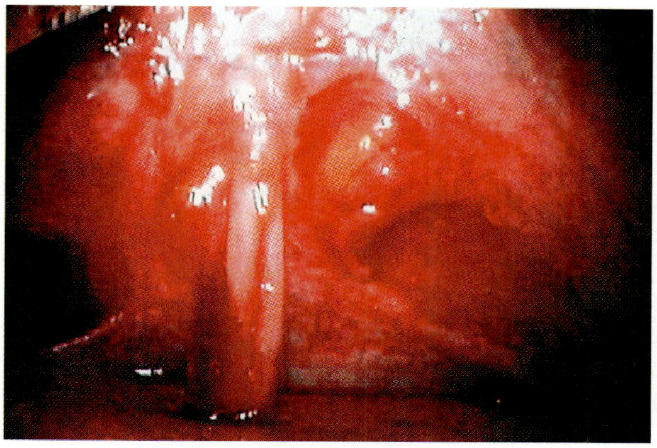

FIG. 5.30. Supraorbital bundle is seen to emerge from a foramen 1.5 cm above the orbital rim. If the surgeon were to blindly undermine to the orbital rim, he or she would avulse the nerve on this side.

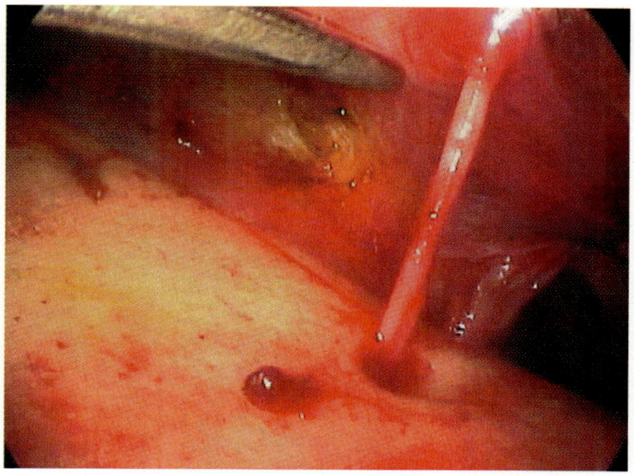

FIG. 5.31. A left lateral supraorbital nerve branch is seen exiting from a foramen 1 cm above the orbital rim. The main supraorbital bundle is seen emerging from a notch below the supraorbital rim.

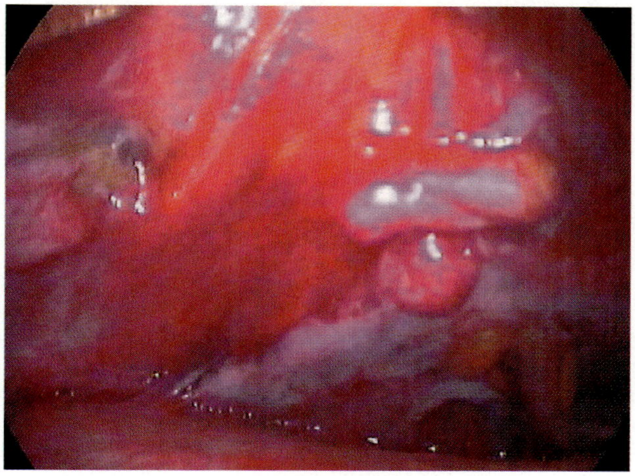

FIG. 5.32. Periosteum is pushed away from the right corrugator muscle.

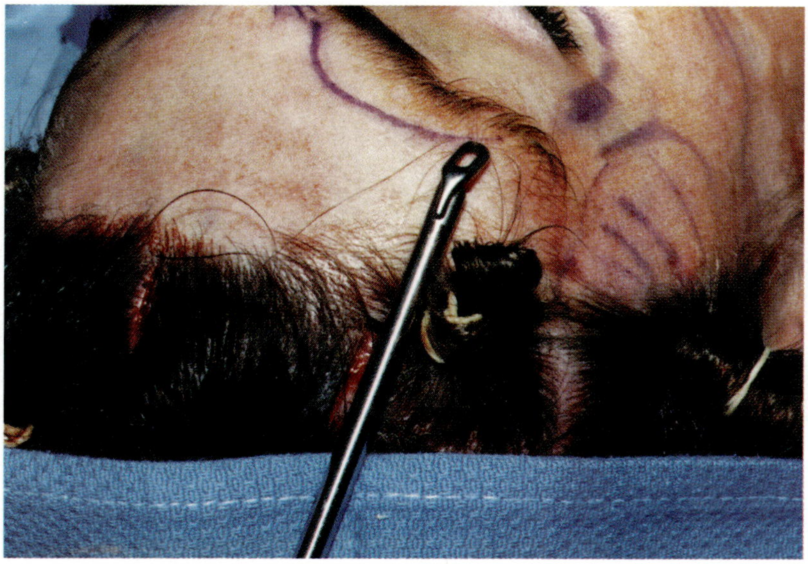

FIG. 5.33. The optical dissector sheath is placed over the right lateral orbital rim to elevate the arcus marginalis.

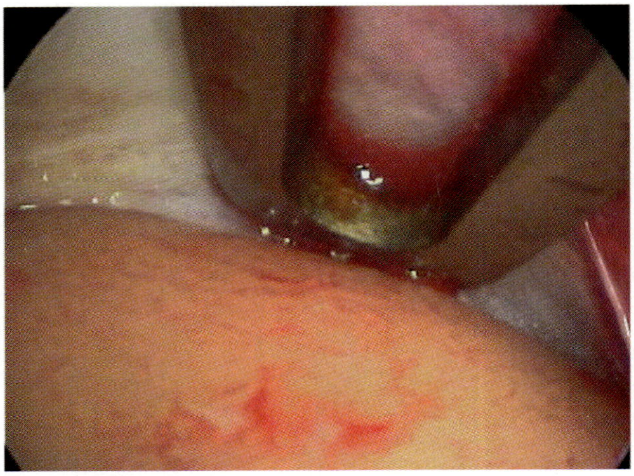

FIG. 5.34. Endoscopic view of the optical dissector sheath, dissecting the periosteum from the frontal bone in the vicinity of the right lateral orbital rim.

(Karl Storz No. 50203SW) are used (Figure 5.38). The laser reduces the amount of postoperative swelling and ecchymosis.

The procerus muscle is a relatively thin muscle that is located between the corrugator insertions that demarcate the supraperiosteal nasal tunnel (Figure 5.39). Its fibers travel vertically upward.

The procerus muscle is normally incised at the level of the nasofrontal suture. However, if a filling in of the nasion is desired to camouflage a nasal hump, the procerus muscle may be incised immediately below the brow, which allows the muscle to retract downward to partially "fill in" the hump (Figure 5.40).

Attention is then turned to the corrugator (Figure 5.41). Because the dissection over the nose is supraperiosteal between the insertions of the corrugator (leaving these insertions intact), the corrugator muscle can

A 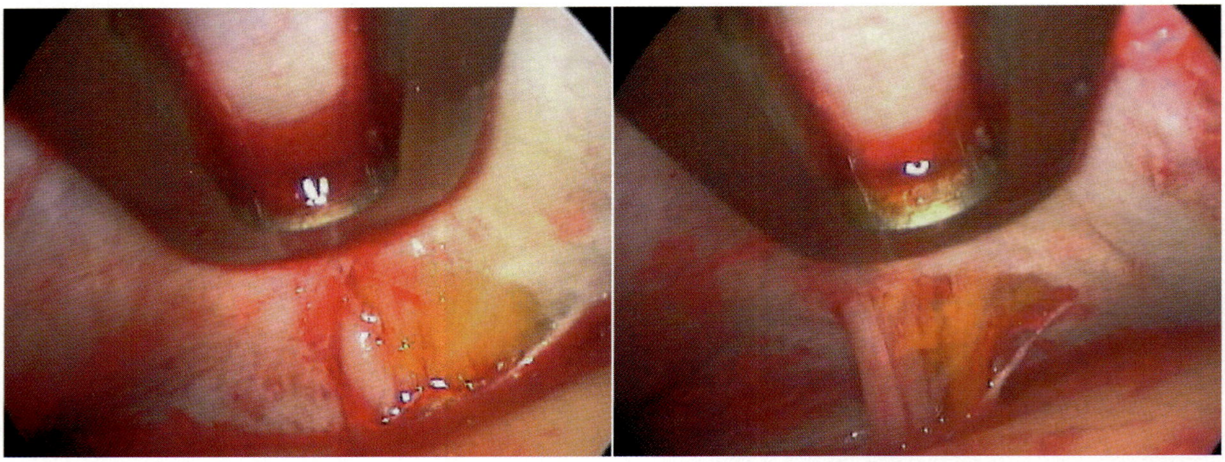 B

FIG. 5.35. **A** and **B,** Optical dissector sheath is used to elevate the periosteum from the right supraorbital bundle, in this instance, emerging from a foramen above the orbital rim.

A 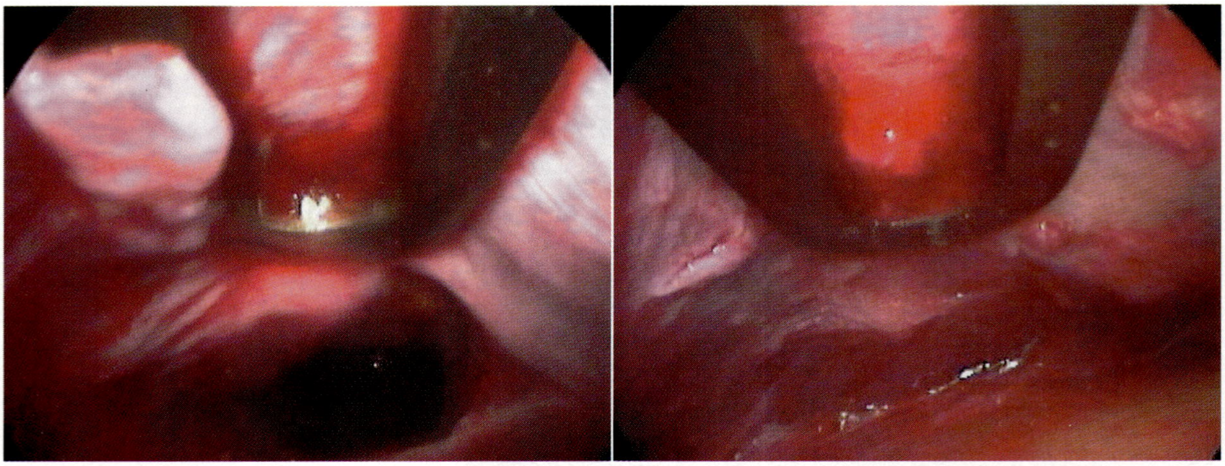 B

FIG. 5.36. **A,** Optical dissector is immediately above the supraperiosteal tunnel that was created over the nose. To the right of the tunnel is the corrugator muscle. Medial edge of this muscle can be seen. **B,** Optical dissector is directed toward the right to sweep the periosteum from the right corrugator.

be found immediately lateral to the supraperiosteal tunnel over the nose. The corrugator is a large red muscle and is not easily missed.

The corrugator muscle fibers travel in a lateral direction. When the optical cavity is tented upward by the endoscopic sheath, these fibers are directed diagonally upward and laterally.

The lateral portion of the corrugator is incised as close to the bony rim as possible with the laser (preferably) or the straight (No. 50203S) or curved vertical endoscopic scissors (Karl Storz No. 50203 SG) (Figure 5.42). Spreading motions with the scissors, followed by cutting of the muscle fibers, allow the supratrochlear

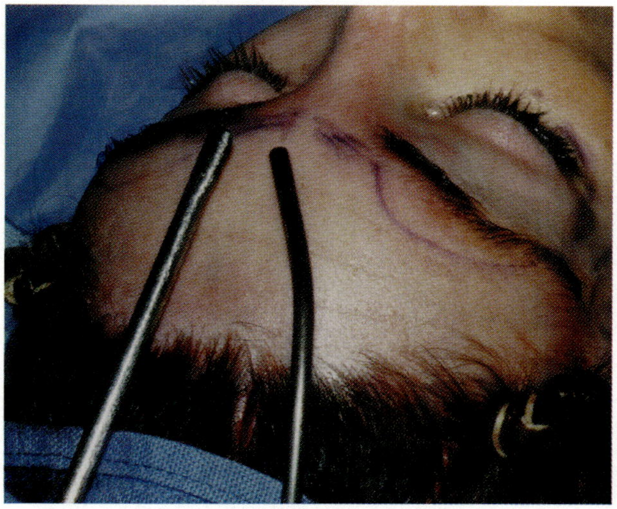

FIG. 5.37. Wide dissector sheath is placed through the left central incision, and the laser fiber waveguide (Sharplan Lasers) is placed through the right central incision.

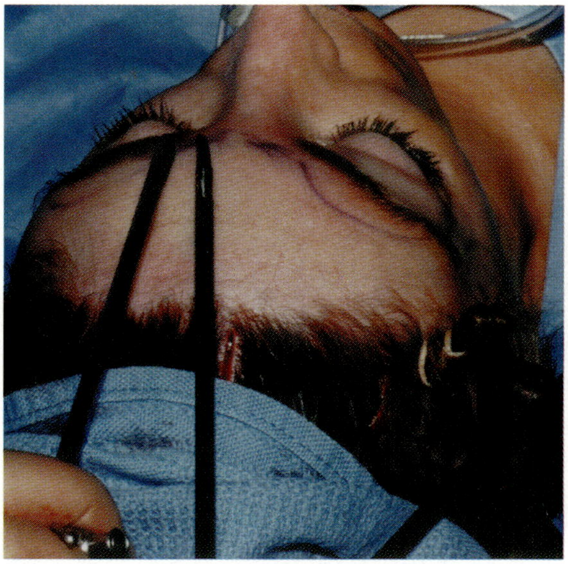

FIG. 5.38. Alternatively, the wide dissector sheath is placed in the left central incision, and the straight endoscopic scissors is placed in the right central incision.

nerves to be exposed as well as arteries and veins to be preserved (Figure 5.43).

When using the laser, a small amount of muscle is incised with two or three pulses from the fiber (Figure 5.44). The remaining muscle is then pushed upward, and the process is repeated until the supratrochlear nerves are exposed.

The supratrochlear nerve can emerge from a single notch or foramen. If this is the case, it can be seen as a single stalk with a bifurcation that, in turn, gives off branches (Figure 5.45) (Sajjad Khan, personal communication, 1996).

Alternatively, the supratrochlear nerve can emerge from the same notch as the supraorbital nerve. In this case, the supratrochlear nerve divides in or immediately outside of the notch into many branches (Figure 5.46) (Sajjad Khan, personal communication, 1996). The surgeon, when incising the muscle, encounters these multiple small branches of the nerve and they must be preserved.

The muscle that remains posterior and medial to the nerve is the depressor muscle. Its fibers travel in a more or less vertical direction that curve laterally. It may be thin or, if hypertrophied, be seen as a thicker bluish muscle. This muscle is also incised with the laser or vertical endoscopic scissors (Figure 5.47).

The muscle that is between the supratrochlear and supraorbital nerves is the corrugator muscle (see Figure 5.47, *A*). If examined closely, the fibers of this muscle travel in a lateral and superior direction. These muscles are also incised, which reveals a fatty layer.

Behind these muscles and fat is the orbicularis muscle, which is adherent to skin. If desired, this muscle is incised with a series of vertical cuts medial to the supraorbital nerve.

If there are deep vertical glabellar rhytids, the con-

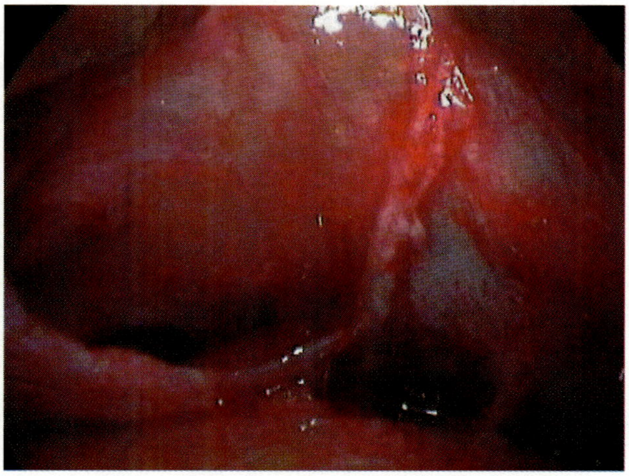

FIG. 5.39. Corrugator muscle is seen above the supraperiosteal tunnel.

A

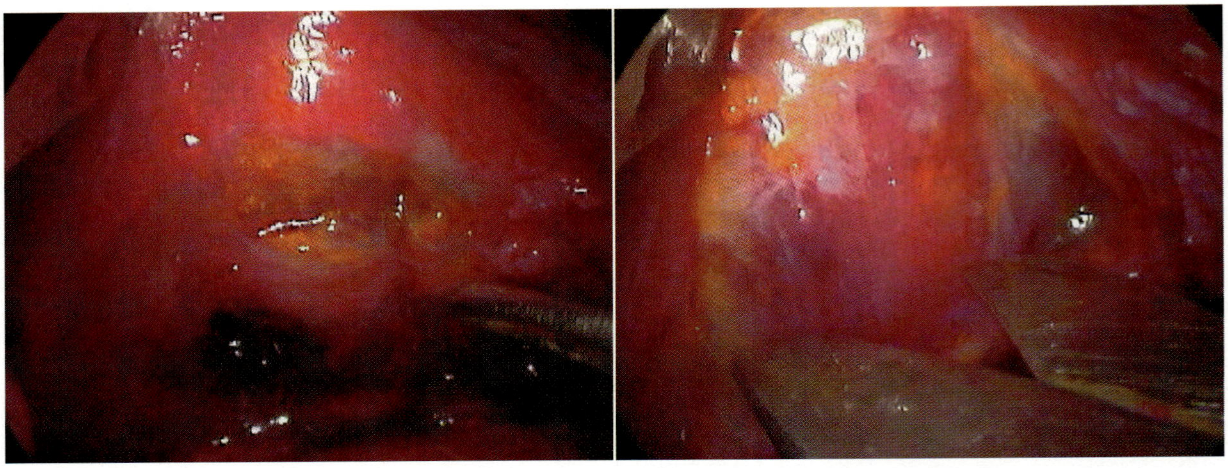

B

FIG. 5.40. **A** and **B,** Incision of the procerus muscle with straight scissors.

A

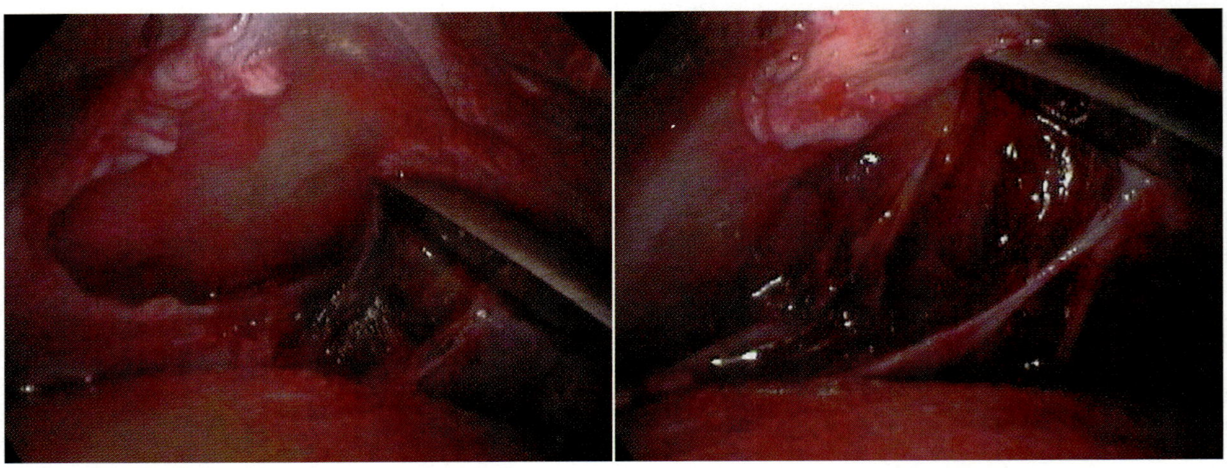

B

FIG. 5.41. **A** and **B,** Corrugator muscle orginates in the midline, at the base of the supraperiosteal tunnel. Its medial edge is located immediately lateral to the supraperiosteal tunnel.

A

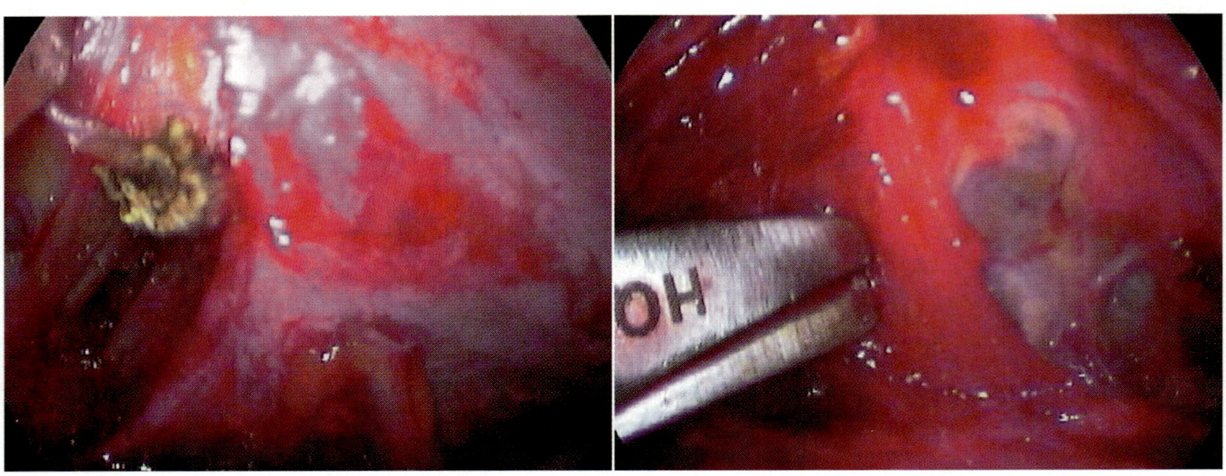

B

FIG. 5.42. **A,** Right corrugator muscle. **B,** Left corrugator muscle.

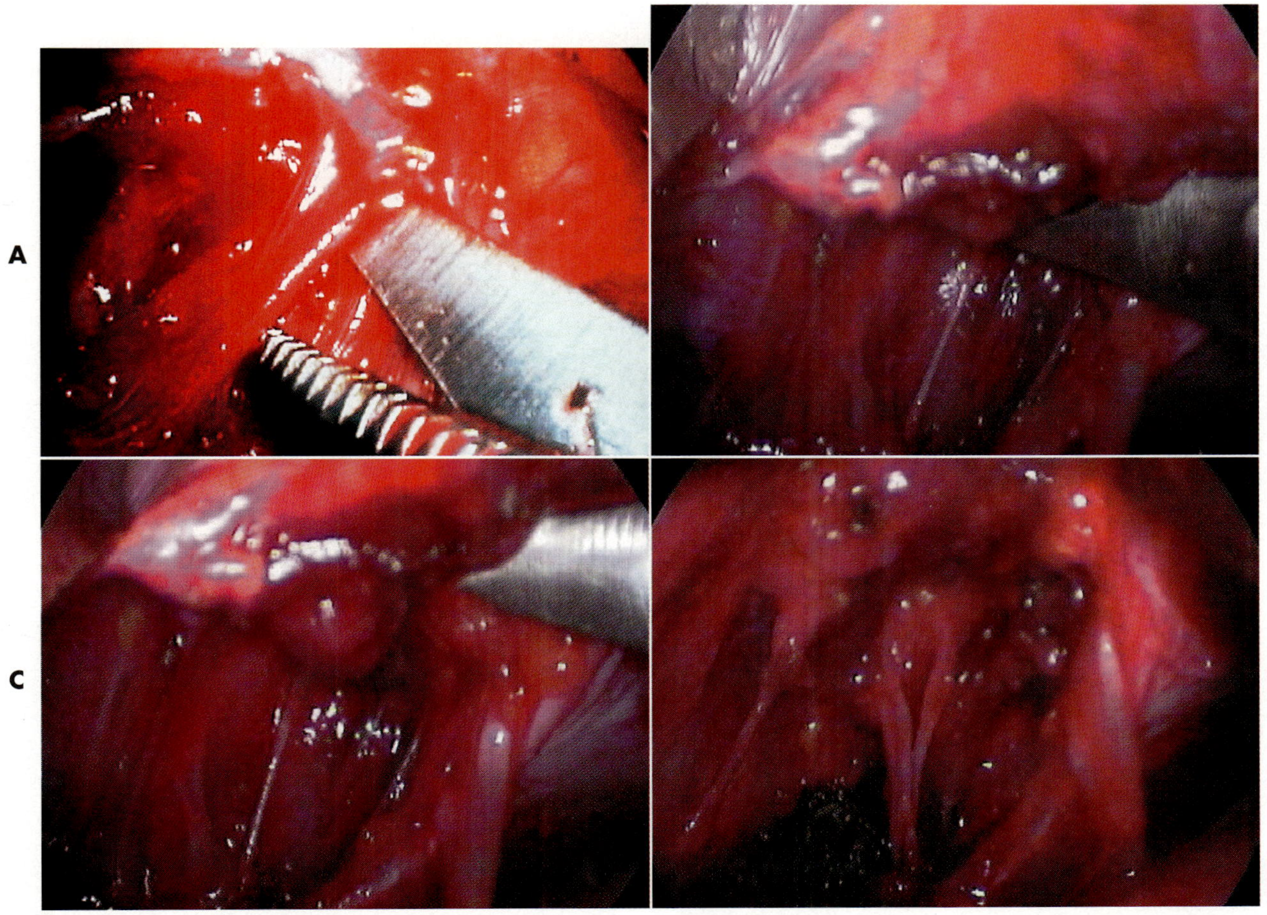

FIG. 5.43. **A,** Spreading motions with the endoscopic scissors are used to dissect the right corrugator. **B** and **C,** As the corrugator is incised, a branch of the supratrochlear nerve comes into view. **D,** Supratrochlear nerve is identified.

fluence of muscles above the medial brow (the "supraorbital wad") normally is hypertrophied. In this instance, the "supraorbital wad" of muscle is crosshatched (Figure 5.48). Although this cross-hatching weakens the muscle (it can be seen to "flatten out"), the cross-hatching may also denervate the muscle, which diminishes its function.

Myotomies are then performed through the orbicularis beneath the brow, circumferentially around the orbital rim (Figure 5.49, *A, B*). These are performed in the direction of the fibers, except when the surgeon lyses a web of orbicularis over the malar eminence.

Fixation. As previously noted, we use a screw technique for backward fixation of the brow. The amount of brow elevation (BE) desired is predetermined and measured according to the physician's judgment and the patient's desires (0.75–3.0 cm; most often, 1.0–1.5 cm).

The previous marking at the anterior end of the lateral incision (point A′) is noted. The incision is then pulled posteriorly and laterally, and the point of screw fixation (point A) is placed at the desired BE distance (Figure 5.50). This allows the direction of pull to be posterior and lateral to the vertical plane of the lateral canthus.

A special hand drill is then used to bore a hole through the outer table of the calvarium, and a self-tapping screw is placed at point A (Figure 5.51, *A*). A skin hook is placed into the posterior portion of the incision and pulled backward until the screw sits at the anterior edge of the incision (Figure 5.51, *B*). A surgical staple is placed immediately behind the screw, fixing the scalp and brow upward (Figure 5.51, *C, D*). Almost immediate contraction of the redundant scalp posterior to the screw is observed.

The temporoparietal fascia is then grasped in the anterior portion of the temporal incision and positioned and sutured posteriorly to the deep temporal fascia. This manuever will usually not elevate the brow, but tends to stabilize the elevation of the brow tail (Figure 5.52).

If the tail of the brow is not sufficiently stabilized, a small stab wound is made in the brow tail with a No. 11 blade. A double-armed Keith needle with a 3-0 Prolene suture is then placed through the stab wound, which

A 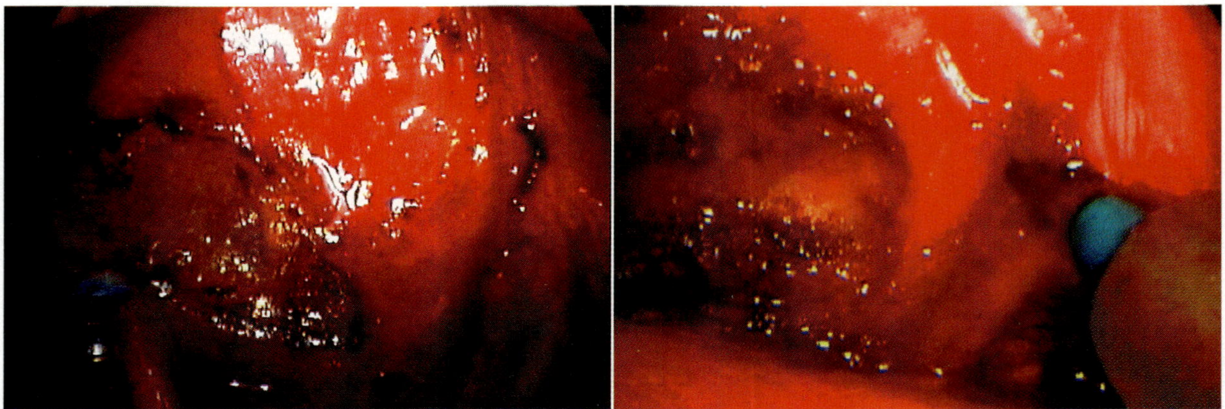 B

C 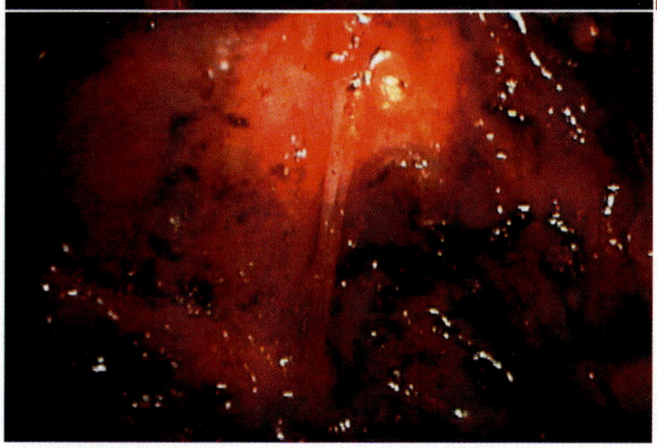

FIG. 5.44. **A,** Procerus muscle and the lateral edge of the corrugator are incised with the laser. **B,** As the laser dissection proceeds laterally, the outline of the supratrochlear nerve is seen. **C,** A branch of the supratrochlear nerve is delineated with the laser.

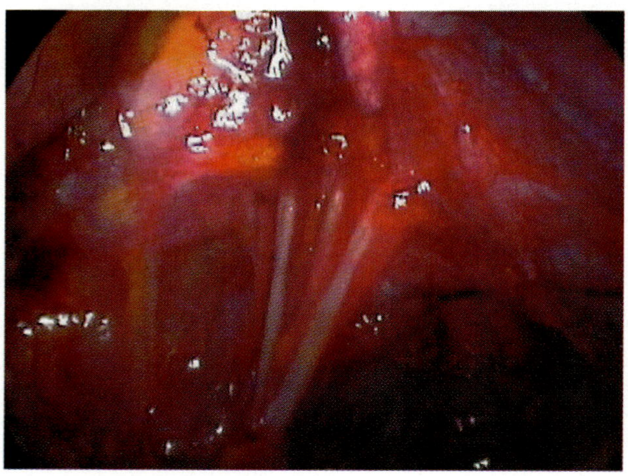

FIG. 5.45. Supratrochlear nerve can emerge from its own foramen. In this instance, it will divide into several branches.

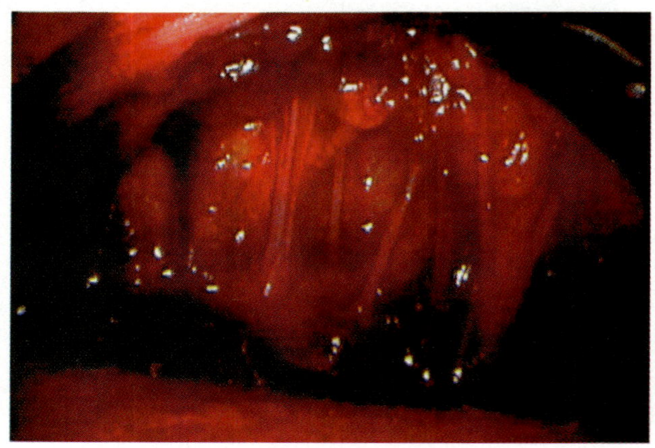

FIG. 5.46. Supratrochlear nerve can emerge from the same notch as the supraorbital nerve and divide immediately. In this instance, multiple nerve branches must be dissected.

grasps the orbicularis oculi muscle between the two arms of the needle. The suture is brought out through the temporal incisions and tied to the deep temporal fascia. Sufficient tension is placed on the brow in order to keep it from falling without creating a pucker (Figure 5.53).

Practical Applications

Our approach to specific patient situations represents a reasoned approach (one of many possible approaches) with reference to our clinical experience. Basically, we try to structure our approach to any patient's problem on an individual basis. We try to alter brow position, forehead height, improve the infrabrow skin overhanging the eyelid, improve forehead and glabellar rhytids, and alter expressive movements based on what best complements an individual's status, rather than to apply a set formula to every patient. Success in these goals is (as was true of large-incision approaches) never absolute. Certain situa-

A

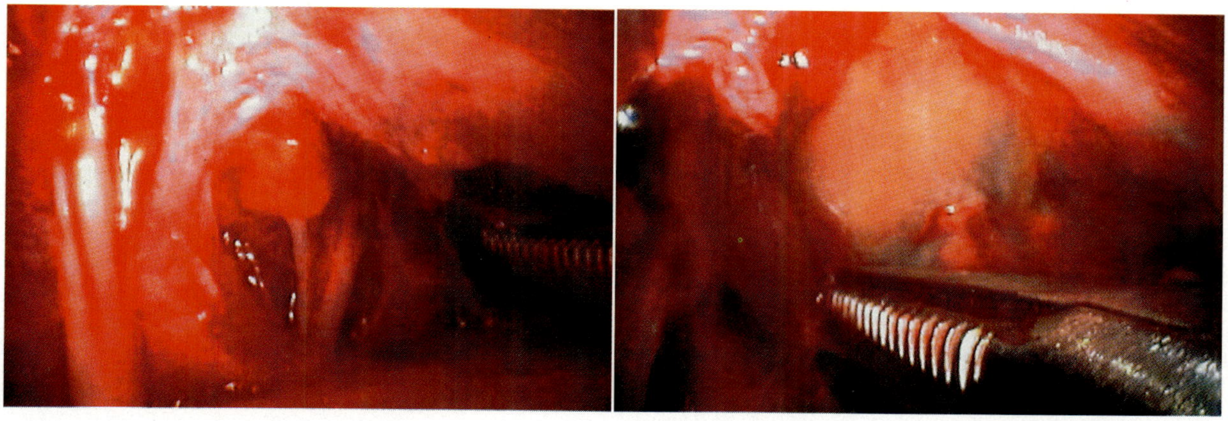

B

FIG. 5.47. **A,** Relationship of the nerves and muscles is illustrated. Supratrochlear nerve travels between the corrugator and depressor supercilii after the lateral edge of the corrugator muscle is incised, the muscle anterior to the supratrochlear nerve is the depressor supercilii (demarcated in this picture by the endoscopic scissors). Muscle between the supratrochlear and supraorbital nerves is corrugator. **B,** Endoscopic scissors is on hypertrophied depressor supercilii muscle, anterior to the supratrochlear nerve.

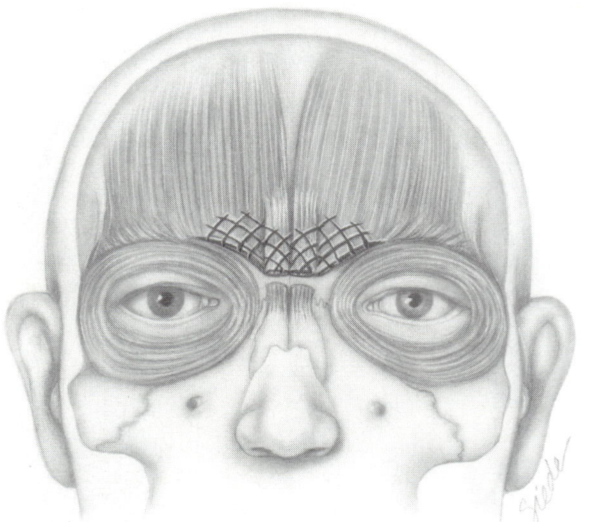

FIG. 5.48. If there are deep glabellar furrows, it is necessary to cross-hatch the region of confluence of glabellar musculature.

tions that have been previously described in this chapter are common. A modification of the "basic approach" to each of these situations can yield an acceptable result; however, an individualized procedure (as described below) can sometimes yield a better result.

Normal aging of the upper face. The typical 40- to 60-year-old patient has components of upper facial aging that are not severe in any one area. Instead, there are aging changes in many different areas.

Brow ptosis and settling have pushed infrabrow skin over the eyelid. Hooding of the eyelid that extends beyond the lateral canthus is a sign that brow ptosis as well as excess eyelid skin is the cause of this hooding. At this time, we refuse to perform a blepharoplasty alone for hooding beyond the lateral canthus. Instead, we perform an endoscopic temple or forehead lift in these situations, along with an optional blepharoplasty, because there is usually a component of brow ptosis present in these patients.

In normally aging patients, there may be horizontal rhytids on the forehead, but these are not deep. These rhytids may be the result of subconscious brow elevation that the patient performs when looking in a mirror or in greeting people, to disguise his or her aging, overhanging eyelids.

For these patients, we perform a subperiosteal/composite forehead lift according to our basic technique. If the patient's medical needs require minimal bruising and swelling, a subgaleal lift may suffice (Figure 5.54).

Frowners and squinters. Patients who are frowners and squinters customarily demonstrate prominent vertical glabellar lines. The medial brows have often fallen together inward and downward. These patients may have had either a single vertical line, twin vertical lines, or three vertical lines in their glabella from a young age. They may also be prone to frowning or squinting because of their occupation (teachers, accountants, and so on).

For these patients, a subperiosteal forehead lift is performed in order to pull the forehead upward and outward with traction on the "stiff" layer of periosteum. In doing so, the "caved in" glabella is "unfurled," pulling the brows and glabellar creases apart.

In addition, it is necessary to cross-hatch (myotomize) the supraorbital "wad" of musculature that represents the confluence of frontalis, corrugator, depressor, and procerus fibers. In these patients, it is common that this medial supraorbital musculature is so hypertrophied from years of frowning or squinting

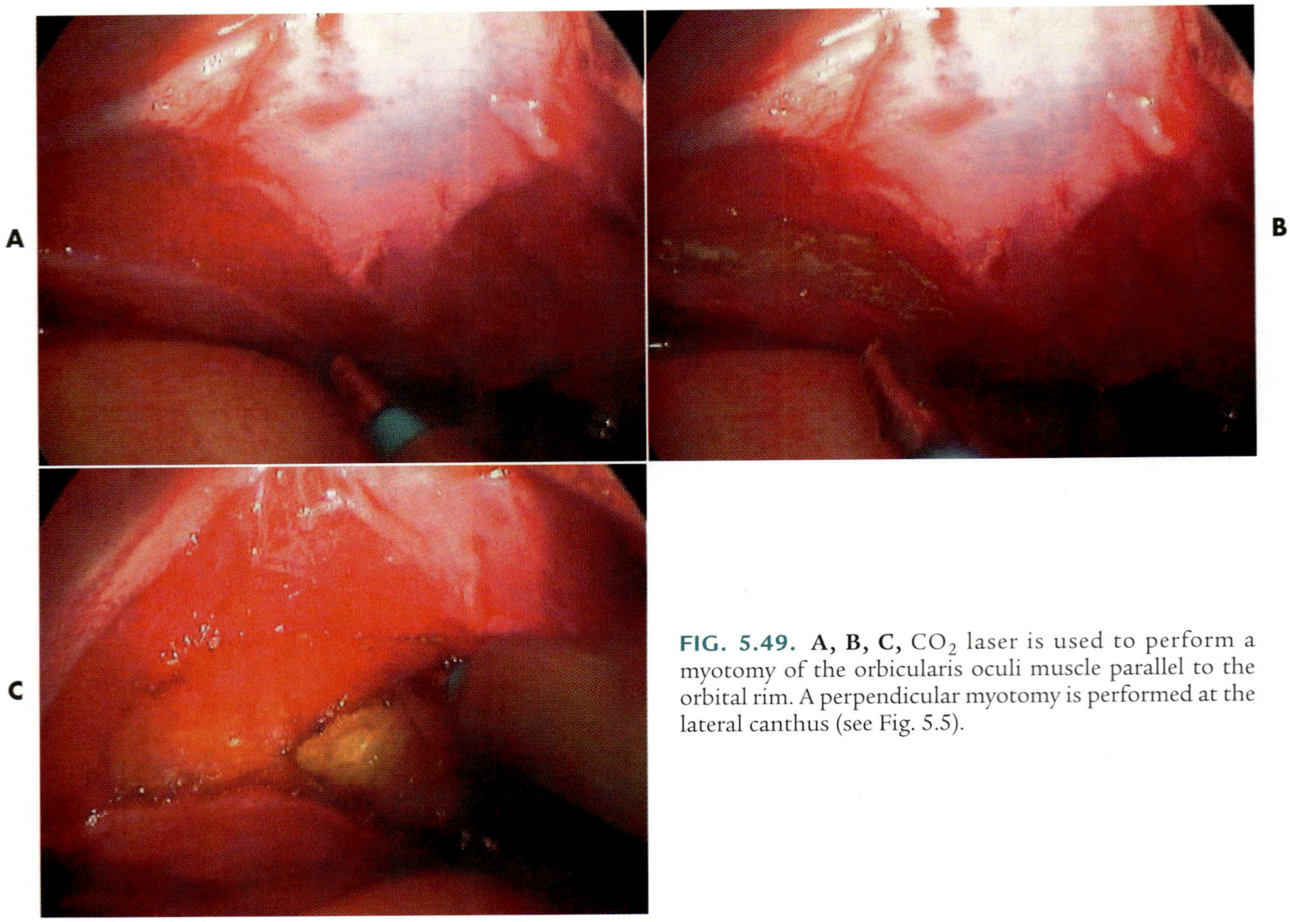

FIG. 5.49. **A, B, C,** CO_2 laser is used to perform a myotomy of the orbicularis oculi muscle parallel to the orbital rim. A perpendicular myotomy is performed at the lateral canthus (see Fig. 5.5).

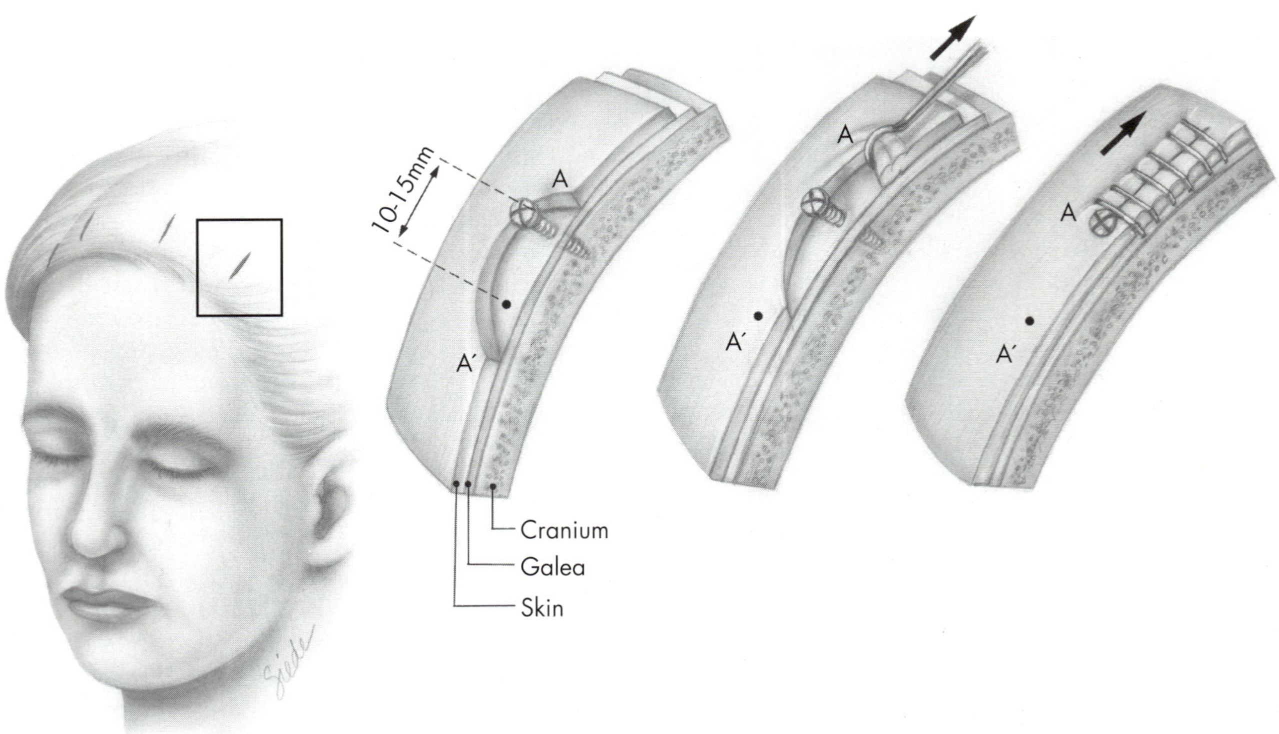

FIG. 5.50. To elevate the brow a predetermined distance (A′–A) a screw is placed at A′, the scalp pulled back, and a staple placed behind the screw to hold the scalp in place.

A B C D
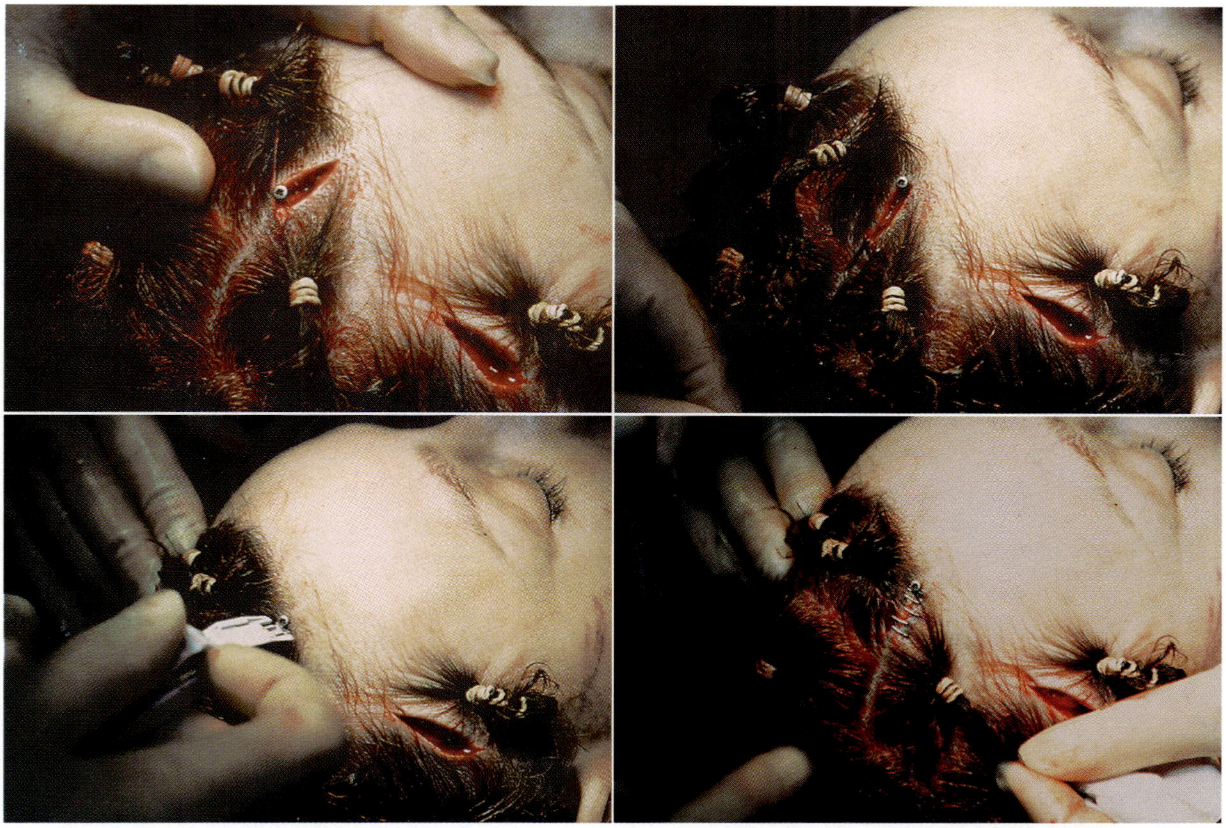

FIG. 5.51. **A,** Titanium screw is placed 1.25 cm posterior to the anterior edge of the vertical right lateral incision. **B,** Hook is placed in the posterior edge of the incision and pulled backward until the screw sits at the anterior edge of the incision. **C,** Staple is used to close the incision behind the screw. **D,** Staples abut screw holding fixation advancement in place.

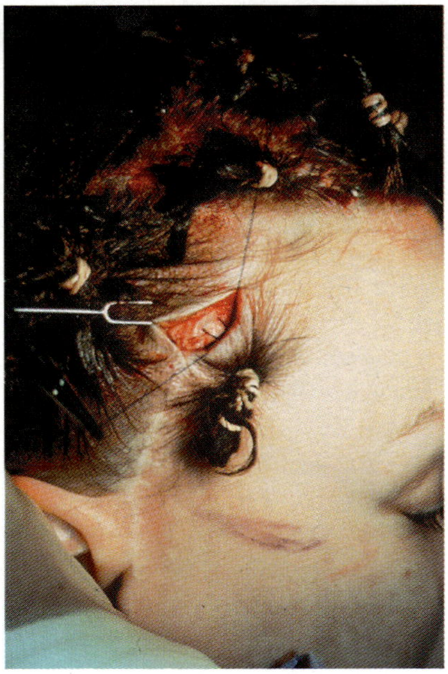

FIG. 5.52. Temporoparietal fascia is retracted backward and sutured to the deep temporal fascia to stabilize the temporal dissection.

that it is easily identifiable even from a distance (Figures 5.55 and 5.56).

Brow elevators. It is not uncommon for patients with brow ptosis to elevate their brows constantly. If the physician asks them to close their eyes and relax, the brows will descend, and the brow ptosis and overhanging eyelid skin becomes immediately apparent.

When the patient is instructed to open his or her eyes, the brows immediately ascend. The brows ascend even further when the patient looks in a mirror, has a photograph taken, or looks at other people.

Usually, these brow movements are subconscious. The movements, however, produce horizontal forehead creases with absent or minimal vertical glabellar furrowing.

Patients with brow ptosis commonly have preoperative and postoperative pictures that appear similar, with the exception of an absence of horizontal forehead furrows. The patients tend to elevate their brow in the preoperative pictures, but they don't in postoperative pictures (after relief of the brow ptosis), which demonstrates a similar preoperative and postoperative brow position in their photographs.

A

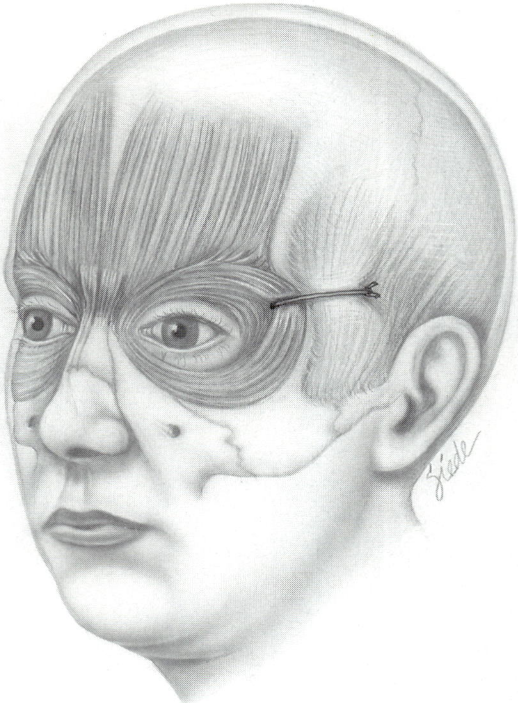

FIG. 5.53. A, If the brow is not adequately stabilized, a small stab wound is made in the brow tail with a No. 11 blade. A double-armed suspension suture is passed through the stab wound and orbicularis oculi muscle in two places and sutured to deep temporalis fascia. **B,** Suspension suture in place. In this case, it is fixed through a blepharoplasty incision.

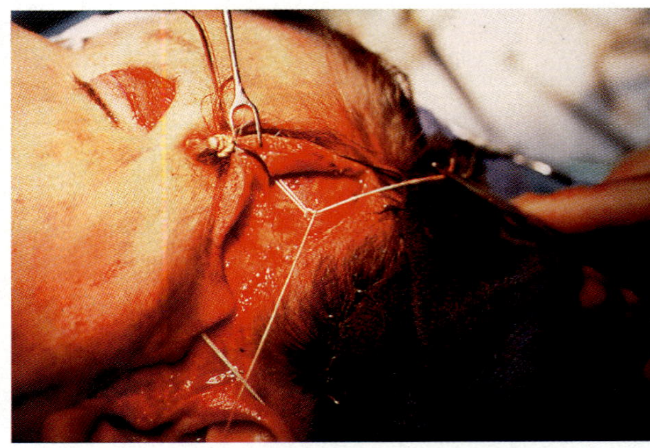

B

A

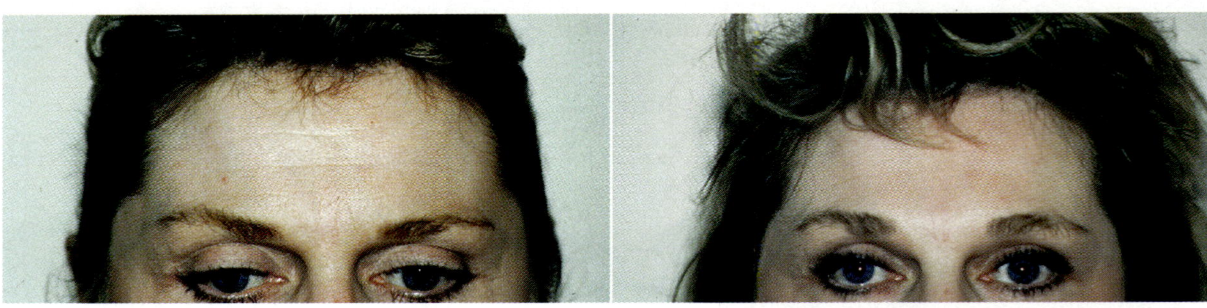

B

FIG. 5.54. A, Preoperative view of patient who has normal aging of the face. Moderate horizontal forehead line, mild vertical glabellar rhytids, and mild-to-moderate brow ptosis are present. **B,** Postoperative view of patient: 1 year.

If pictures of these patients at a younger age can be obtained, they can often be seen to have straight horizontal brows with a low, almost oriental-style eyelid fold. Often, they will have plucked the inferior lateral portions of their brow as they age to give the brow a higher appearance.

Commonly, patients with brow ptosis have already had a blepharoplasty, or one has been suggested to them, in order to deepen their brow fold. At times, these patients may elect to have a blepharoplasty, instead of brow elevation.

When large incision forehead lifting was the only option for these patients, many surgeons would accede to these patient preferences for blepharoplasty only. With the diminished morbidity that has occurred with endoscopic forehead lifting, it has become our practice to insist that a patient with overhanging eyelid folds that extend beyond the lateral canthus have a brow lifting procedure (either temple or brow). A conservative blepharoplasty may be performed at the same operation.

A standard endoscopic forehead lifting technique, either in the subgaleal or subperiosteal plane, can be effective in the correction of brow ptosis. If the forehead is "high," a subperiosteal lift is preferable. If it is "low," a subgaleal lift may be performed if the patient wishes minimal swelling and ecchymosis (Figures 5.57 and 5.58).

Round brows. It is not uncommon to see patients with brow ptosis of the brow tail. These patients can have this condition genetically (in which event, the condition is extremely difficult to treat) or they may

FIG. 5.55. **A,** Patient who "squints" because of sun exposure. She has prominent vertical glabellar lines, as well as brow ptosis. **B,** Postoperative view of patient: 1 year. A lateral suspension stitch has also been placed at the brow tail, in addition to the endoscopic forehead lift. Cross-hatching of glabellar musculature at the "supraorbital" was also performed. This patient had not undergone a blepharoplasty.

A

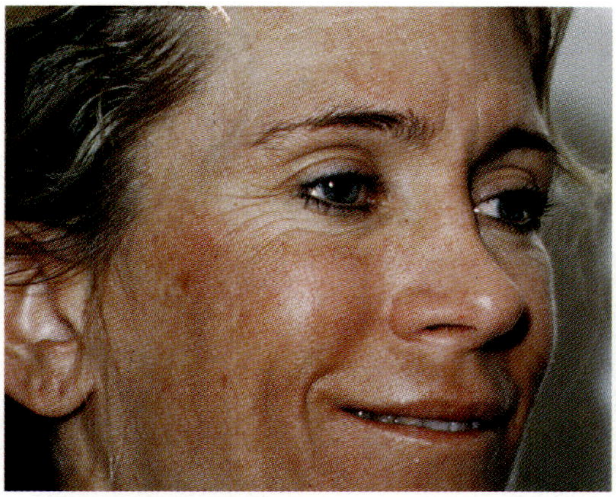

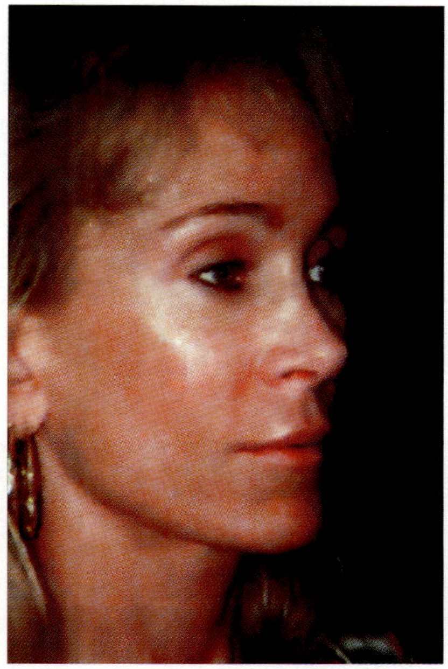

B

A

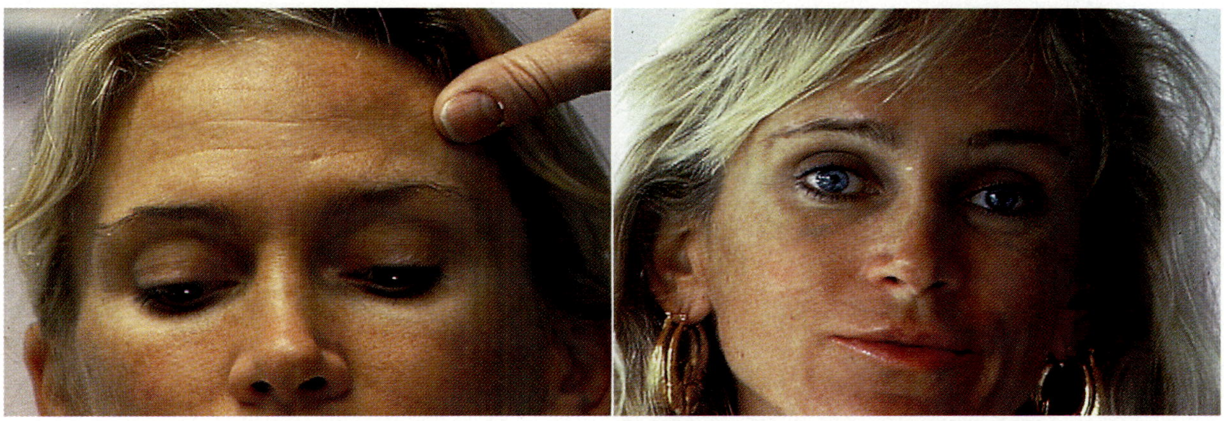

B

FIG. 5.56. **A,** Same patient as in Fig. 5.55 during assessment of desired brow position. **B,** Postoperative view of patient 1 year later.

A

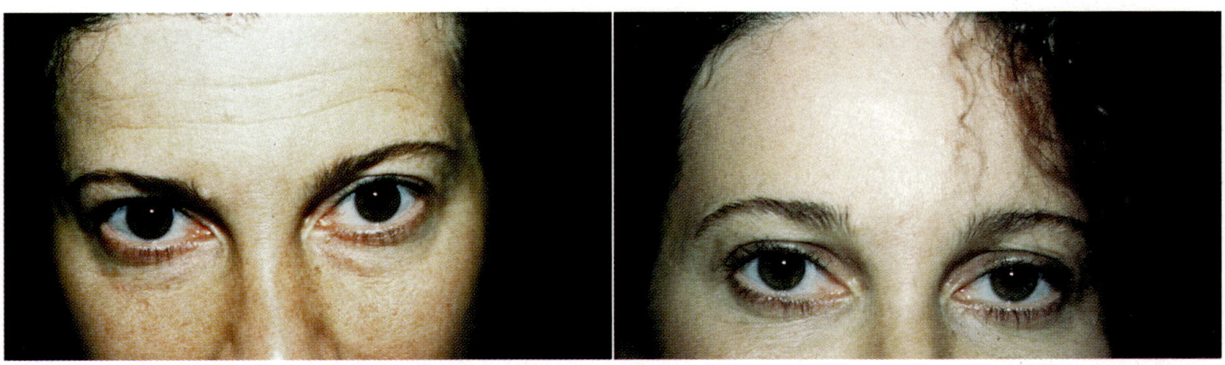

B

FIG. 5.57. **A,** Preoperative example of a patient who is a brow elevator. Prominent central forehead rhytids and brow ptosis are present. **B,** Postoperative patient: 6 years. This patient underwent surgery early in our series. At this time, larger horizontal incisions were used with limited scalp excisions. Note that there is a small amount of forehead elevation due to the scalp excision. No blepharoplasty was performed.

have ptosis of the lateral brow that occurs with the aging process (Figure 5.59).

An isolated temple lift may be performed in these patients, if they lack central forehead aging. The forehead lift procedure is performed without the central incisions, and the area between the corrugator is not blindly undermined. The central musculature also remains untouched.

An additional form of temple fixation—a suspension suture—is performed in these (and other) patients, as previously described in this chapter. A double-armed suspension suture is placed through a needle-size stab wound at the very lateral portion of the brow and brought out through the temple incision. The two arms are placed through the brow to grasp the orbicularis immediately beneath the brow.

After screw fixation through the lateral incisions on the forehead, the suspension suture is tightened only enough to suspend the brow and hold its position. To avoid a pucker where the suspension suture grasps the orbicularis muscle, no attempt is made to elevate the brow with the suspension suture.

A B C

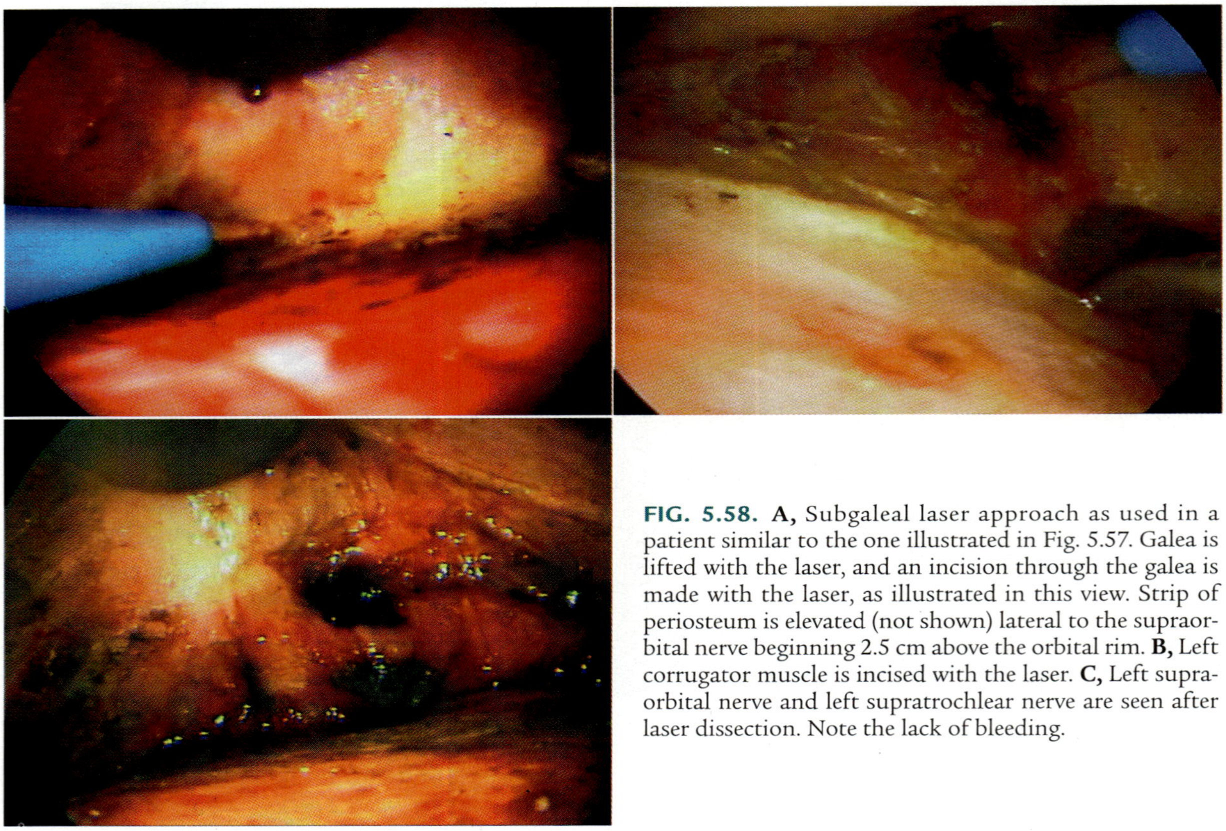

FIG. 5.58. **A,** Subgaleal laser approach as used in a patient similar to the one illustrated in Fig. 5.57. Galea is lifted with the laser, and an incision through the galea is made with the laser, as illustrated in this view. Strip of periosteum is elevated (not shown) lateral to the supraorbital nerve beginning 2.5 cm above the orbital rim. **B,** Left corrugator muscle is incised with the laser. **C,** Left supraorbital nerve and left supratrochlear nerve are seen after laser dissection. Note the lack of bleeding.

A B

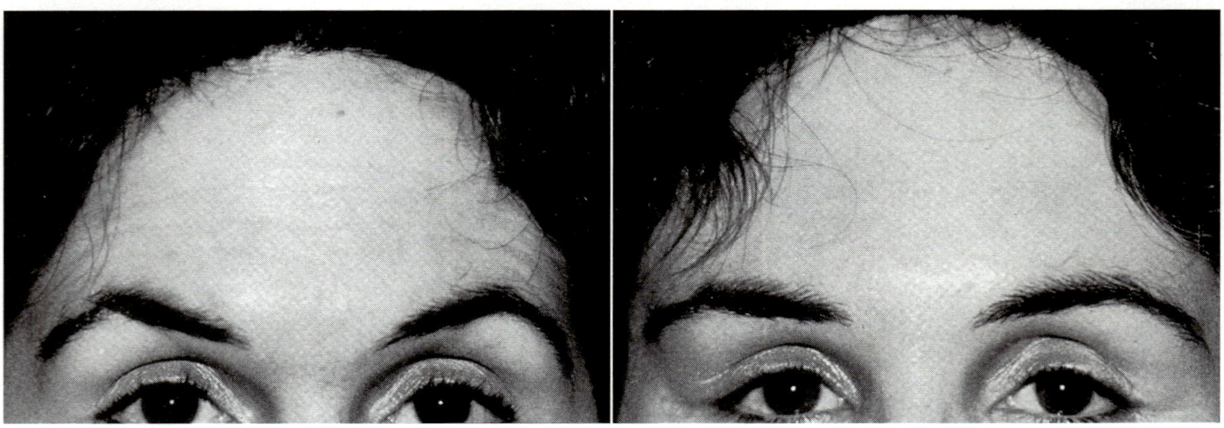

FIG. 5.59. **A,** Preoperative view of patient with "round brows." **B,** Postoperative (18 months) view of correction with forehead/temple lift. A lateral suspension suture was used.

The suspension suture is fastened to the deep temporal fascia, at the level of the incision. The temple is then fixated and closed as previously described. This temple lift may be performed in the subcutaneous plane or on top of the deep temporal fascia (see Figure 5.53). Even with suspension suture fixation, however, it is still difficult to adequately change the configuration of the congenitally round brow.

High forehead. Most patients who have high foreheads can undergo an endoscopic subperiosteal lift. By placing the lateral incisions at the lateral canthus as far lateral as possible and angling them outward as described previously, a central forehead elevation of only 2.5 to 4 mm may be achieved, with a lateral brow elevation of 5 to 10 mm.

Some patients' forehead height requires lowering, however. If this is the case, a pretrichial or trichophytic incision of 2.5 to 5 cm can be made between the supraorbital nerve corridors. A subcutaneous dissection is then performed for 2 cm. An incision is then made through the frontalis muscle and the dissection becomes subgaleal. A standard brow release and temple dissection is then performed. The frontalis muscle is advanced over itself and sutured into the advanced positions. An ellipse of redundant skin is incised, which reduces the central forehead (Figures 5.60 and 5.61).

Medial brow ptosis. A subperiosteal forehead lift may be used to correct medial brow ptosis. Screw fixation is used in the central as well as the lateral incisions to provide an upward vector of lift to the medial brow. This approach is described in Chapter 9.

Another approach that is used for this situation in patients with high foreheads is a composite subcutaneous/subgaleal plane lift as described previously in the high forehead section. When the frontalis is sutured over itself, the medial brow is elevated (see Figures 5.60 and 5.61).

A

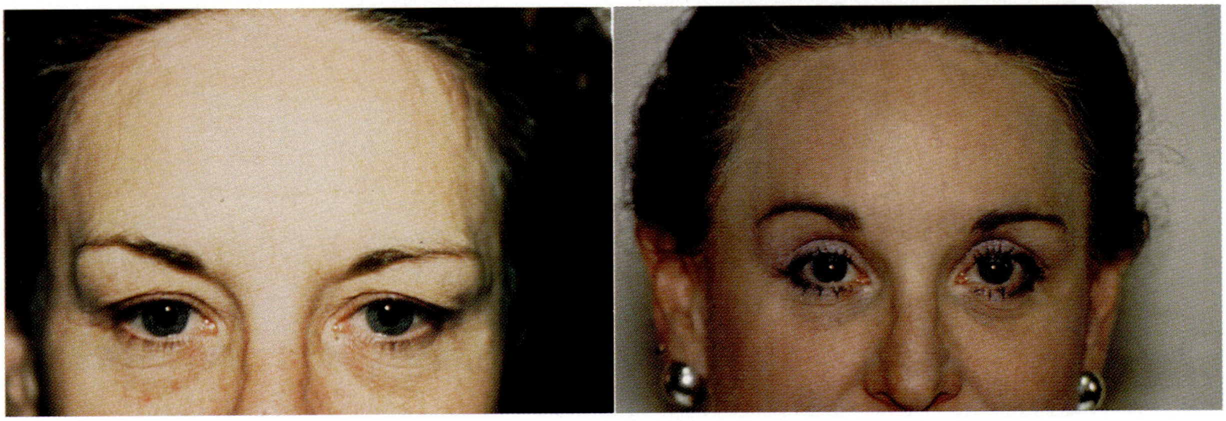

B

FIG. 5.60. **A,** Preoperative view of patient who has medial brow ptosis and a high forehead. **B,** Postoperative view (2 years) of the same patient. A small pretrichial incision with subcutaneous dissection converted to subgaleal dissection was used. Excess forehead skin was excised. Concurrent blepharoplasty was performed.

A

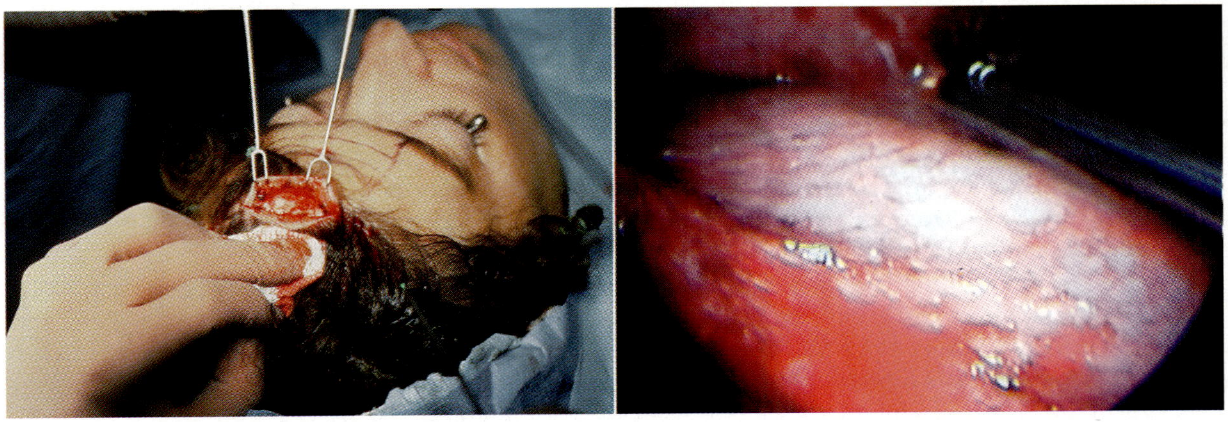

B

FIG. 5.61. **A,** Example of the subcutaneous incision as used in the patient in Fig. 5.60 is shown. **B,** Incision through frontalis muscle and transition to a subgaleal plane is illustrated. Myotomies of the corrugator with visualization of the supratrochlear nerve are shown.

A 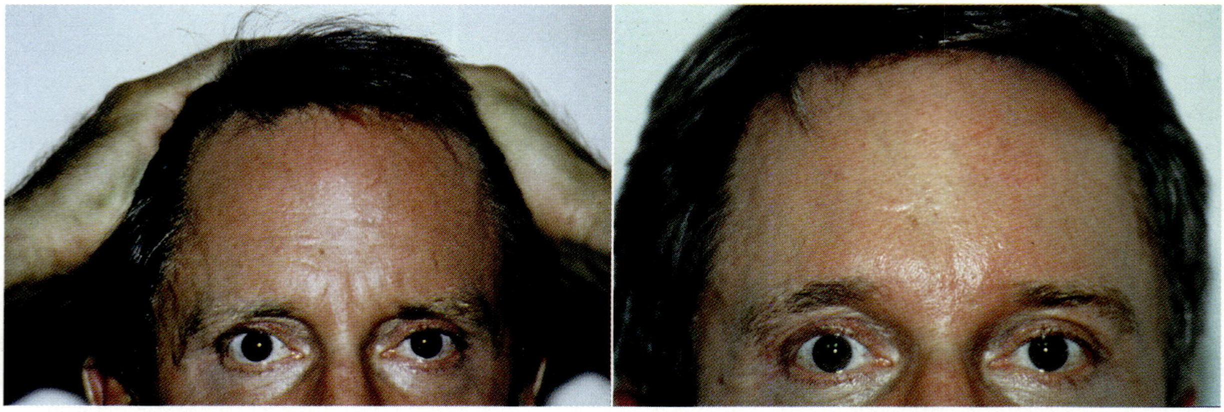 B

FIG. 5.62. **A,** Preoperative view of a patient with male pattern baldness. **B,** Postoperative view of the same patient: 1 year. A single central incision vertically oriented was used (as illustrated in Fig. 5.2).

A 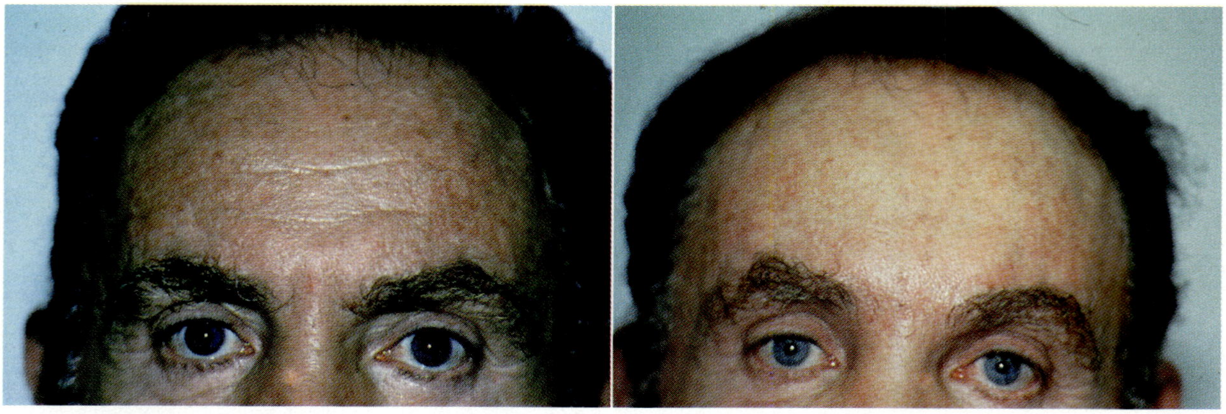 B

FIG. 5.63. **A,** Patient with more advanced male pattern baldness. Incisions are as illustrated in Fig. 5.3. **B,** Postoperative view of patient: 1 year. Access to the corrugators was via the blepharoplasty incision.

Male pattern baldness. For patients who have male pattern baldness, a subperiosteal lift may be used, but the incisions may need to be modified. In men with a stable tuft of frontal hair, a single central 1 cm vertical incision may be constructed for elevation and access (Figure 5.62). Care must be taken to fixate only laterally to avoid medial forehead elevation.

In men who have total frontal baldness, a central incision may cause an unacceptable scar. Therefore, access is often limited to incisions at the fringe or larger temple incisions. In this event, the dissecting endoscopic sheath (Karl Storz No. KST 521) is especially useful. When access is limited to temple incisions, a subcutaneous approach is often used for several centimeters and then transitioned to an approach over the superficial layer of deep temporal fascia. This allows an excision of a small ellipse of skin, if necessary.

If the surgeon is unable to reach the central muscles (corrugator, procerus, depressor) through the above incisions, access to these muscles may be provided via a blepharoplasty incision approach similar to that used in a transblepharoplasty brow suspension.[35] This approach is described in Chapter 7 (Figure 5.63).

Bony abnormalities. The endoscopic approach can be used to drill down many bony abnormalities. Forehead bossing, osteomas, and other bony abnormalities can be drilled down with long shaft drills and smoothed with sinus or arthroscopic shavers (Figure 5.64). Abnormalities of the bony orbital rim that are not amenable to a superior approach can often be reached through a transblepharoplasty approach.

A

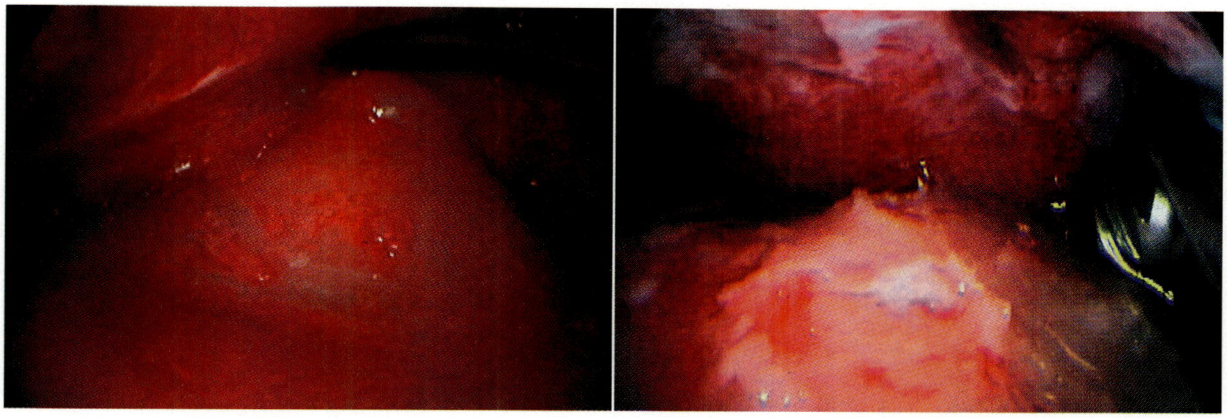

B

FIG. 5.64. **A,** Osteoma of the frontal bone in a patient undergoing endoforehead lift. **B,** Drilling and planing the osteoma can be performed through the endoscope.

SUMMARY

In summary, concepts that are unique to endoscopic forehead lifting are: (1) the use of small incisions rather than a single large incision, (2) the creation of an optical cavity, (3) release of the brow along with myotomy and/or denervation, and (4) elevation of the brow through posterior fixation of the scalp. These concepts provide the framework of principles that enable the surgeon to lift the brows, diminish rhytids, and diminish brow ptosis to achieve the goal of forehead rejuvenation (see Box 5.2).

In our practice, we have not performed a coronal frontal rhytidectomy in more than 3 years, because of the effectiveness of the endoscopic procedures. As our technical expertise has increased over the past 6 years, we have noted that our endoscopic techniques are actually more effective than our open techniques had been, particularly in elevating the brow tail, reducing lateral canthal skin overhang, and achieving brow symmetry.

Recently, Sasaki[30] has evaluated by questionnaire the satisfaction of 93 plastic surgeons with endoscopic forehead lifting procedures. The surgeons queried only had an average of 11 months of experience with the procedure. They reported performing an average of 4.9 surgeries during the first half of their experience and 12.7 cases during the second half (approximately 18 surgeries, on average, per year). Most of the surgeons felt that both their expertise and desire to perform the procedure increased over this time. A variety of techniques and methods of fixation were used.

The majority of the surgeons (69%) subjectively felt that the endoscopic procedure was less effective than open procedures, but most (74%) also felt that there were less complications with endoscopic surgery. Decreased complications probably explained why 66% of the surgeons interviewed felt that the endoscopic forehead procedure was supplanting open surgical techniques in their practices.

Sasaki[36] has also attempted to objectify which groups do best with the endoscopic forehead lift for brow ptosis. The criterion for the presence of brow ptosis that he uses is the measurement of the distance from midpupil to the top of the brow (the frame height), as described by McKinney. If this distance is less than 2.0 to 2.5 cm, brow ptosis can be assumed to exist, and an endoscopic forehead lift is indicated.

Sasaki combines the frame height measurement with the "glide test" to try to predict the effectiveness of the alleviation of brow ptosis by the endoscopic forehead lift. The glide test is a measurement of brow excursion in the medial, central, and lateral portions of the brow.

The examiner lifts the brow and measures its excursion from the resting position in each portion. This test is repeated three times in order to eliminate patient resistance to the procedure. The maximum glide is then taken at each position and averaged.

Sasaki found that the best improvement in brow position from endoscopic forehead lifting occurred when the patient's frame height was between 1.5 to 2.0 cm and the glide test values were between 2 to 3 cm.

Younger patients or ethnic (especially Asian) patients usually have higher frame heights (2–2.5 cm) and minimal glide indices. Their brows are in a relatively high position, and brow ptosis is often minimal. Their skin is elastic and tight, and the brows do not glide easily.

These patients usually are seeking a change in the shape of the brow, a goal that is relatively harder, in our experience, to achieve. This subclass of patients is generally more difficult to please.

A
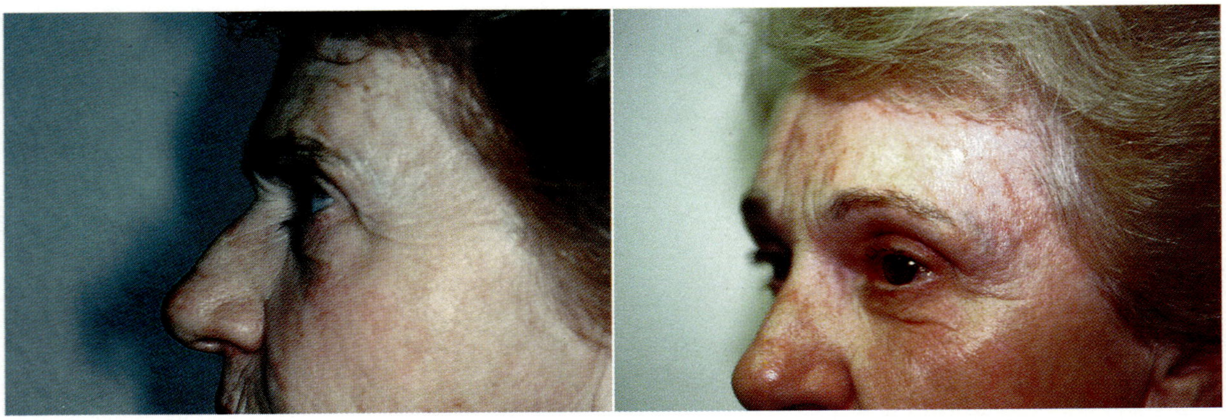
B

FIG. 5.65. **A,** Patient with a glide test > 3.25 cm. **B,** Postoperative view of the same patient: 1.5 years.

Older (> 60 years old) patients who have loose skin often have a great deal of brow ptosis. Extreme examples of these can manifest a frame height less than 1.5 cm and a glide test of 2 to 3 cm. Sasaki found it difficult to obtain brow correction without skin excisional techniques (Figure 5.65). We have found suspension sutures to be helpful in these patients (see the Round Brows section of this chaper).

In Sasaki's series, improvement of forehead rhytids could be surmised to occur in all patients, because corrugator and procerus function was noted to be successfully diminished in all groups treated. In our series, all patients' forehead and glabellar rhytids were improved. Myotomy remains a cornerstone of the endoscopic forehead procedure.

As noted previously, more than two thirds of the surgeons surveyed reported that they noticed decreased morbidity and a decreased incidence of complications when using endoscopic as opposed to coronal or other large-incision techniques. Nonetheless, side effects and complications occur with this procedure, as with any other surgical exercise.

Seroma, ecchymosis, numbness, paresis, stitch abscess, relapse of brow ptosis, neuropraxia of the temporal branch of the facial nerve, skin burns from cautery, transient alopecia, hematoma, hypertrophic scar, irregularities, pruritis, and asymmetrical brows have all been reported as side effects or complications. Most of these have been reported as minor problems that resolve with time. No permanent paralysis of the temporal branch of the facial nerve was reported.[37-40]

Despite these complications (which are also present in coronal and pretrichial lifting procedures), it has been our experience (as well as the experience of the group surveyed by Sasaki[30]) that there is a reduced incidence and severity of complications with the endoscopic procedures as compared with large-incision procedures. The endoscopic frontal lift avoids the hair-bearing scalp resections and supraorbital nerve interruption that is present in the larger procedure. It is also our experience that patient acceptance of the endoscopic forehead lift has been much better than that for the coronal forehead lift.

The negative aspects of endoscopic forehead lifting are the expense of the equipment and the extra training required to become proficient. Although not insignificant, it is the authors' personal bias that the added expense and training is balanced by increased acceptability of endoscopic forehead rejuvenative procedures by patients.

REFERENCES

1. Keller GS: US Patent No. 5,370,642, Endoscopic Facial Plastic Surgery, Applied 1991, Awarded 1994.
2. Keller GS: Small incision frontal rhytidectomy with the KTP laser. Paper presented at the American Academy of Cosmetic Surgery, World Congress, October 13, 1991, Scottsdale, Ariz.
3. Keller GS: Use of the KTP laser in cosmetic surgery, Am J Cosmetic Surg 9:177-180, 1992.
4. Keller GS: Endolaser excision of glabellar frown lines and forehead rhytids. Paper presented at the American Academy of Facial Plastic and Reconstructive Surgery, February 1, 1992, Los Angeles, Calif.
5. Core GB, Vasconez LO, Askren C, Yamamoto Y, Gamboa M: Coronal face-lift with endoscopic techniques, Plast Surg Forum 15:227-228, 1992.
6. Liang M and Narayanan K: Endoscopic ablation of the frontalis and corrugator muscles—a clinical study, Plast Surg Forum 15:58-60, 1992.

6a. Khan SH: Nerve block anesthesia of the scalp. In Stough D and Haber R, editors: Hair replacement: Medical and surgical, St. Louis, 1996, Mosby-Year Book.

7. Keller GS, Razum N, et al: Small incision laser lift for forehead creases and glabellar furrows, Arch Otolaryngol Head Neck Surg 119:632-635, 1993.
8. Keller GS: KTP laser rhytidectomy, Facial Plast Surg Clin North Am, 1(2):153-162, 1993.
9. Isse NG: Endoscopic facial rejuvenation: endoforehead, the functional lift, Aesthetic Plast Surg 18:21, 1994.
10. Daniel RK and Ramirez OM: Endoscopic-assisted aesthetic surgery, Aesthetic Surg 14:14, 1994.

11. Ramirez OM: Endoscopic options in facial rejuvenation: An overview, Aesthetic Plast Surg 18:141-147, 1994.
12. Ramirez OM: Endoscopic full face lift, Aesthetic Plast Surg 18:363-371, 1994.
13. Fodor PB: Endoscopic plastic surgery, a new milestone in plastic surgery (editorial), Aesthetic Plast Surg 18:31, 1994.
14. Toledo LS: Video-endoscopic facelift, Aesthetic Plast Surg 18:149, 1994.
15. Chajchir A: Endoscopic subperiosteal forehead lift, Aesthetic Plast Surg 18:269, 1994.
16. Vasconez LO, Core GB, Gamboa-Bobadilla M, et al: Endoscopic techniques in coronal brow lifting, Plast Reconstr Surg 94: 788-793, 1994.
17. Keller GS and Cray J: Laser-assisted surgery of the aging face. Facial Plast Surg Clin North Am 3(3):319-341, 1995.
18. Nahai F, Eaves F, Bostwick J: Forehead lift and glabellar frown lines. In Bostwick J, Eaves F, Nahai F, editors: Endoscopic plastic surgery, St. Louis, 1995, Quality Medical Publishing, pp 166-230.
19. Core G, Vasconez L, Graham HD: Development and current status of endoscopic browlifting, Clin Plast Surg 619-631, 1995.
20. Graham HD and Core G: Endoscopic forehead lifting using fixation sutures, Operative Techniques Otolaryngology–Head Neck Surg 6(4): 245-252, 1995.
21. Matarasso A and Matarasso SL: Endoscopic surgical correction of glabellar creases, Dermatol Surg 211:695-700, 1995.
22. Ramirez OM: Endoscopically assisted biplanar forehead lift, Plast Reconstr Surg 96:323-333, 1995.
23. Song IC, Pozner JN, KSadeh AE, Shin MS: Endoscopic-assisted recontouring of the facial skeleton: the forehead, Ann Plast Surg 34:323-325, 1995.
24. Fuente del Campo A: Subperiosteal facelift: open and endoscopic approach, Aesthetic Plast Surg 19:149-160, 1995.
25. Hamas RS: Reducing the subconscious frown by endoscopic resection of the corrugator muscles, Aesthetic Plast Surg 19:21-25, 1995.
26. Aiache A: Endoface-lift: subcutaneous approach. In Ramirez O and Daniel R, editors: Endoscopic plastic surgery, New York, 1996, Springer-Verlag
27. Abramo AC: Forehead rhytidoplasty, endoscopic approach, Aesthetic Plast Surg 19:463-467, 1995.
28. Isse N: The endoscopic forehead lift, Presentation at Interdisciplinary Facial Plastic Surgery Symposium, Santa Barbara, Calif, November 12, 1995.
29. Isse N, Fodor P: Forehead rejuvenation. In Fodor P, Isse N, editors: Endoscopically assisted aesthetic plastic surgery, St. Louis, 1996, Mosby-Year Book, pp 55-56.
30. Sasaki G: Questionnaire analysis for endoscopic forehead lift procedures. In Sasaki G, editor: Endoscopic, aesthetic, and reconstructive surgery, Philadelphia, 1996, Lippincott-Raven, pp 80-89.
31. Becker W, Buckingham R, Holinger P, et al: Reference to the work of Brubaker and Brubaker. In Becker W, Buckingham R, Holinger P, et al, editors: Atlas of otorhinolaryngology and bronchoesophagology (preface), Philadelphia, 1969, WB Saunders (English edition).
32. Klein JA: The tumescent technique, Dematol Clinics 8:425, 1990.
33. Strahan R: Personal communication, 1995.
34. Nahai F: Personal communication. Interdisciplinary Approaches to Facial Rejuvenation Course, Vail, Colo, Harvard University (sponsor), March 1996.
35. Keller GS: Transblepharoplasty brow suspension with the KTP laser, Int J Aesthetic Restorative Surg 1:101-105, 1993.
36. Sasaki, G: Brow ptosis. In Sasaki G, editor: Endoscopic, aesthetic, and reconstructive surgery, Philadelphia, Lippincott-Raven, 1996, pp 19-28.
37. Ibid: pp 72-79.
38. Isse N, Fodor P: Forehead rejuvination. In Fodor P, Isse N, editors: Endoscopically assisted aesthetic plastic surgery, St. Louis, 1996, Mosby-Year Book, pp 57-61.
39. Eaves F: Basics of endoscopic plastic surgery; Forehead lift and glabellar frown lines. In Bostwick J, Eaves F, Nahai F, editors: Endoscopic plastic surgery, St. Louis, 1995, Quality Medical Publishing, pp 78-79, 228-229.
40. Daniel R: Endoforehead and subperiosteal approach. In Ramirez O and Daniel R, editors: Endoscopic plastic surgery, New York, 1996, Springer-Verlag, pp 65-67.

chapter six

Endoscopic Forehead Lifting Using Fixation Sutures

H. Devon Graham III and Grady B. Core

Endoscopic brow and forehead lifting has become increasingly popular recently as both surgeons and patients alike search for techniques that reduce morbidity and recovery time, yet maintain the ability to achieve excellent results.

Endoscopic, or endoscopically assisted brow and forehead lifts, show great promise in the area of facial rejuvenation surgery. Although this technique will never completely replace the traditional open techniques, endoscopic brow lifting has a definite place in the armamentarium of the facial plastic surgeon because of its decreased morbidity and excellent patient satisfaction. One problem around which major variations and techniques center is soft-tissue fixation of the elevated brow and forehead. We will review the various techniques for suspension in use today as well as our preferred technique.

Endoscopic brow lifting, as with any of the open techniques, ideally should correct tissue ptosis, eliminate rhytids, and weaken any hyperdynamic action of the underlying musculature without creating additional deformity. It is imperative that facial plastic surgeons understand the aesthetic importance of treating the upper face and forehead in order to achieve overall facial rejuvenation. The skin of the face, through the process of aging, weather damage, and other factors gradually loses elasticity and creates redundancy and ptosis. The upper third of the aging face, especially the brow and glabellar complex, is one of the areas that first shows the early signs of aging. Deep vertical glabellar frown lines, along with horizontal forehead rhytids, are caused by a combination of weakened, inelastic skin acted upon by the contractile forces of the frontalis, procerus, corrugator, and depressor supercilii muscles. Once this scenario occurs, patients often exhibit a tired, sad, or even angry look when they in fact feel quite happy and rested. These patients will often present requesting a blepharoplasty when in fact the majority of their problem stems from ptotic brows and forehead and hyperactivity of the brow depressor muscles. Thus, when evaluating these patients preoperatively, the entire forehead, brow, and orbital complex must be taken into consideration, working from the top downward.

Aesthetic ideals of brow position as well as the available options of open techniques are well documented in the literature, and although fashion trends come and go, the "ideal" aesthetic brow has changed little during the last 15 years.[1-7]

INDICATIONS AND CONTRAINDICATIONS

The indications for endoscopic brow lifting are the same as those for the open technique and include patients who have brow ptosis, lateral canthal ptosis, and forehead and glabellar rhytids. The most favorable candidates for endoscopic brow lifting are thin-skinned Caucasian women. The least favorable candidates include patients who have thick, heavy sebaceous skin and marked brow ptosis. All patients in between these extremes, including Orientals, Hispanics, and men, who typically have thicker skin than women, can be acceptable candidates. These patients, however, may occasionally require additional maneuvers to obtain the best results, and as with any procedure, they should be evaluated on a case-by-case basis.

The contraindications for this technique are relative and include patients with very thick sebaceous skin and marked brow ptosis, where skin excision as well as support would probably be needed. This would include all patients with complete loss of frontalis muscle function on one or both sides as a result of facial nerve paralysis. In our experience we have not found the endoscopic technique completely satisfactory for adequate elevation of the brow in these patients probably because of complete loss of muscle tone. These patients would be better served by using a subcutaneous or subgaleal dissection with skin excision and/or direct muscle suspension. Additionally, patients with a pre-existing high frontal hairline, where brow elevation is needed, are not ideal candidates, because the endoscopic technique does move the hairline somewhat superiorly. The relationship between the brows and the hairline, however, remain relatively constant as compared to the traditional coronal technique. Thus, in the endoscopic subperiosteal procedure the entire brow forehead complex is advanced superiorly as a complete unit, repositioning the brows and forehead together in the desired position. With the traditional coronal technique the dissection is performed in the subgaleal plane and the skin of the anterior scalp and forehead is stretched posteriorly, excising a hair-bearing portion. This skin stretching technique changes the relationship between the brows and anterior hairline causing elongation of the forehead.

The advantages of the endoscopic versus the open technique include minimal incisions with decreased bleeding, decreased sensory neuropathy, and no need for drains. In addition, less postoperative discomfort, more rapid recovery, decreased alopecia problems, and excellent visualization may be achieved.

The disadvantages are mainly the need for specialized training in the use of endoscopes and endoscopic instrumentation if the surgeon is not yet familiar with this equipment. Also, if the surgeon or his or her operating facility is not equipped with the endoscopes, camera, and video equipment or the endoscopic instrumentation, these must be obtained.

Work-up and Preparation of the Patient

As with any facial plastic surgery procedure, patient selection is critical for a good surgical result. Factors both physical and mental must be taken into consideration when selecting patients for any facial aesthetic procedure.

The ideal candidate is in good mental and physical health without any systemic conditions existing in an uncontrolled state. A thorough and complete history and physical examination still remain the most important preoperative screening mechanisms for diseases and conditions that could adversely affect the patient's surgical experience. Along with the physical preparation, patient education is a vital element and one of the most powerful and effective tools in reducing anxiety and establishing realistic postoperative goals.

A full series of photographs, both full face and close-up of eyes and forehead, should be taken. These should be taken with the patient's hair pinned back in order to see the entire frontal and temporal hairlines. In order to maintain continuity for critical postoperative evaluation, magnifications should be fixed and documented for each patient so that the preoperative and postoperative photos will coincide. When taking photos, the patient must be educated in how to relax and pose in a normal anatomic position, because the tendency for patients during any photographic event is to open their eyes widely, which raises the brows. When the patients are positioned and the camera is set, they should close their eyes and relax their forehead for 10 to 15 seconds, concentrating on complete relaxation of the brows. After this is accomplished, the patients are instructed to open their eyes slowly, just enough to see clearly straight ahead, while maintaining the relaxation of their brows. They should feel as though they have heavy, tired eyes in this position. By using this maneuver in every patient, the frontalis muscle, which is the major elevator of the brows, will be in its most relaxed and natural anatomic position.

SURGICAL ANATOMY

The prerequisite for any facial plastic surgeon is a working knowledge of the functional and static anatomy of the forehead. The functional anatomy of the brow/forehead complex consists of paired muscles that act in conjunction or opposition, creating a myriad of facial expressions. These muscles are divided into elevators and depressors.

The major elevator of the brow/forehead complex is the paired frontalis muscle, which along with the paired occipital muscles and the interconnecting galea aponeurotica form the epicranium. These muscles, acting in concert, draw the scalp superiorly to raise the eyebrows. The frontalis muscle is by far the major elevator of the brow, although the corrugator muscles have a very small role in elevation of the medial portion of the brow upon contraction. The antagonistic depressor muscles include the strong orbital portion of the orbicularis oculi muscle, the central procerus, the paired corrugators, and depressor supercilii. An excellent anatomic study of the function of these muscles can be found in the work of G.B. Duchenne from 1862.[8]

The static forehead anatomy includes the skin, subcutaneous tissue and adnexa, and the underlying layers of fascia that overlie, underlie, or envelop the facial musculature. Also included in the static anatomy are the sensory and motor nerves as well as the accompanying arterial and venous supply to these muscles and the overlying soft tissue. An excellent description and demonstration of these structures as well as their pertinence and relationships in terms of surgical procedures may be found in the work of Larrabee and Makielski.[9] One of the debatable aspects of the endoscopic approach is the plane of dissection used. As we know, the classic bicoronal forehead lift is performed in the subgaleal, supraperiosteal plane. Thus, when we first began working with the endoscopes in the forehead, this was the approach we used. The theoretical advantages are: (1) these are quick, safe planes that are traditionally used in open procedures, (2) dissection is relatively avascular, and (3) direct access to muscles of the brow and forehead is obtained.

As the evolution of our technique has progressed, we have moved to the subperiosteal plane of dissection for various reasons. These reasons include the fact that the subperiosteal plane is a quicker, easier, and safer plane than others and that minimal bleeding is seen while working in this plane. When viewing through the scope, the bone of the frontal skull and the undersurface of the periosteum are gleaming white and virtually bloodless, which allows for excellent visualization. With this approach, the forehead and midface dissection can be carried out in the same plane, thus overcoming the so-called zygomatic arch barrier.

The surgeon can achieve in continuity vertical lifting and suspension of the soft tissues of the upper as well as midface with the subperiosteal approach. The flaps theoretically have better vascularity, and fibrosis and scarring is not created in the plane over which the frontalis muscle glides. The rigid inflexible periosteum does not stretch, so that the brow ptosis correction achieved is better maintained over time. Finally, this approach more safely allows additional superficial procedures such as liposuction or skin resurfacing.

SURGICAL TECHNIQUE

Instrumentation used for the endoscopic approach to the forehead and brows includes 4- or 5-mm, 0- and 30-degree endoscopes with attached camera and video monitor. These scopes and equipment are probably already available and in use by many otolaryngologists and facial plastic surgeons either in their offices or surgical facilities. Along with the scopes and video equipment, specially designed endoscopic instruments, some of which are still in their evolutionary stages, are also used.

The evolution of our present technique, the first method that we employed was simply wide undermining from the superior orbital rims posteriorly to several centimeters beyond the coronal suture line, combined with an external compression dressing (Figure 6.1). Severance or release of the corrugator and procerus muscles was included in this approach. This remains an important part of our technique today; however, we found that this method lacked control and predictability for elevating the brows. If glabellar furrows caused by hyperactive corrugators and procerus muscles are the sole problem in a particular patient, then this approach, along with correction of the hyperdynamic musculature, is still the method of choice.

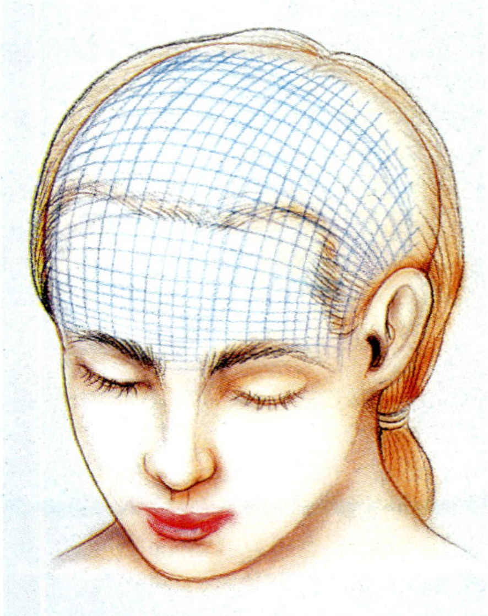

FIG. 6.1. Original technique involving wide undermining as illustrated, combined with an external compression dressing.

The next technique we used was an attempt to suspend the skin to the superficial layer of the deep temporal fascia with a large transcutaneous suture. This was tied in the hair-bearing skin and remained in place for approximately 2 weeks (Figure 6.2). This method also appeared to lack control and elicited patient complaints of moderate-to-severe pain. An offshoot of this attempt at fixation was our present method of augmenting lateral brow fixation and reducing lateral periorbital wrinkling by dissection and suspension of the lateral orbital/temporal region. This is done via a small incision in the temporal hairline and dissection in the plane between the temporoparietal fascia and the superficial layer of the deep temporal (intermediate) fascia (Figure 6.3).

Our next attempt at soft-tissue suspension was a more direct approach with two different modifications. First, we placed a suture directly through the galea to the orbicularis oculi muscle at the desired peak in the arch of the brow; second, we secured this permanent suture to the skull using a small bone anchor

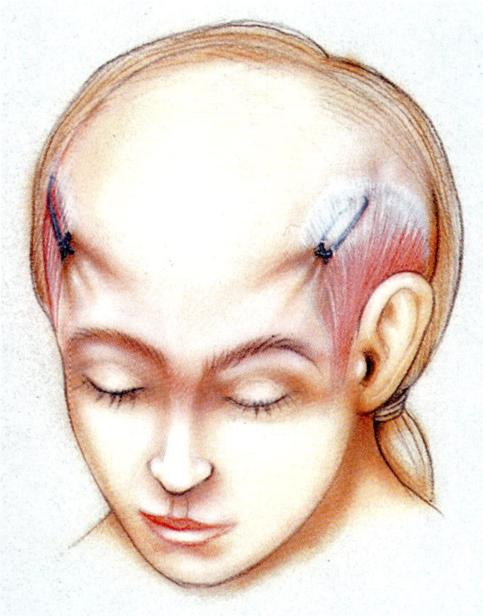

FIG. 6.2. Early technique involving bilateral transcutaneous sutures suspending the overlying skin to the underlying temporal fascia.

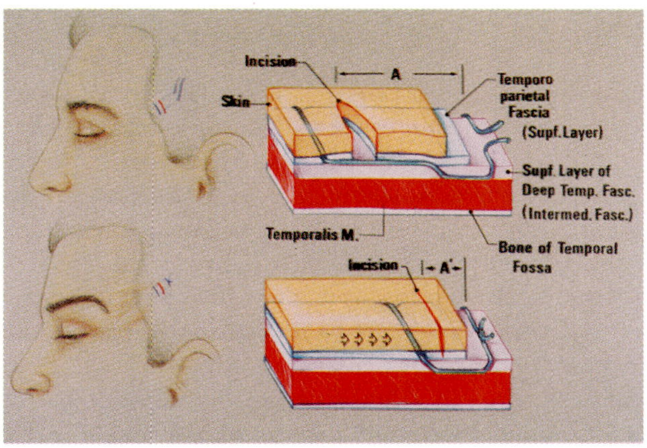

FIG. 6.3. Lateral brow suspension as part of our present technique.

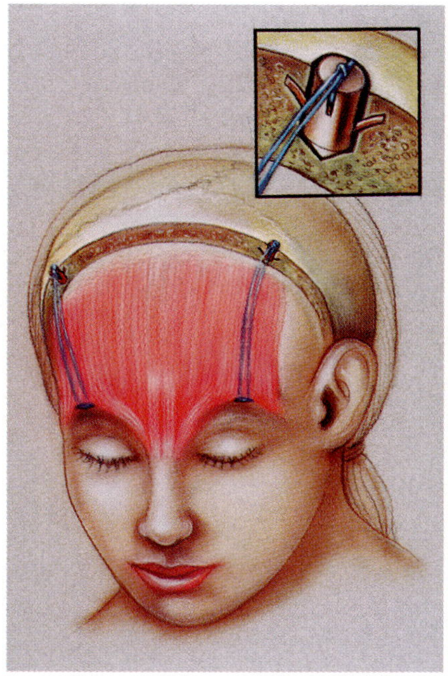

FIG. 6.4. Early technique involving attempted direct suspension of the orbicularis oculi muscle via permanent suture to a small bone anchor.

(Figure 6.4). Problems we encountered using this technique included dimpling of the skin at the point of insertion in the orbicularis muscle and the inability to rethread a suture through the bone anchor should the suture break during tying. At this point, after returning to the laboratory for further anatomic studies and dissections, we determined that the best way to predictably support the brow and forehead would be to suspend it superiorly by the entire frontal occipital aponeurosis (galea aponeurotica). Because the skin of the forehead and scalp, due to the increased number of adnexal structures, is firmly attached through a dense connective tissue layer to this aponeurosis, we believed that suspension of this structure superiorly would afford us more control and predictability of results. By including the periosteum in the suspension we have an added layer that is strong, that does not stretch, and that readily readheres to the underlying frontal bone. Thus, we began using our present technique of periosteum, galea, and frontalis suspension to cranial bone via permanent sutures and a titanium microplate as described next.

During the time period in which we were developing our suspension technique, methods of fixation were taking other paths in the hands of other practitioners. Initially, internal methods of suspension and fixation were not considered, and an external dressing was all that was used. As was the case with our experience, however, it became apparent that external compression for a few days was inadequate to properly maintain brow elevation. Thus, various techniques were developed to aid in this task. These included plication of the scalp to itself in the hair-bearing region as a "scalp crown" (Aiache);[10] inverted T-V skin advancement along with placement of various layers of paper and foam tape (Bostwick);[11] and finally, deep sutures from the galeal-periosteal layer to microscrews along with external tied-over dressings (Daniel & Ramirez)[12] (Figures 6.5, 6.6, and 6.7, *A*, *B*). Another nonfixation technique relies on simply releasing the brow depressors (procerus, corrugators, and depressor supercilii), leaving the only brow elevator (frontalis) unopposed (Isse).[13] Some of these techniques have been discarded, and some remain in use either in their original or slightly modified form.

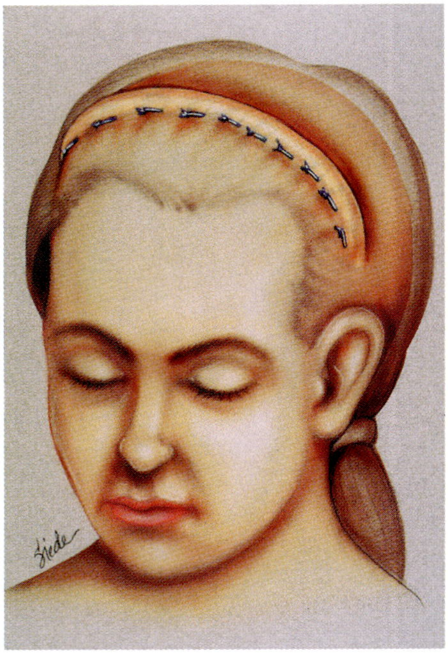

FIG. 6.5. Additional suspension technique involving scalp plication.

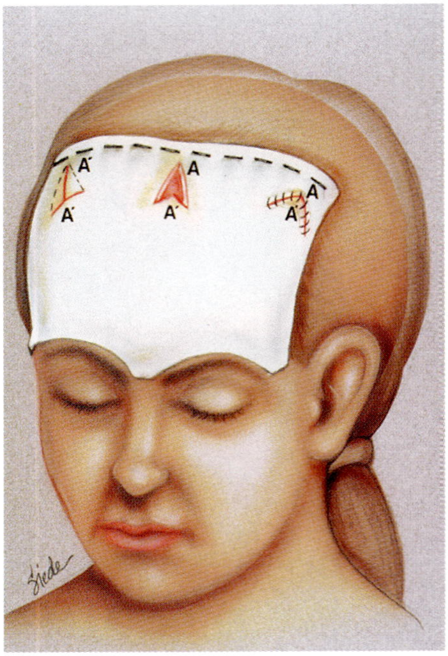

FIG. 6.6. Suspension technique involving T-V skin advancement along with tape suspension.

In our present technique, the patient is first seen in the holding area, and the necessary vectors of pull are marked with the patient in the upright sitting position (Figure 6.8). The patient is then moved to the operative suite, where neuroleptanesthesia is initiated. Infiltrative local anesthesia and nerve blocks are administered.[14] After intravenous (IV) sedation has been achieved and the area has been localized, we create our portals approximately 1 to 1.5 cm posterior to the anterior hairline, in the midline, and in the paramedian areas, with the incisions oriented vertically, corresponding to the desired vectors of pull (Figure 6.9). These minimal incisions can be compared with the extensive bicoronal excision of the traditional open technique (Figure 6.10). The optic cavity is then created in the subperiosteal plane using the larger endoscopic elevators in a blind, yet controlled, dissection. An important surgical point here is that when the elevation is begun at the incision sites, one should use a small, sharp dissector such as a Cottle elevator or the small endoscopic elevator, taking care to ensure that the continuity and integrity of the periosteum beyond the small incision is maintained, because this will be vitally important when the time comes to place the suspension sutures.

The central optic cavity is created blindly down to 1.5 to 2 cm above the orbital rims inferiorly, to the temporal lines laterally, and several centimeters beyond the coronal suture line posteriorly (Figure 6.11). After this is completed, the 30-degree endoscope is introduced, and the dissection proceeds inferiorly under direct vision. Note the almost bloodless plane of dissection, with excellent contrast between the underlying bone and overlying periosteum (Figure 6.12). The periosteum is elevated first in the interbrow area down to the root of the nose. Dissection is then carried laterally, using the fine endoscopic elevator down along the orbital rim, taking care to identify and preserve the supraorbital neurovascular bundles, which will typically exit through palpable notches approximately 2 to 2.5 cm lateral to the midline bilaterally (Figure 6.13, *A*). In 10% of patients, however, the supraorbital neurovascular bundles will exit the frontal bone from true foramina. These can be located up to 2 cm superior to the supraorbital rims, thus the reason for ceasing the blind dissection of the central pocket 2 cm above the orbital rims and introducing the endoscope for direct visualization (Figure 6.13, *B*). At this point, the elevation is carried over the orbital rim, releasing the periosteum at the level of the arcus marginalis (Figure 6.14). As this occurs, the periosteum appears to gently separate, and the overlying brow fat pad or retro-orbicularis oculus fat (ROOF) becomes easily visible (Figure 6.15). We have not found the need to make a distinct incision in the periosteum at this level because it separated easily and precisely using the small, sharp, slightly arched endoscopic periosteal elevator designed for this purpose. As the periosteum is separated medial to the supraorbital neurovascular bundles, the obliquely oriented fibers of the corrugator muscle become distinctly

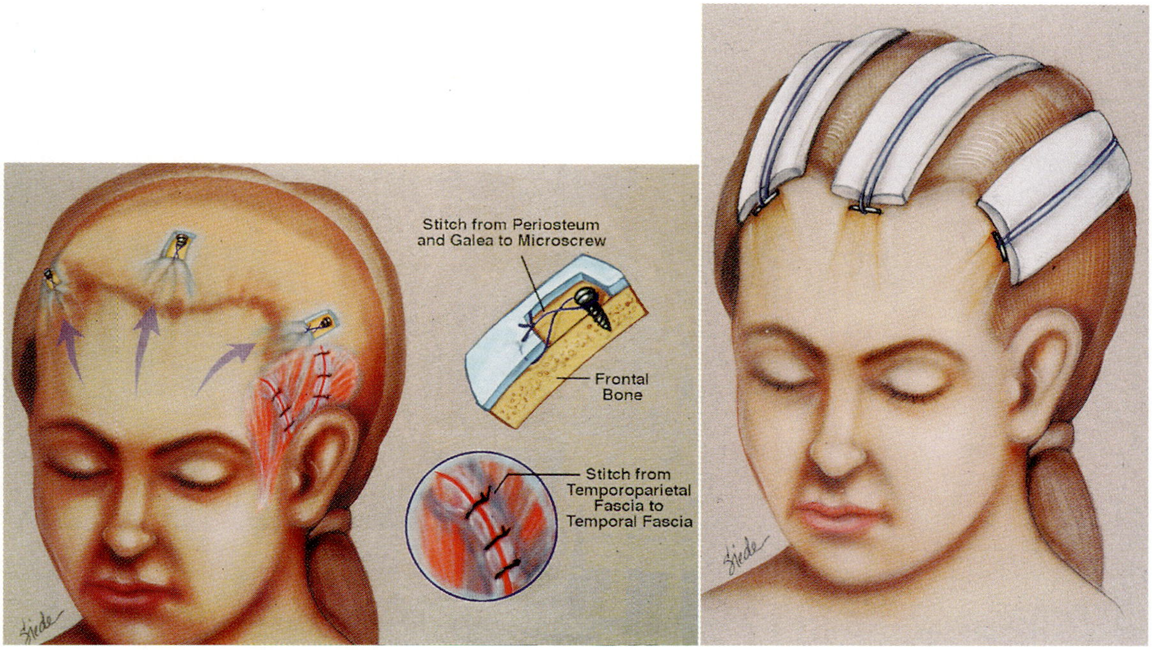

FIG. 6.7. **A** and **B,** Suspension technique involving suspension sutures to microscrews along with external tied-over dressings.

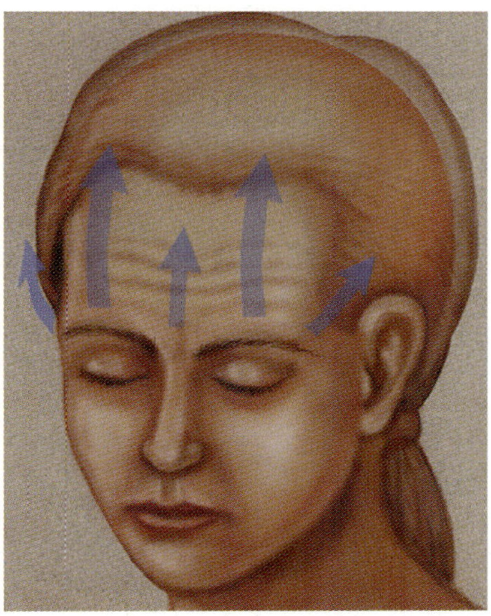

FIG. 6.8. Desired vectors of pull are marked with the patient in the upright position before the procedure is begun.

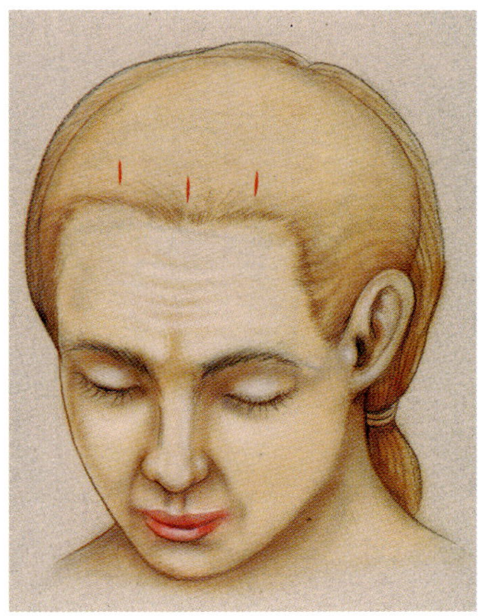

FIG. 6.9. Central and paramedian incisions are made 1 to 1.5 cm posterior to the anterior hairline, which correspond to the desired suspension vectors.

apparent (Figures 6.16 and 6.17). As the separation progresses into the interbrow area, the periosteum becomes much more dense and may require a direct incision or a muscle punch, which we have most recently been using, to incise and remove a portion of the periosteum and the procerus muscle. Once the periosteum is released at the arcus marginalis bilaterally, attention is turned to the corrugator musculature and any remaining intact procerus fibers.

The fibers of the corrugator muscles are isolated using an endoscopic right-angled blunt hook, and are then divided using either an endoscopic hook knife, muscle punch forceps, or biting forceps (Figures 6.18, 6.19, and 6.20). Care is taken to identify and preserve the supratrochlear nerve fascicles that will typically enter the forehead through the fibers of the corrugator muscle. Thus, the muscle fibers must be isolated in sections

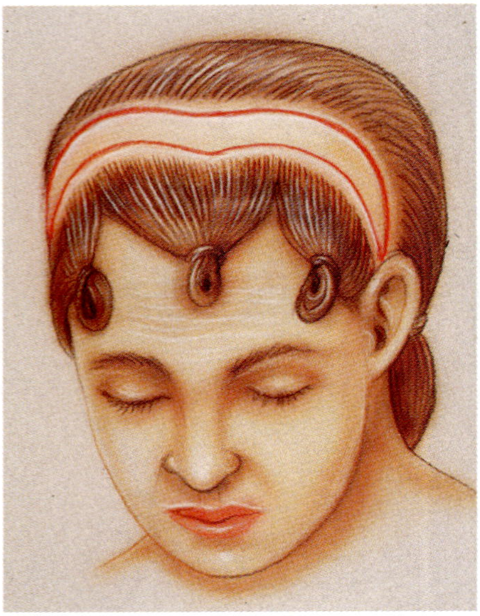

FIG. 6.10. Excision of hair-bearing scalp involved with traditional open coronal technique.

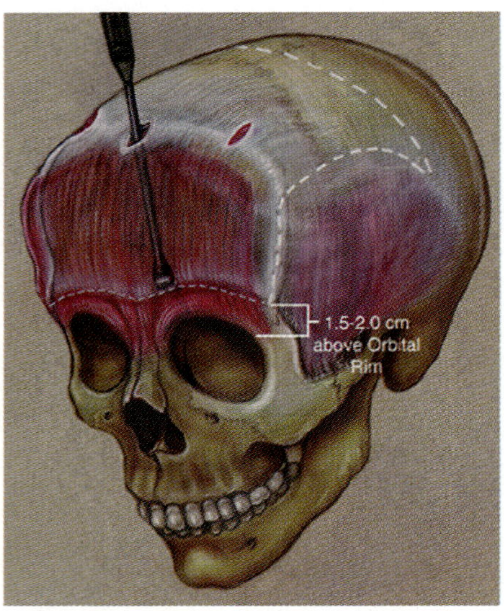

FIG. 6.11. Central optical cavity is bounded by the orbital rims inferiorly and the temporal lines bilaterally.

from around the supratrochlear neurovascular bundle, and then carefully incised. Often, the supratrochlear and occasionally the supraorbital nerves will exit the skull through multiple nerve roots rather than a single branch. In any event, if the supratrochlear nerve is injured, it will result only in a small area of decreased sensation overlying the glabella. Once the muscle fibers of the corrugator have been completely incised, the remaining retracted stump is debulked using Weil-Blakesly forceps. This is done to prevent bunching of the muscle, which can cause an external bulge, or reconnection of the distal ends through fibrosis. The tougher central area of periosteum and procerus muscle is addressed using WeilBlakesly forceps or a muscle punch in order to remove a strip oriented horizontally. This strip of periosteum and muscle is removed down to the subcutaneous fat. This will address any hyperactivity of this muscle and the resultant horizontal creasing in the area of the nasal root.

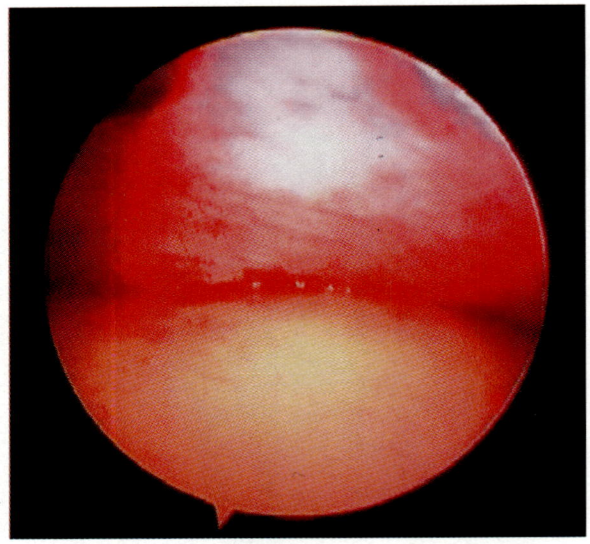

FIG. 6.12. Endoscopic view of the initial dissection oriented with bone inferiorly and periosteum superiorly.

Rarely is any further muscle work needed; however, each patient should be evaluated individually, and occasionally a patient with very deep horizontally oriented central forehead creasing is encountered. In the past in a case such as this, we would divide the periosteum only in a horizontal fashion corresponding to the overlying areas, confining this to a narrow area in the midline between the origins of the two supratrochlear neurovascular bundles. We have since abandoned this maneuver for two reasons. First, if we score and thus weaken the periosteum of the central forehead, we are weakening the very structure that we are relying on for tissue repositioning and predictable fixation. Second, we have found that in patients who first were seen to have some horizontal forehead rhytids but did not have any periosteal incisions to specifically address these, the rhytids resolved or were markedly improved after simply repositioning the brows in a more superior natural anatomic position. This presumably occurs as a result of the gradual relaxation of the frontalis muscle hyperactivity (or even spasticity), because the need for it is no longer present due to the superior repositioning of the brows.

At this point, the central portion of the procedure is completed, and attention is turned to the temporal area in preparation for creation of the temporal pock-

A 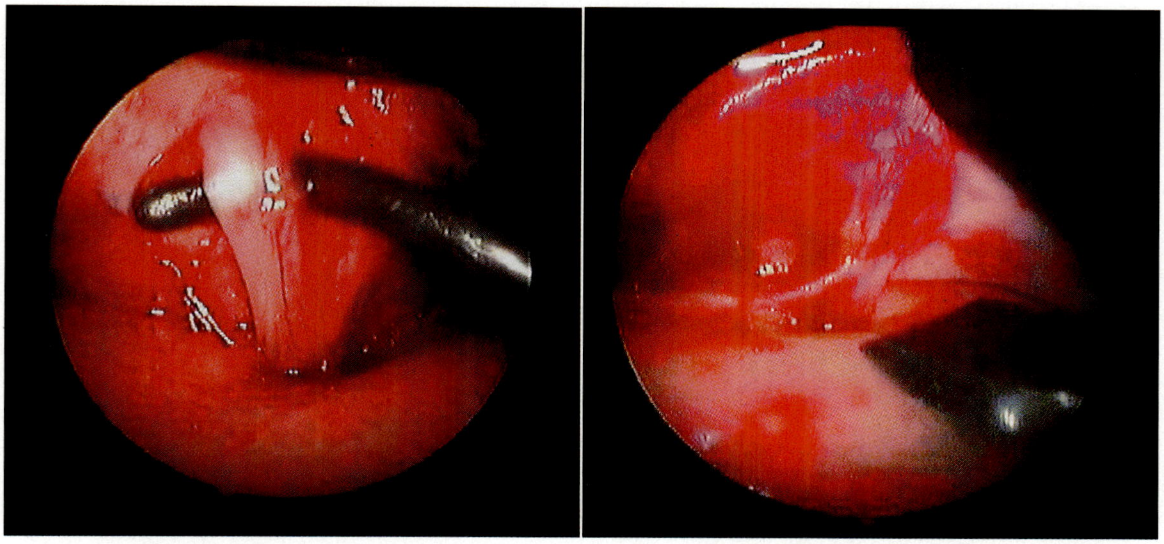 B

FIG. 6.13. **A,** Endoscopic view of the supraorbital neurovascular bundle exiting the supraorbital notch. **B,** Endoscopic view of the supraorbital bundle exiting through a true foramen.

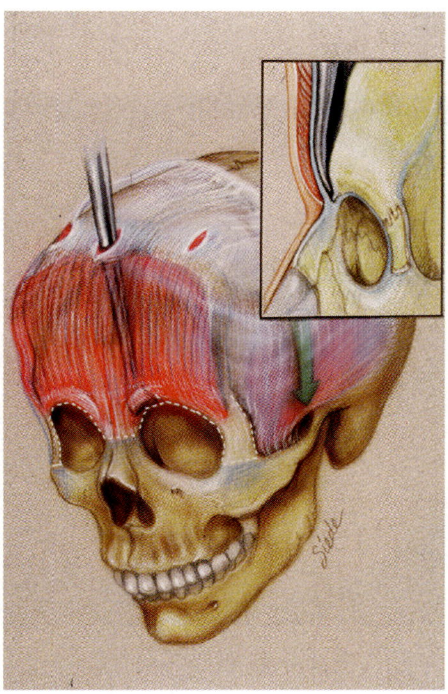

FIG. 6.14. Illustration of the position of periosteal release at the arcus marginalis.

ets bilaterally. The temporal pocket is located over the temporalis muscle and is bounded by the temporal line superiorly, the cephalic edge of the zygomatic arch inferiorly, and the orbital rim anteriorly (Figure 6.21). It is important to understand the anatomy of this region because the frontal branch of the facial nerve spans this area, and care must be taken to preserve this

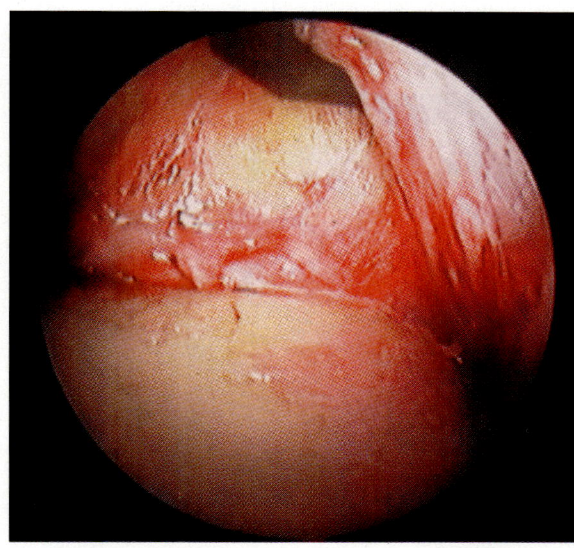

FIG. 6.15. As the periosteum is released, the yellow retro-orbicularis oculus fat (ROOF) becomes apparent.

structure. The anatomy of the area from superficial to deep may be seen in Figure 6.22. Access to the temporal pocket is obtained through a 1- to 1.5-cm incision within the hairline above the ear usually just posterior to the temporal tuft of hair and on an approximate line from the lateral nasal alar margin through the lateral canthus (Figure 6.23).

This incision is carried down through the skin and subcutaneous tissue and through the temporoparietal (superficial) fascia. The proper plane is easily identified as the edges of the incision are slid inferiorly and superiorly while viewing the depth of the incision. If there is

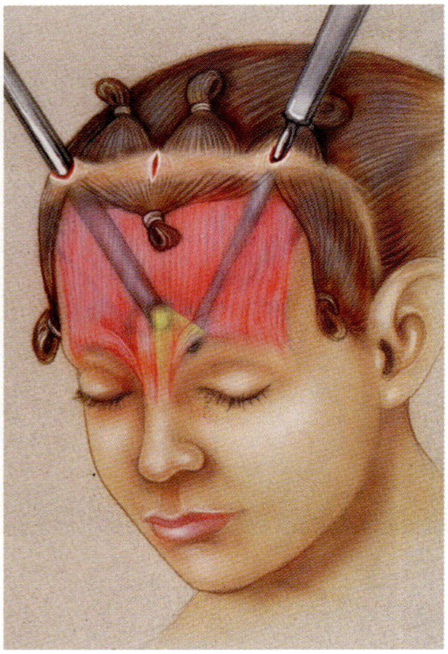

FIG 6.16. Illustration of the endoscopic location and examination of the corrugator musculature.

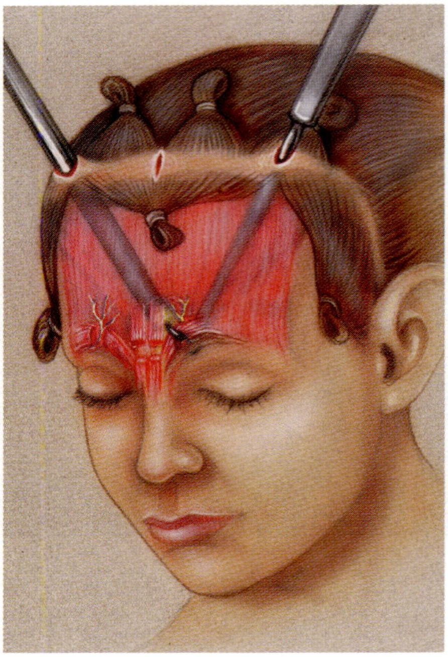

FIG. 6.18. Illustration of the release of the corrugator and procerus muscles.

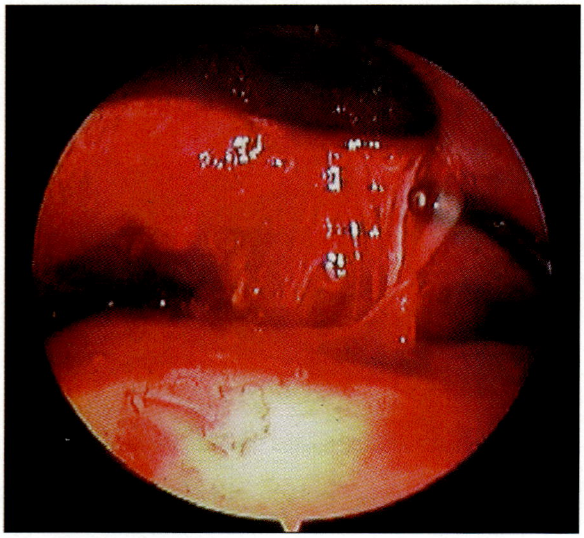

FIG. 6.17. Corrugator musculature located just medial to the supraorbital nerve, which is being retracted laterally.

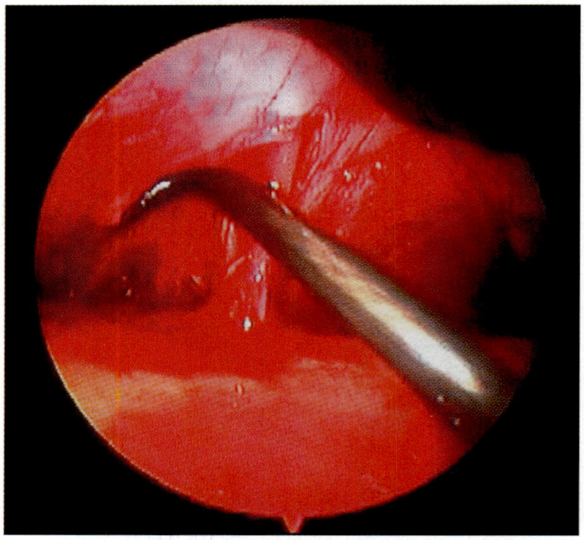

FIG. 6.19. Several instruments may be used to identify, isolate, and release the corrugator muscles, including blunt right angle (shown), endoscopic knives, forceps, or laser.

a layer of tissue not incised that still glides freely over the deeper white fascia, the dissection through the superficial fascia is not yet complete. When the correct depth has been achieved, the gleaming white fascia of the superficial layer of the deep temporal (intermediate) fascia will be clearly seen as a stationary layer directly covering muscle that does not move when sliding the overlying tissues up and down. At this point, we make a small incision through the intermediate fascia, which reveals the red underlying muscle, with the patient in repose so that the spot of incision can be marked before elevation (Figure 6.24). Then, using the flat round-tipped endoscopic elevator and the endoscope, the dissection is carried anteriorly and inferiorly over the lateral temporal/orbital area in the plane between the more superficial temporoparietal fascia and the underlying superficial layer of the deep temporal fascia (Figure 6.25).

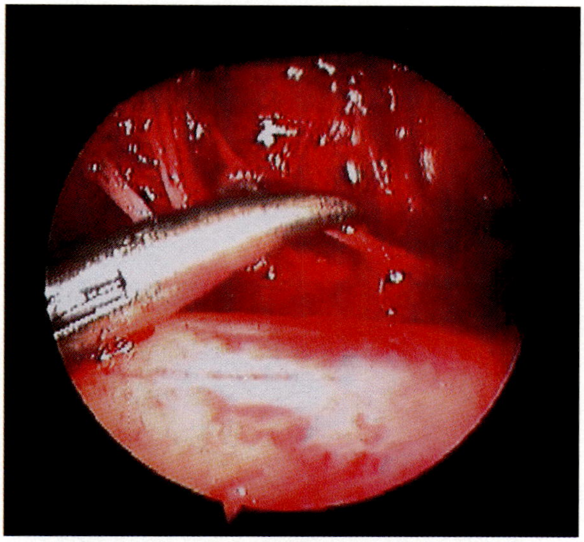

FIG. 6.20. Insulated electrocautery forceps may be used to remove portions of the corrugator and procerus musculature and/or to cauterize any bleeding vessels.

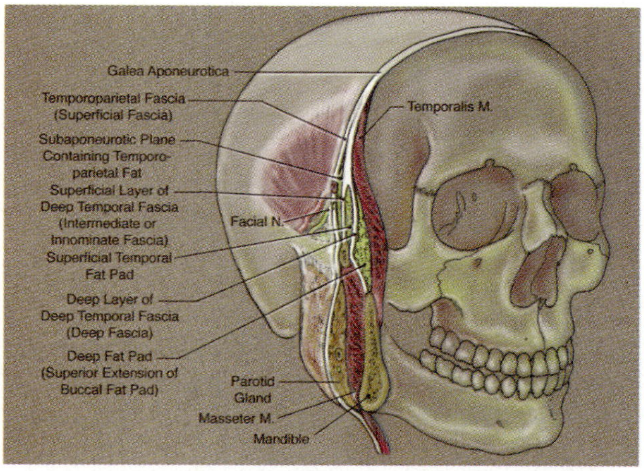

FIG. 6.22. An understanding of the anatomy of the temporal area is critical, because this is the region where the frontal branch of the facial nerve is most at risk.

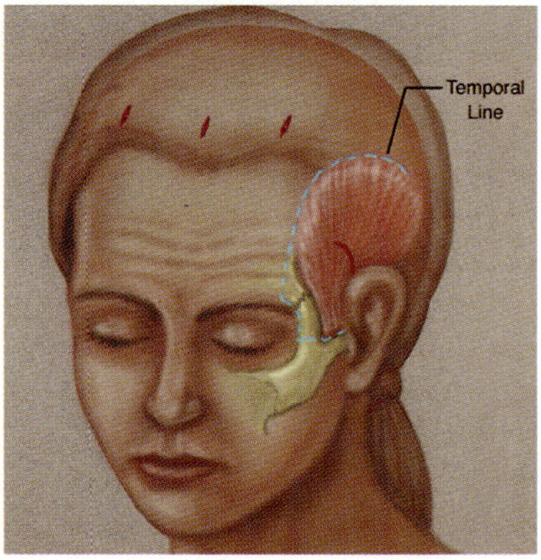

FIG. 6.21. Temporal pocket is bounded by the temporal line superiorly, the cephalic edge of the zygomatic arch inferiorly, and the orbital rim anteriorly.

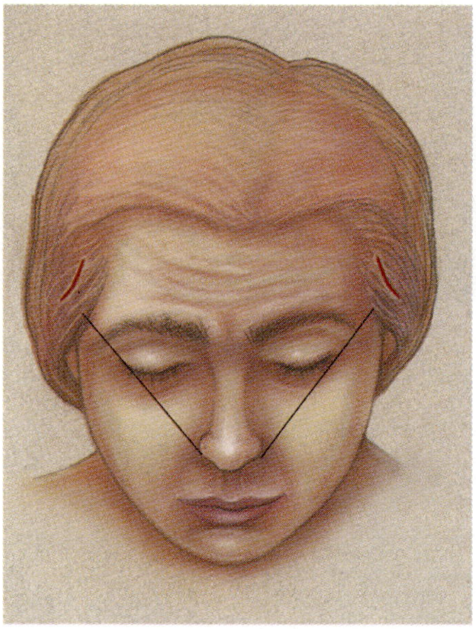

FIG. 6.23. A general rule of thumb for the location of the temporal incision is on a line from the lateral nasal alar margin through the lateral canthus. This gives an approximate location for the lateral brow suspension in women, although adjustments must be made on a case-by-case basis. In men, the incision lies on a more lateral plane.

The temporoparietal fascia corresponds to the superficial musculoaponeurotic system layer in the face and contains the superficial temporal artery and vein as well as the frontal branch of the facial nerve. Thus, inferior elevation should be cautious and delicate, because this motor nerve lies on the undersurface of the fascia above the zygomatic arch. Inferior dissection is continued carefully to the area of the fusion line of the superficial and deep layers of the deep temporal fascia. A landmark that is often encountered is the so-called sentinel vein, which represents the zygomaticotemporal vein and is predictably between 5 to 10 mm lateral and slightly inferior to the frontozygomatic suture line (Figure 6.26). For the standard forehead and brow lift, this marks the most inferior level of dissection. Once the temporal pocket elevation has been completed, it is connected with the central pocket through the temporal line. The temporal line lies on the parietal bone and represents the area of fusion of the galea aponeurotica, temporoparietal fascia, deep temporal fascia, and frontal periosteum (see Figure 6.21). This line of fusion forms a dense, firm area of attachment that must be sharply and carefully divided in order to connect the central and lateral pockets. The release is best performed from lateral to medial under endoscopic control by placing the endoscope through a paramedian incision and angling it toward the temporal pocket. Using the flat, rounded endoscopic dissector, dissection is carried anteriorly over the superficial layer of the deep temporal fascia to the temporal line (Figure 6.27). At the transition from underlying fascia and muscle to parietal bone, the sharp edge of the elevator is used to free the attachments at the temporal line. Through the endoscopic view, the surgeon will see the elevator approaching his scope from lateral to medial (Figure 6.28).

Once a connection has been established, dissection is carried inferiorly along the temporal line using the sharp edge of the elevator, as well as various endo-

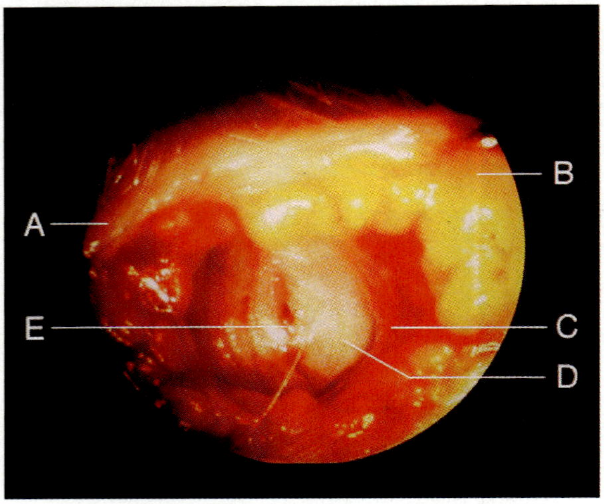

FIG. 6.24. Anatomy in the area of the temporal incision as seen through the endoscope. **A,** Skin. **B,** Subcutaneous fat. **C,** Temporoparietal fascia. **D,** Superficial layer of the deep temporal fascia (temporalis fascia) (intermediate fascia). **E,** Temporal muscle seen through incision in intermediate fascia.

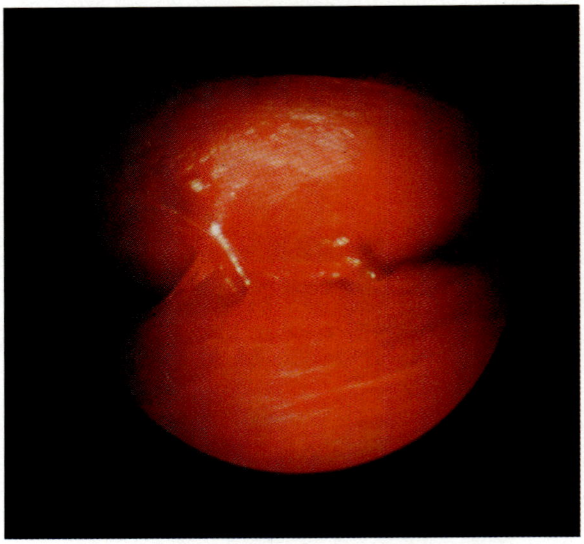

FIG. 6.26. "Sentinel vein," which is the zygomaticotemporal vein, is between 5 to 10 mm lateral and slightly inferior to the frontozygomatic suture line and represents the inferiormost extent of dissection in the standard procedure. In this example, two veins are present.

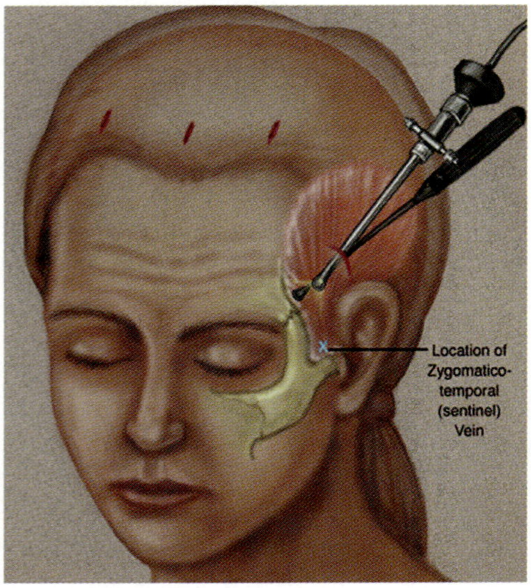

FIG. 6.25. Temporal pocket is dissected in the plane between the temporoparietal fascia superiorly and the underlying temporal fascia covering the temporalis muscle.

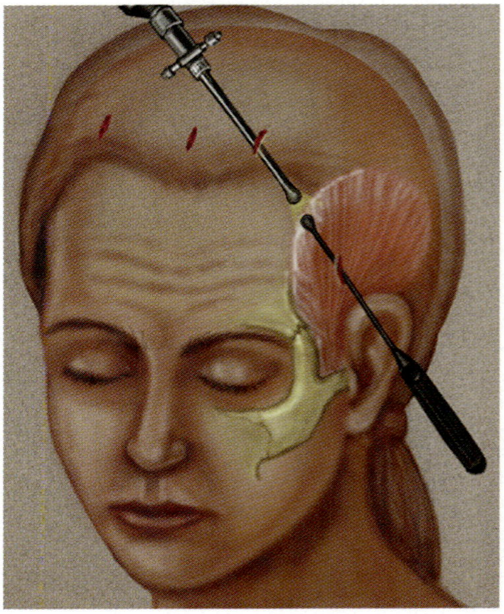

FIG. 6.27. Illustration of the maneuver used to connect the temporal pockets with the central optic cavity.

scopic scissors and blades, taking care to stay directly on the bone of the temporal ridge in the subperiosteal plane. This is carried inferiorly to the area of the lateral orbital rim, where further dense connective tissue attachments to the bone are encountered. These are sharply elevated in the subperiosteal plane using the curved, sharp endoscopic dissectors, scissors, or knife (Figure 6.29). Once this dissection has been completed in its entirety on both sides, palpation and manipulation of the forehead and brow will reveal marked excursion of the entire soft-tissue complex over the underlying bone. A final check for hemostasis using the endoscope in the entire optical cavity is made. If any bleeding vessels are encountered, they are cauterized using the special endoscopic cauterization forceps.

At this point, attention is turned to the fixation portion of the procedure; 2-0 nylon sutures are placed approximately 1 cm anterior to the portals of the central pocket through the periosteum, galea, and frontalis to obtain a good, solid purchase of tissue (Figure 6.30). These sutures may number anywhere from three to six and are placed corresponding to the desired vector of upward pull, which can vary from patient to patient. Typically, three sutures are placed to obtain the needed support. A separate incision is then made approximately 6 to 8 cm posterior to the central portal, where a 5-holed, T-shaped microplate is fixed to the cranium with two 3-mm screws (Figure 6.31). If needed, two separate microplates may be used and placed lateral to the midline, although in the typical case one will suffice. In unilateral or asymmetric ptosis cases a single plate is used in a more lateral position, depending on the vectors of pull required. The nylon suspension sutures are then passed from the anterior portals under the intact but elevated scalp flap and are loosely secured to the horizontal bar of the T plate (Figure 6.32). The patient is then raised on the operating room table to a sitting position, and the brow height is evaluated. Final adjustments are made, if needed, and the sutures are secured (Figure 6.33). After

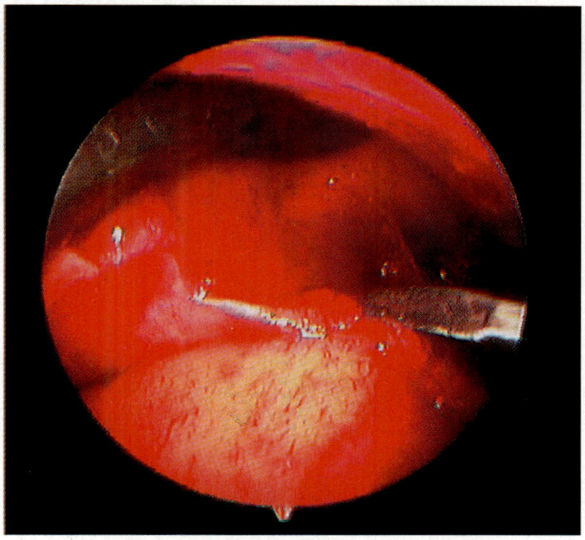

FIG. 6.29. At its inferior end, the temporal line is composed of dense connective tissue attachments to the lateral orbital rim. It is often necessary to elevate these sharply in the subperiosteal plane using endoscopic dissectors or knife (shown).

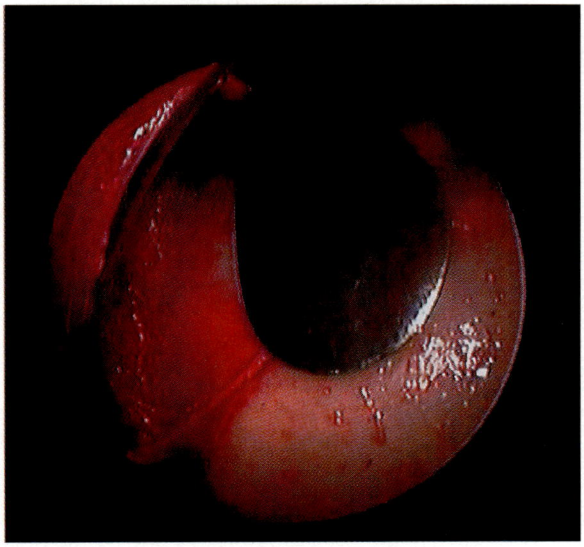

FIG. 6.28. Temporal line is elevated from lateral to medial under direct vision in order to maintain the proper plane of dissection.

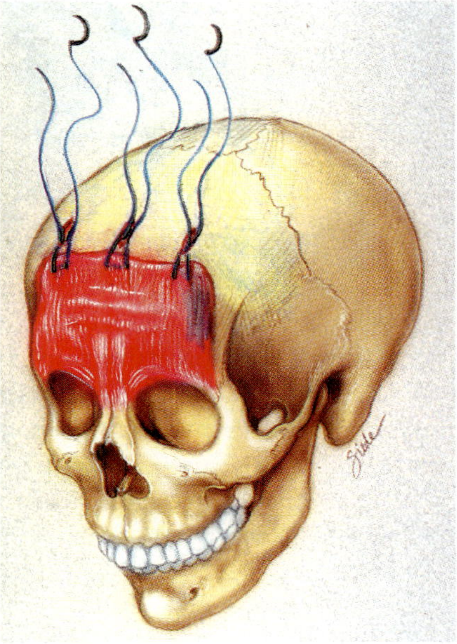

FIG. 6.30. Nylon suspension sutures are placed encompassing the periosteum, galea, and frontalis muscle, obtaining a strong solid purchase of tissue.

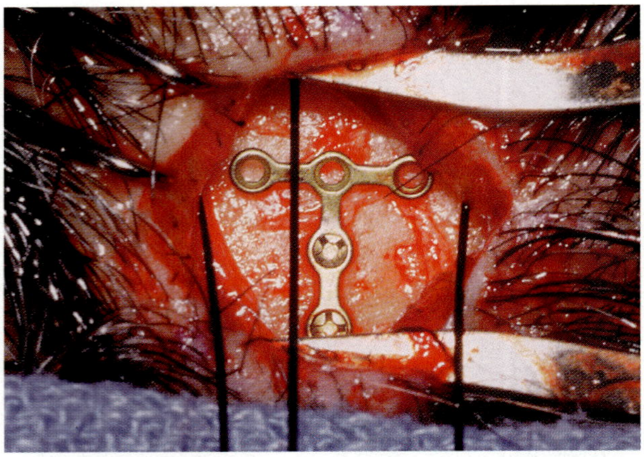

FIG. 6.31. A T-shaped microplate is fixed to the cranium just off the midline approximately 6 to 8 cm posterior to the central portal.

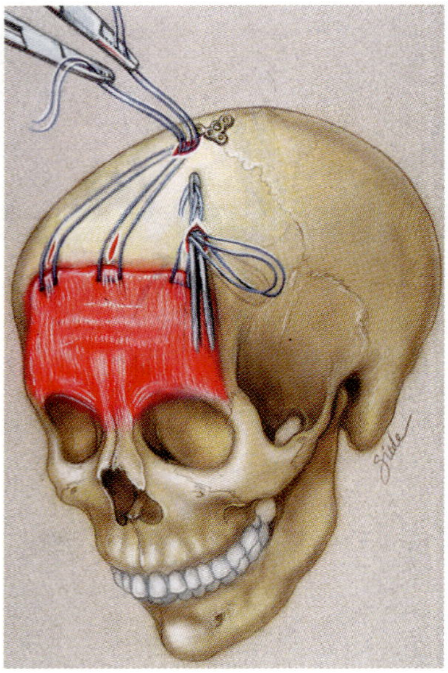

FIG. 6.32. Suspension sutures are passed under the intact, elevated scalp flap and loosely secured to the T plate.

the sutures have been tied and cut, the knots are tucked under the plate so that the relatively stiff 2-0 nylon suture ends will not be pressing outward on the relatively thin scalp. We had one suture extrusion 6 months postoperatively before we incorporated the technique of burying the suture knot under the plate. The same patient complained of palpation of the plate through the scalp, which we removed under local anesthesia 1 year postoperatively. This is the only patient who required either suture or plate removal.

Other complications have included varying degrees of mild, localized numbness and two cases of occasional recurrent tingling pain for up to 6 months postoperatively. Two cases of forehead and scalp itching

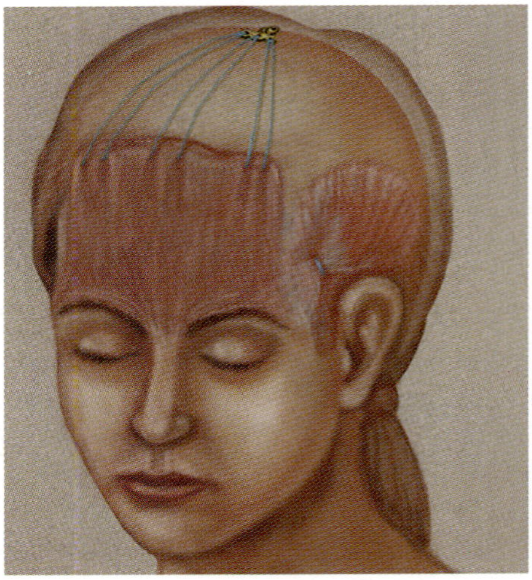

FIG. 6.33. With the patient in the upright position, the brow height is evaluated, and final adjustments are made before the sutures are secured.

were also reported. Two patients experienced a temporary paresis of the frontalis muscle unilaterally, which lasted for 1 week and 1 month, respectively. No patients experienced marked swelling, and most experienced very mild-to-moderate edema of the forehead tissues. One patient did experience some bleeding that manifested not as a hematoma but as bruising through the dependent portion of her face down to her neck area.

Of note is that several patients seemed to experience some slightly prolonged nausea sensations, with occasional vomiting postoperatively. These patients all underwent local anesthesia with IV sedation and thus this may have experienced a galeal stretching reflex phenomenon.

CONCLUSION

Endoscopic brow and forehead lifting with soft-tissue fixation using permanent suture and microplate technique appears to be a safe and predictable means of permanently suspending the upper third of the aging face, in our experience. We have found this procedure well suited to patients with a variety of deformities, including predominant medial brow ptosis with vertical glabellar and horizontal forehead rhytids (Figure 6.34), generalized brow ptosis with asymmetry (Figure 6.35), and predominant lateral brow ptosis with vertical glabellar creases and horizontal forehead rhytids (Figure 6.36). We believe that endoscopic brow lifting represents clear advantages over the open technique in selected patients, which include avoidance of the long transverse incision and its secondary sequelae.

A 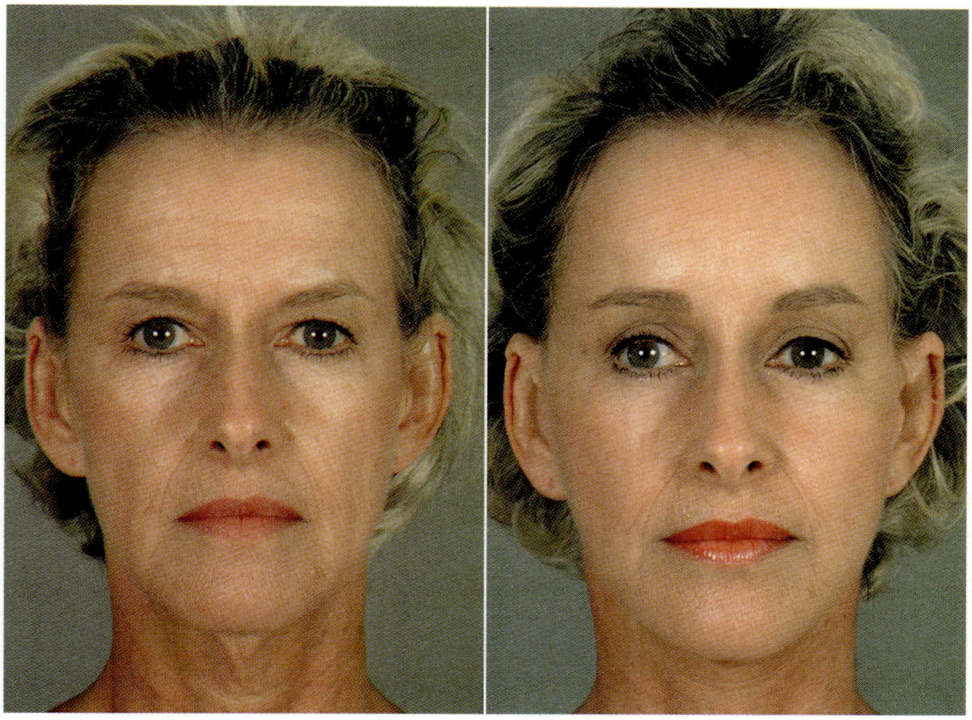 B

FIG. 6.34. **A,** Preoperative view of patient with predominant medial brow ptosis along with vertical glabellar and horizontal forehead rhytids. **B,** One year postoperative view of patient after endoscopic forehead/brow lift, upper blepharoplasty, and rhytidectomy.

A 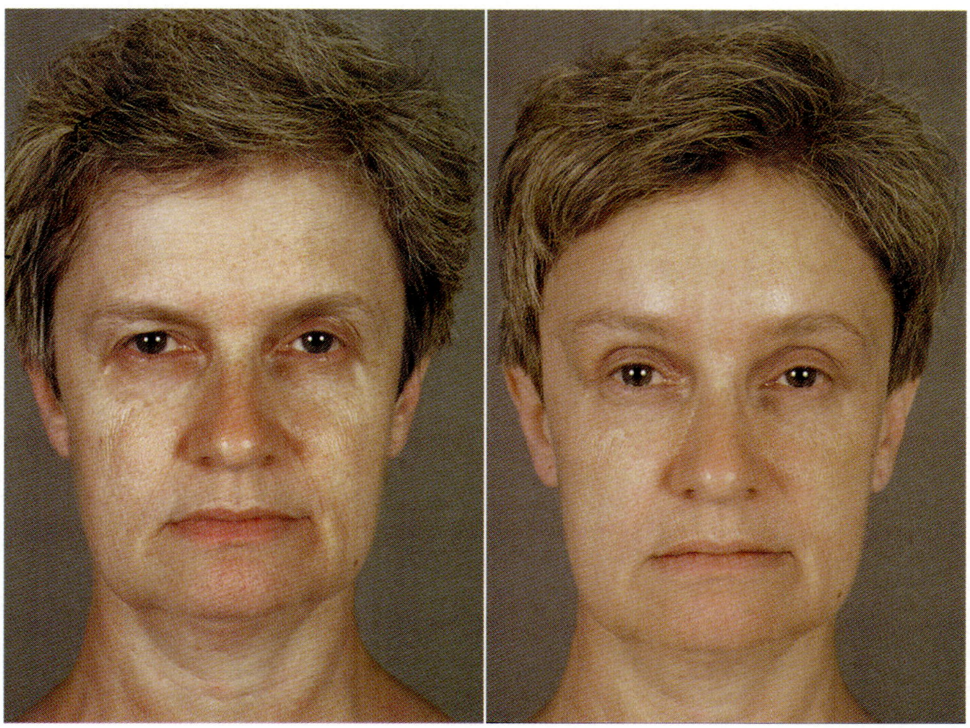 B

FIG. 6.35. **A,** Preoperative view of patient with generalized brow ptosis with asymmetry. **B,** One year postoperative view of patient after endoscopic forehead/brow lift.

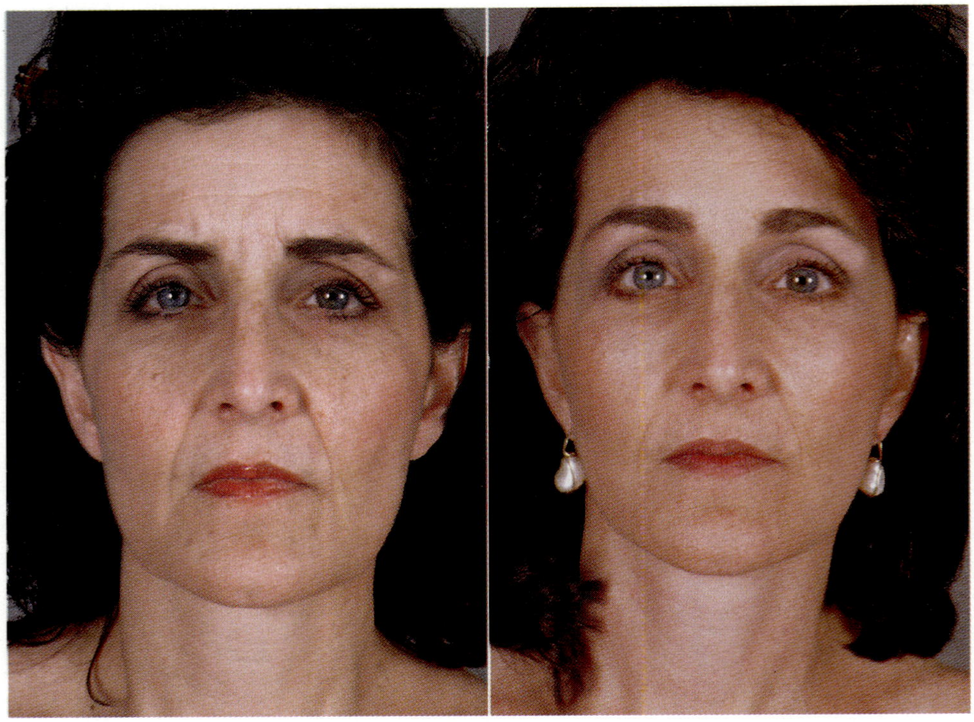

FIG. 6.36. **A,** Preoperative view of patient with predominant lateral brow ptosis with vertical glabellar creases and horizontal forehead rhytids. **B,** One year postoperative view of patient after endoscopic forehead/brow lift, endoscopic midface lift and rhytidectomy.

Additionally, improved magnification and visualization of small structures is a secondary advantage. Long-term follow-up of patients in whom this technique is used will help determine the full range of possible complications as well as the durability and permanency of this suspension technique as compared to others. We believe that this technique will continue to be refined and will achieve a permanent place among the armamentarium of the facial plastic surgeon.

REFERENCES

1. Brennan HG: Correction of the ptotic brow, Otolaryngol Clin North Am 13(2):265-273, 1980.
2. Brennan HG: The forehead lift, Otolaryngol Clin North Am 13(2):209-223, 1980.
3. Tardy ME and Tom LWC: Aesthetic correction of the ptotic brow. In Putterman A, editor: Cosmetic oculoplastic surgery. New York, 1982, Grune and Stratton, pp 147-176.
4. Johnson CM and Waldman SR: Midforehead lift, Arch Otolaryngol 109:155-159, 1983.
5. Becker FF and Johnson CM: Surgical treatment of the upper third of the aging face, Otolaryngol Head Neck Surg 1:475-485, 1986.
6. Cook TA, Brownrigg PJ, Wang TD, Quatela VC: The versatile midforehead browlift, Arch Otolaryngol Head Neck Surg 115:163-168, 1989.
7. Kerth JD and Toriumi DM: Management of the aging forehead, Arch Otolaryngol Head Neck Surg 116:1137-1142, 1990.
8. Duchenne GB, Cuthbertson RA (translator, editor): The mechanism of human facial expression, New York, 1990, Cambridge University Press.
9. Larrabee WF and Makielski KH: Surgical anatomy of the face, New York, 1993, Raven Press.
10. Aiache AE: Endoscopic facelift. Paper presented at Endoscopy in Plastic Surgery: A Consensus Multi-Disciplinary Symposium, Birmingham, Ala, July 20-24, 1994.
11. Bostwick J III, Eaves FF III, Nahai F: Foreheadlift and glabellar frown lines, Endoscopic Plastic Surgery, St. Louis, 1995, Quality Medical Publishing, pp 166-230.
12. Ramirez OM: Endoscopic full facelift. Paper presented at Endoscopy in Plastic Surgery: A Consensus Multi-Disciplinary Symposium, Birmingham, Ala, July 20-24, 1994.
13. Isse NG: Endoscopic facial rejuvenation. Endoforehead: The functional lift case report, Aesthetic Plast Surg 18:21-29, 1994. Also presented at Endoscopy in Plastic Surgery: A Consensus Multi-Disciplinary Symposium, Birmingham, Ala, July 20-24, 1994.
14. Graham HD: Anesthesia in facial plastic surgery. In Waldman SR and Willet JM, editors, Practical aspects of facial plastic surgery, Norwalk, Conn, Appleton & Lang (in press).

chapter seven

Subperiosteal Forehead Lift: Modification of the Endoscopic Technique Using a Transpalpebral Approach

Ronald W. Strahan and David H. Perrott

Characteristic findings of the aging upper face include brow ptosis, forehead rhytids, and glabellar skin creases. Treatment of these findings has included an open forehead lift with excision of the corrugator supercilii and procerus muscles.[1-8] Although this treatment has been successful, complications have included large scars, loss of hair, alterations in sensation, facial nerve injury, and elevation of the frontal hairlines.

Introduction of the endoscopic subperiosteal foreheadplasty (ESFP) has reduced or eliminated many of these potential complications.[9-11] The early results of this technique are favorable, but there are some disadvantages of ESFP. The surgeon must have access to expensive endoscopic equipment and obtain specialized training. Long-term failure of ESFP can occur if there is inadequate transection of the periosteum at the level of the brows and inadequate excision of the corrugator, deep supercilii, and procerus muscles. In addition, the standard ESFP with five incisions in the anterior hair-bearing scalp could not be used in some individuals (e.g., patients with baldness or thin hair).

The purpose of this chapter is to describe a foreheadplasty with brow lift that has four features. First, there should be a complete division of the glabellar structures of the procerus, deep supercilii, and corrugator muscles with direct vision via an approach through the upper eyelid incision. Second, subperiosteal division should be made at the bony brow and subperiosteal elevation should be made over the frontal bone via the same approach. Third, division of the conjoint tendon and anterior dissection of the temple area over the temporalis fascia should be made via the same incision. Last, subperiosteal dissection of the occipital area and over the temporalis fascia dissection of the temporal areas should be made via two small incisions in the crown hair. This procedure can be accomplished without endoscopic equipment, and exposure is provided with lighted retractors.

TECHNIQUE

Preoperatively, the supraorbital foramen and the two paramedian crown hair incisions are marked. In addition, the lower horizontal line of the upper blepharoplasty incision site is marked. The midline scalp incision and temporal incisions used in the standard ESFP technique are not needed. The brow areas and incision sites are injected with 1% lidocaine with epinephrine (1:100,000), and the remaining scalp and forehead areas are injected with 0.25% lidocaine with epinephrine (1:400,000).

Blepharoplasty Incision

The lower horizontal limb of the upper blepharoplasty incision is made through the skin and the fibers of the obicularis oculi muscle. A skin-muscle flap is developed that exposes the septum orbitale (Figure 7.1). A small curved rake retractor (Van Sickle Instrument Co, Bedford, Tex) is used to facilitate elevation of the orbicularis oculi muscle of the septum orbitale superiorly to the supraorbital rim. Maintaining the integrity of the septum orbitale is important. If removal of excessive fat (medial and lateral fat pads) is necessary, it is postponed until the end of the procedure and is conservatively completed through small holes. An incision is made through the lateral supraorbital periosteum at the frontozygomatic suture and extended slightly above the orbital rim to a point approximately 5 mm lateral to the supraorbital foramen. Using a periosteal elevator, the periosteum is elevated off of the lateral and inferior aspect of the frontal bone (Figure 7.2). A vertical releasing incision is made in the periosteum at the frontozygomatic suture.

Attention is then directed to dissection of the medial supraorbital rim. Medially, the first structure identified is the large corrugator muscle (Figure 7.3). The muscle has a bluish hue and is darker than other surrounding tissues. Once identified, the corrugator muscle is transected at the level where it passes between the frontalis and orbicularis oculi muscles. Elevation of this portion of the muscle permits direct

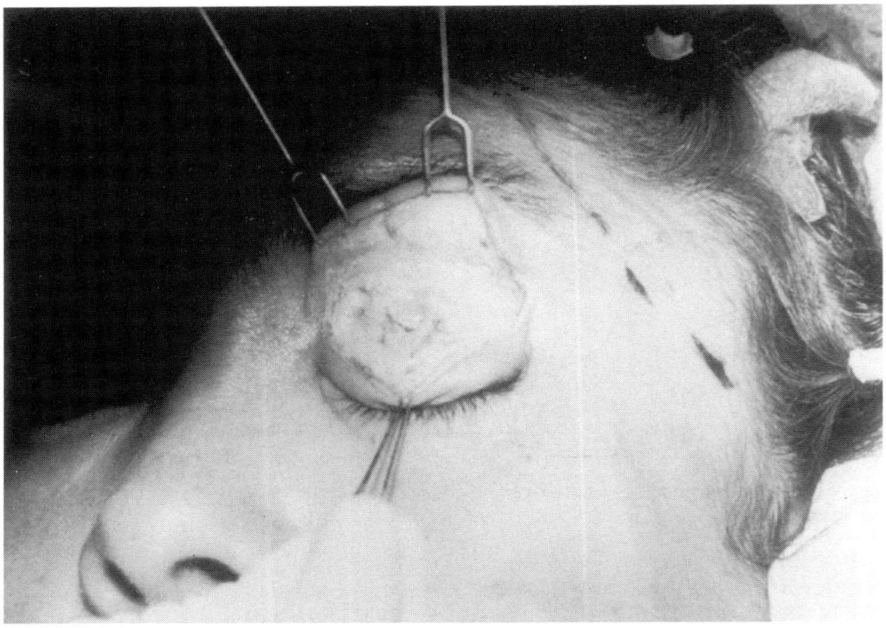

FIG. 7.1. Elevation of the skin-muscle flap through an upper blepharoplasty incision.

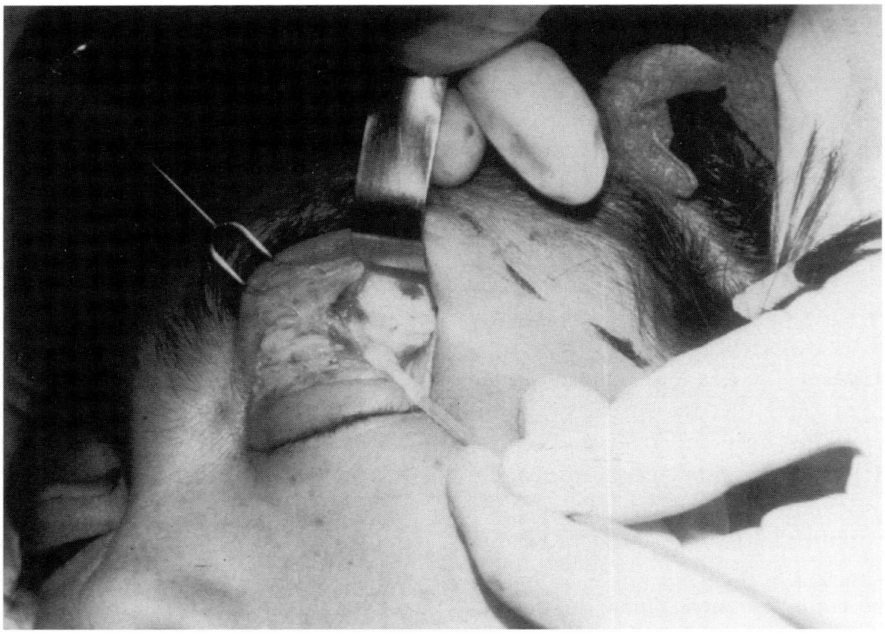

FIG. 7.2. Dissection of the lateral supraorbital periosteum approximately 5 mm lateral to the supraorbital foramen.

palpation of the supraorbital foramen. The foramen location is also identified by the presence of the dark, engorged supraorbital vein. Visualization of the remaining neurovascular bundle can be seen with magnification. Dissection is then completed medial to the neurovascular bundle until the remaining fibers of the corrugator and lighter colored depressor supercilii muscle are incised. Medially, the supratrochlear nerve can be identified and preserved. Following identification of these vital structures, the remaining medial orbital periosteum is carefully incised, and superior elevation of the periosteum is completed, with preservation of the supraorbital neurovascular bundle and the supratrochlear nerves (Figure 7.4). The same dissection is completed on the contralateral side.

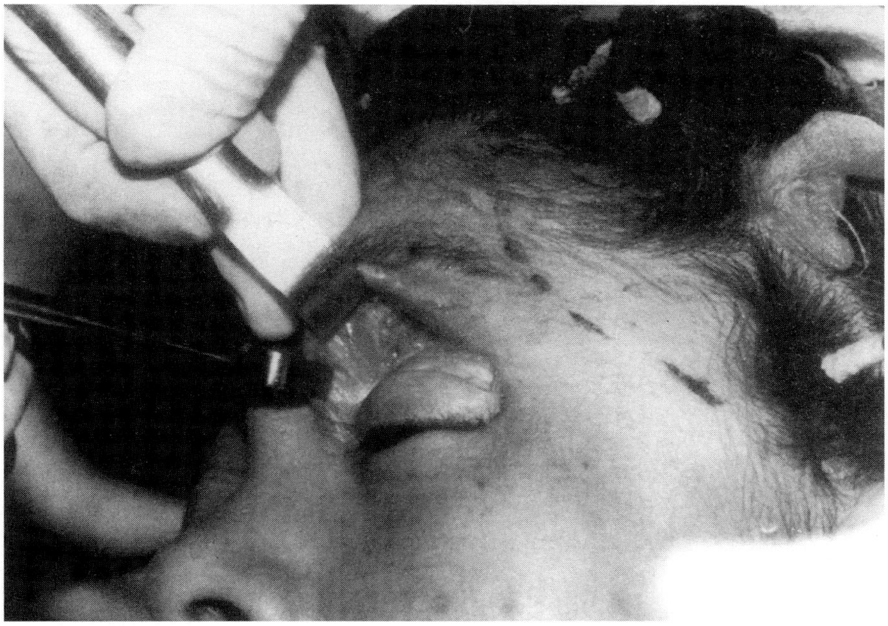

FIG. 7.3. Identification of the corrugator muscle.

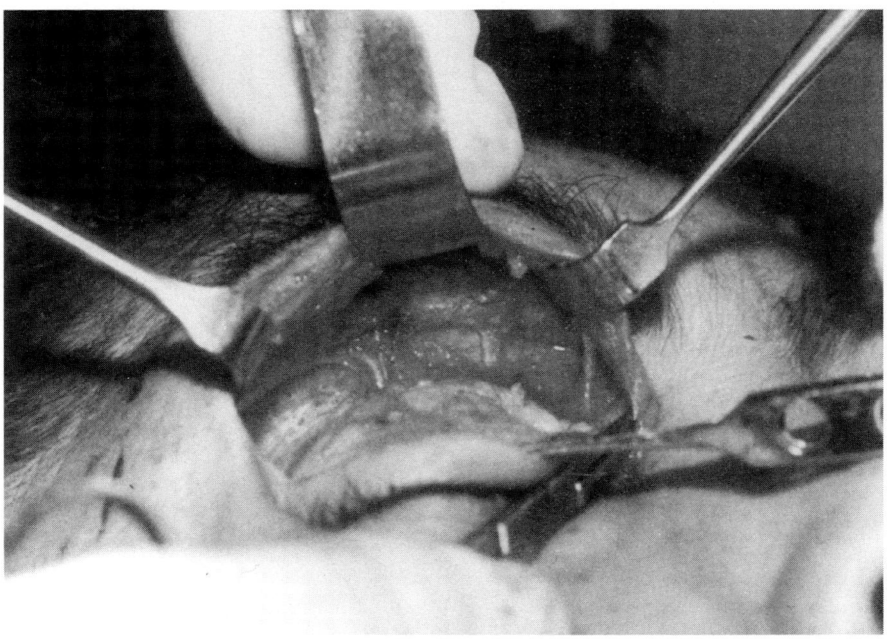

FIG. 7.4. Supraorbital dissection completed with preservation of supraorbital and trochlear nerves.

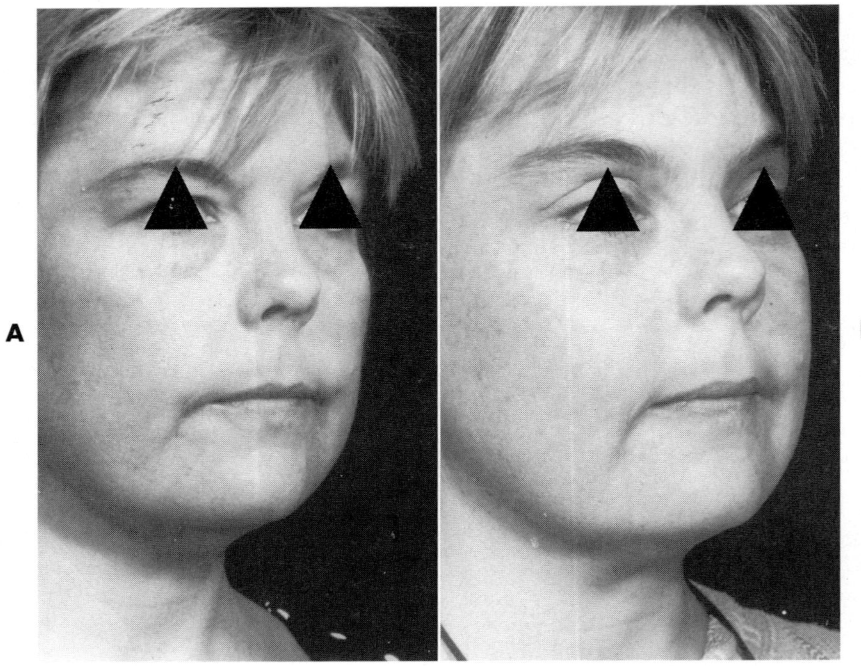

FIG. 7.5. Preoperative (**A**) and 6-month postoperative (**B**) lateral photographs.

Following bilateral supraorbital dissection, only the midline skin and underlying procerus muscle remain attached. To assist in dissection of this area, a small lighted retractor (ESI Co, Rochester, N.Y.) is placed in the medial aspect of the blepharoplasty incision. This allows direct vision of the procerus muscle, which is divided with a laser or electrocautery. Electrocautery is recommended, because the procerus muscle contains several large veins. Dissection from the contralateral side is completed in a similar fashion until all fibers of the procerus muscle have been divided. At this point, the midline periosteum at the nose-forehead junction can be elevated in a superior direction. Following completion of this step, the entire frontal bone periosteum can be elevated through the blepharoplasty incision sites. Through the lateral portion of this upper eyelid incision, the frontozygomatic bony suture line is reidentified. Posterior and superior dissection from here allows division of the conjoint tendon and dissection over the anterior half of the temporalis fascia. This dissection is completed on the contralateral side.

Scalp Elevation and Fixation

The remainder of the dissection is completed through two small incisions that are just medial to the superior most attachment of the temporalis fascia and transect a line that runs from ear to ear. These landmarks keep the small incisions within the crown hair. The subperiosteal dissection adjacent to the incision is done with a straight dissector, such as a Henahan dissector (Walter Lorenz Surgical, Inc, Jacksonville, Fla). The subperiosteal dissection over the remainder of the occiput is done with a curved dissector, such as the Branson Scalp Dissector (Tulip Co, San Diego, Calif). This dissection extends posterior to meet the supreme nuchal line. This same curved dissector is used laterally to complete the dissection over the posterior half of the temporalis fascia.

These maneuvers totally free the scalp from the supreme nuchal line to the supraorbital rim and from ear to ear. Simultaneous observation of the level of the brow and skin hook retraction of the scalp incision permit determination of the fixation point. A cortical bone tarmel is completed at the desired location and fixation is completed by passing a permanent suture through the galea, periosteum, and cortical bone tunnel. Layered closure of these scalp incisions completes this phase of the operation.

Attention is returned to the eyelid incision. If removal of upper lid fat is indicated, it is done through very small perforations of the septum orbitale. If indicated, removal of excessive upper lid skin and orbicularis oculi muscle is conservatively completed.

A

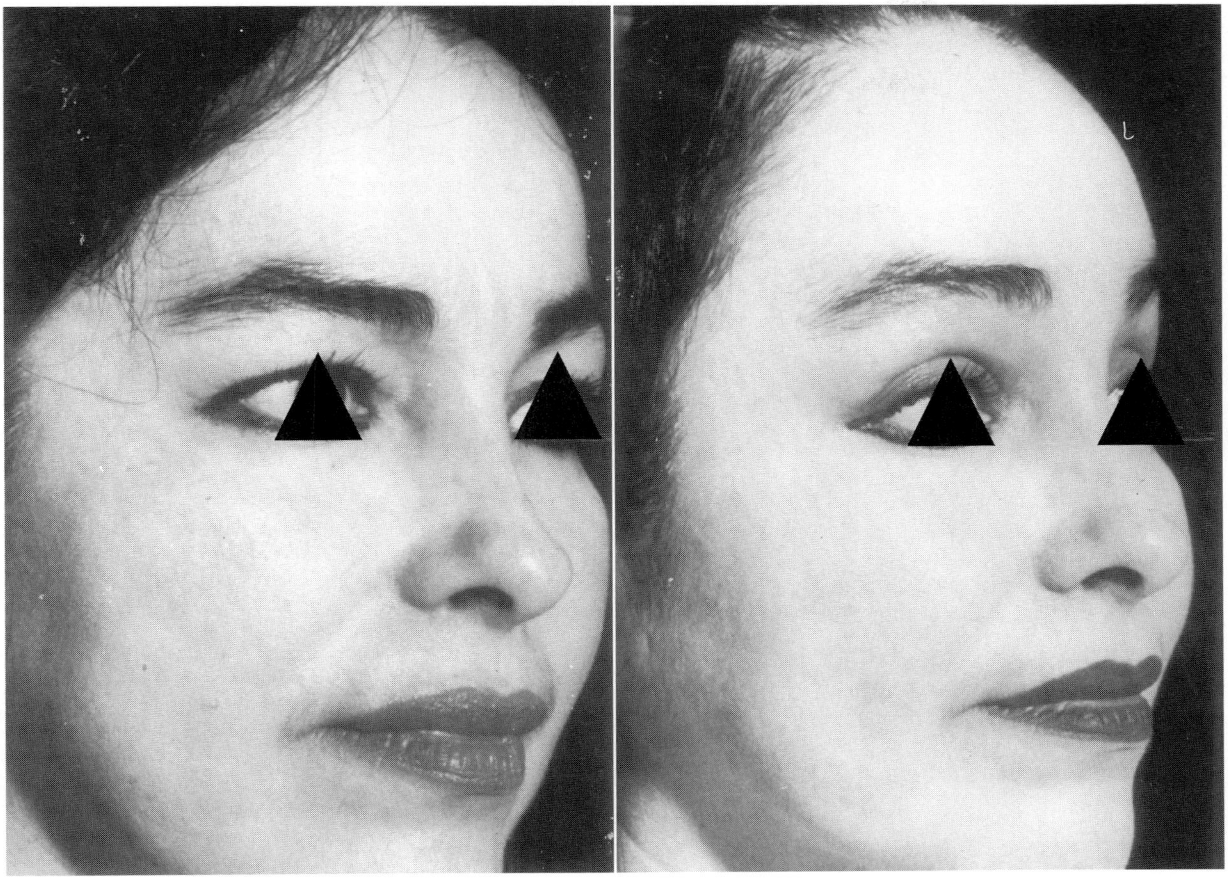

B

FIG. 7.6. Preoperative (**A**) and 8-month postoperative (**B**) lateral photographs.

RESULTS

This technique has been used in 21 patients (Figures 7.5 and 7.6). Average follow-up has been 18 months. No long-term sensory deficits, motor nerve deficits, or brow relapse have been noted. However, it has been noted that the majority of patients have an increased rate of ecchymosis and swelling when compared to patients who undergo the standard ESFP.

DISCUSSION

The ESFP is an increasingly popular alternative to the coronal approach for treating the aging forehead. The modification of the ESFP described in this chapter is especially appropriate for the aging forehead patient who is bald or has extremely thin hair. This technique could also be considered in any patient being treated for an aging forehead who also requires upper blepharoplasty. In these patients, this modification offers the advantages of enhanced long-term results because of completeness of strategic maneuvers at the brow and glabellar sites, ease of these strategic maneuvers and preservation of critical structures with direct exposure, camouflage of only two scalp scars in the crown hair, and a minimal amount of specialized equipment.

Patients who have had this operation do have prolonged upper eyelid ecchymosis and swelling compared to those patients who have surgical treatment of the aging forehead by standard ESFP. This short-term increase in morbidity needs to be presented to the patient before the operation.

REFERENCES

1. Brennen HG: Correction of the ptotic brow, Otolaryngol Clin North Am 13:265, 1980.
2. de Benito J: Aesthetic incision in the subcutaneous forehead lift, Aesthetic Plast Surg 17:239, 1993.
3. Gasperoni C, Salgarello M, and Gargani G: Subperiosteal lateral browlift and its relationship to upper blepharoplasty, Aesthetic Plast Surg 17:243, 1993.
4. Guyuron B and Davies B: Subcutaneous anterior hairline forehead rhytidectomy, Aesthetic Plast Surg 12:177, 1988.

5. Johnson CM, Jr and Waldman SR: Midforehead lift, Arch Otolaryngol 109:155, 1983.
6. Knize DM: Transpalpebral approach to the corrugator supercilii and procerus muscles, Plast Reconstr Surg 95:52, 1995.
7. McKinney P, Moddir RD, Zulkowski MI: Criteria for the forehead lift, Aesthetic Plast Surg 15:141, 1991.
8. Ortiz-Monasterio F, Barrera G, Olmedo A: The coronal incision in rhytidectomy and the brow lift, Can Plast Surg 5:167, 1978.
9. Chajchir A: Endoscopic subperiosteal forehead lift, Aesthetic Plast Surg 18:269, 1994.
10. Isse NG: Endoscopic facial rejuvenation: endoforehead, the functional lift. Case reports, Aesthetic Plast Surg 18:21, 1994.
11. Rameriz OM: Endoscopic techniques in facial rejuvenation: an overview, Part I. Aesthetic Plast Surg 18:141, 1994.

chapter eight

Alternative Endoscopic Approaches for Glabellar Myectomies with Placement of Expanded Polytetrafluoroethylene Augmentation Material

Larry D. Schoenrock, Mark M. Oyama, and W. Gregory Chernoff

The brow and glabella are a common source of concern for persons who seek consultation for surgical facial rejuvenation. Hyperactive glabella musculature creates deep vertical and horizontal creases in repose, and with animation, conveys an unfavorable "scowl" or "mean" look. The goal of correction for this hyperanimation is to restore the smooth, flat contour that is associated with a more youthful, pleasant appearance.

Current treatment modalities involve ablation of the muscular activity of the corrugator and procerus muscles, either surgically during conventional or endoscopic brow lift procedures, or pharmacologically. Botox and collagen injections offer temporary improvement; however, repeated treatments are required to sustain an effect. Even surgical myectomy can have limitations, because resection of the corrugators often produces a contour deficit at the brow, which creates a dilemma for the surgeon and less-than-ideal results for the patient. Replacement of the defect with autogenous tissue, such as fat and fascia, has been tried and reported.[1, 2] Moreover, even after corrugator myectomy, deep glabellar rhytids can persist or reoccur over time, along with reactivation of muscle activity.

Custom-designed, expanded polytetrafluoroethylene (PTFE) subcutaneous augmentation material can be a valuable adjunct in brow lift surgery and glabella myectomy to improve and refine the final aesthetic result. We have much experience with the documented safety and reliability of a variety of facial applications, such as soft-tissue alloplast, nasolabial crease, perioral enhancement, and malar and nasal augmentation.[3]

The PTFE glabellar augmentation patch (GAP) is soft, pliable, and fabriclike, and is available in 1- , 2- , or 4-mm thicknesses (Figure 8.1). The safety of this alloplastic augmentation material has been well established and documented in over 2000 implantation sites by Schoenrock and Reppuci.[4]

Contemporary advances in endoscopic brow lift surgery and instrumentation have created another opportunity to approach and treat glabella frown lines. We now routinely use PTFE GAP in conjuction with corrugator and procerus resection in nearly all endoscopic brow lift procedures. Anatomically designed GAP specifically addresses two goals: First, glabella contour can be improved by effacement of deep creases with the GAP, as well as augment the iatrogenic soft-tissue deficit created at the brow after corrugator myectomy. Second, interposing PTFE at the bony origin of the corrugators and procerus muscles can minimize return of muscle activity by inhibiting reattachment to the frontal bone. Thus, the use of the custom GAP as an adjunct to glabella myectomy can improve the resolution of deep glabellar creases and maximize the potential for long-lasting results.

Occasionally, the situation arises where the patient desires treatment of only the glabellar rhytids. In this chapter, we describe an alternate endoscopic transbrow approach for the glabella when a patient wishes to have these frown lines treated without a full brow lift procedure. This approach allows complete glabellar dissection and myectomy under endoscopic visualization and facilitates placement of the PTFE GAP. The instrumentation is more direct, and the morbidity of a full forehead dissection is avoided. The incision within the brow heals with virtually no visible scarring. Introduction of 2.0-mm endoscopes and smaller instru-

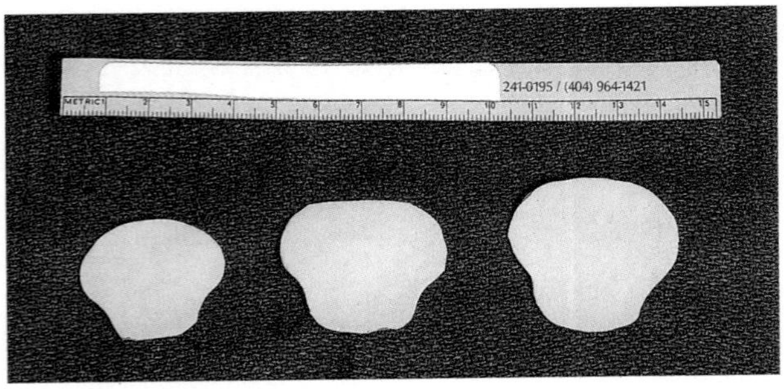

FIG. 8.1. Polytetrafluoroethylene glabellar augmentation patch.

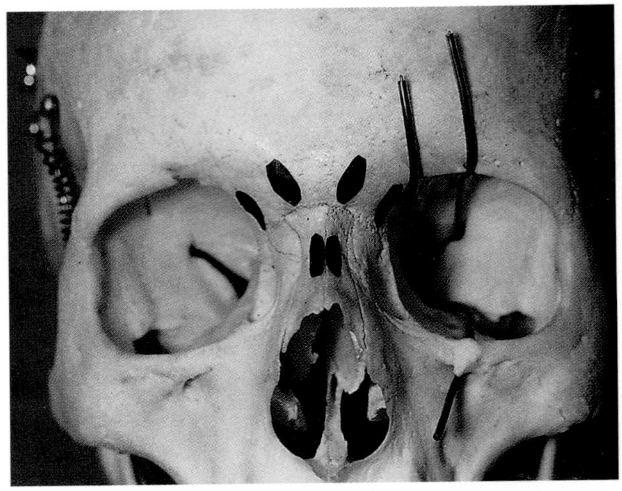

FIG. 8.2. Relationship of the supratrochlear and supraorbital nerves to the brow musculature.

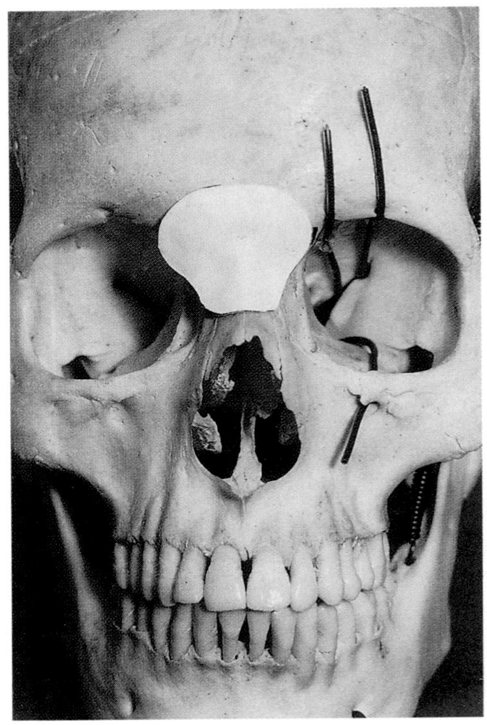

FIG. 8.3. Anatomic placement of the polytetrafluoroethylene glabellar augmentation patch, interposed at the muscle attachments.

mentation will allow further refinement and development of minimally invasive endoscopic aesthetic surgery.

Similarly, the endoscopic-assisted treatment of the glabella can be performed in conjunction with a blepharoplasty incision, as well as a transnasal approach during rhinoplasty.

SURGICAL ANATOMY

Covered elsewhere in this text in greater detail is the glabellar anatomy. However, recognizing landmarks specific for glabellar myectomy and GAP placement through a brow incision are essential in anticipation of this procedure. Injury to the supratrochlear and supraorbital neurovascular bundles can be avoided, and the glabellar musculature must be adequately undermined and resected before placement of the GAP.

The supratrochlear nerve arises from the medial aspect of the superior orbital rim, which supplies sensation to a limited portion of the middle forehead. The sensory supraorbital nerve serves the greater portion of the forehead and scalp, and arises from a foramen or notch central to the superior orbital rim. Externally, the supratrochlear nerve emerges directly vertical to the medial palpebral commissure, and the supraorbital nerve is vertically aligned with the medial half of the limbus. This relationship defines the limits of the surgical dissection and approach. By placing the incision and limiting dissection to the most medial aspect of the eyebrow, the two neurovascular bundles can be avoided. Moreover, injury to the supratrochlear nerve results in less morbidity than that to the supraorbital nerve.

The corrugator supercilii is a thin muscle with bone attachment at the nasofrontal suture line, medial to the superior orbital rim and the supratrochlear nerve (Figure 8.2). The muscle penetrates the frontalis muscle to insert onto the medial half of the eyebrow, terminating at the supraorbital nerve. Contraction draws the brows inferomedially, which creates the vertical glabellar creases. The procerus muscle is an extension of the frontalis muscle, with insertion onto the dorsum of the nasal bone at the nasal frontal angle of the nose. Fibrous attachments to the skin create transverse creases with contraction. The orbicularis oculi superioris attaches medially at the inner aspect of the superior orbital rim, and also contributes to the inferomedial contraction of the eyebrow. Thus, the boundary of the glabellar musculature and the surgical zone of dissection is the supraorbital nerve bilaterally, the superior orbital rim, and the root of the nose. After complete extirpation of the periosteum and glabellar musculature, the GAP is inserted to conform and occupy this space, thereby inhibiting reattachment of the muscles and enhancing the postsurgical contour (Figure 8.3).

CASE PRESENTATION AND SURGICAL PROCEDURE

A 62-year-old Caucasian woman was bothered by her deep glabellar furrows. She had no prior treatment to her brow. In her consultation, the brow position was felt to be adequate, but there was a need to de-emphasize the glabellar frown lines (Figure 8.4). An endoscopic transbrow glabellar myectomy with placement of a PTFE GAP was decided upon.

The procedure is performed with intravenous sedation, and local anesthesia using nerve block and regional infiltration with 0.5% lidocaine and 1:200,000 epinephrine. Before the incision and dissection, the appropriate-sized GAP is selected for the patient, and its position is marked off onto the skin (Figure 8.5). Two small horizontal stab incisions were made at the medial aspect of the eyebrows, beveled to the direction of the brow hair follicles. Blunt dissection with a mosquito clamp avoids and displaces the supratrochlear neurovascular bundle laterally; then the periosteum is incised sharply (Figure 8.6). A sharp elevator or Freer is used for subperiosteal dissection to detach the procerus and corrugator supercilii muscles. A 4-mm 30% endoscope with a hooded sheath is introduced to create the optical cavity. The image is transmitted to a three-dimensional, high-resolution monitor via a triple-chip camera (Figure 8.7).

A cauterizing right-angle hook is introduced through the contralateral incision, and the corrugator and procerus muscles are resected under direct vision to avoid nerve injury. When using a cauterizing hook, care must be taken to avoid thermal injury to the overlying skin. Additional resection may be completed with a biting forceps. Alternatively, an Ultrapulse CO_2 laser can be used for the myectomy; however, the laser poses greater risk for nerve or skin injury.

Triangulation of suture placement allows for precise localization of the GAP (Figure 8.8). The suture at the inferior pole of the GAP is fixated through the skin over the nasion, where the inferior end of the GAP will lie. The other suture is passed through both incisions; then the furled GAP is gently pulled through the incision and into position. The endoscope is reintroduced, and final adjustment and positioning of the patch is performed. Care is taken to ensure that the GAP is completely unfurled and smooth. Finally, the sutures can be secured over a dental roll, which is left in place for 3 days. The incisions are closed with 6-0 Prolene sutures.

Postoperative results reveal a marked improvement with these glabella frown lines; the incisions are not visible, and there is no alopecia (Figure 8.9). In the event a blepharoplasty is being performed, endoscopic glabellar myectomy can be approached through the upper lid incision. A subcutaneous flap over the orbicularis oculi at the medial aspect of the incision affords more exposure. The endoscope and sheath is then introduced through the skin flap, up to the orbital rim, which creates the optical cavity (Figure 8.10). The cor-

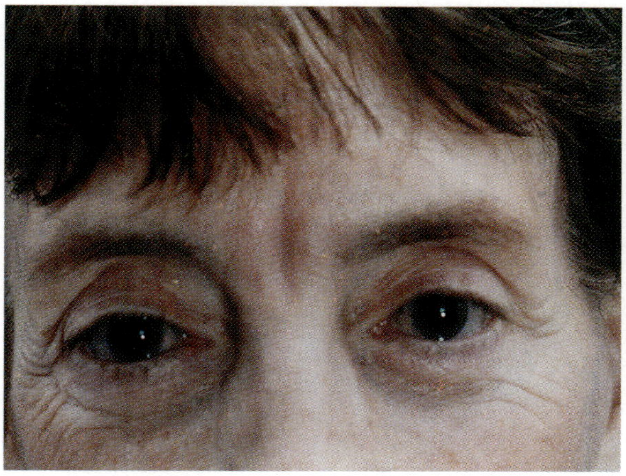

FIG. 8.4. Preoperative photo: 62-year-old woman who has deep glabellar frown lines.

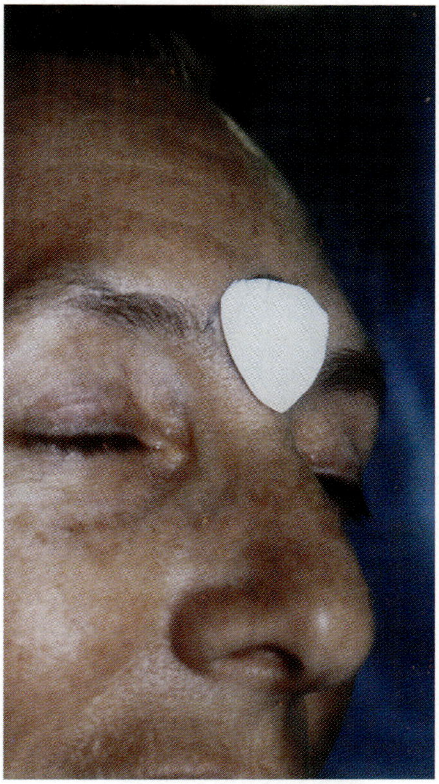

FIG. 8.5. Correct placement of the glabellar augmentation patch is marked off over the glabella.

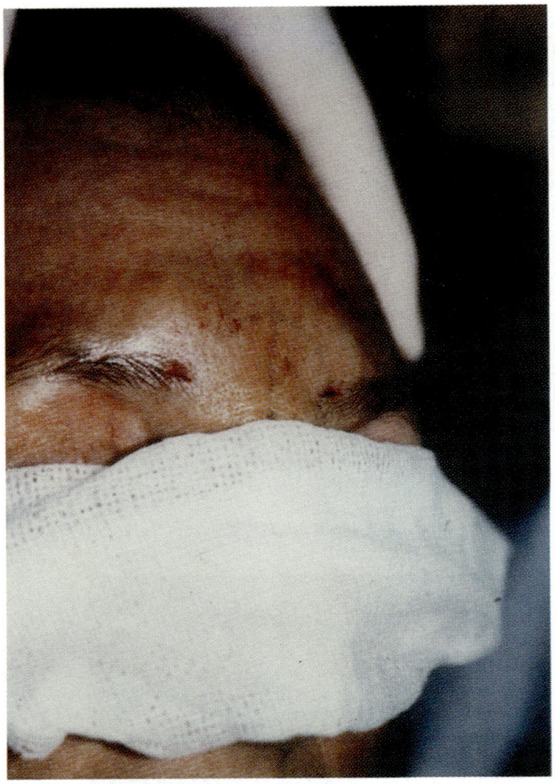

FIG. 8.6. Incisions are made at the medial edge of the brow, and dissection proceeds medially down to the periosteum.

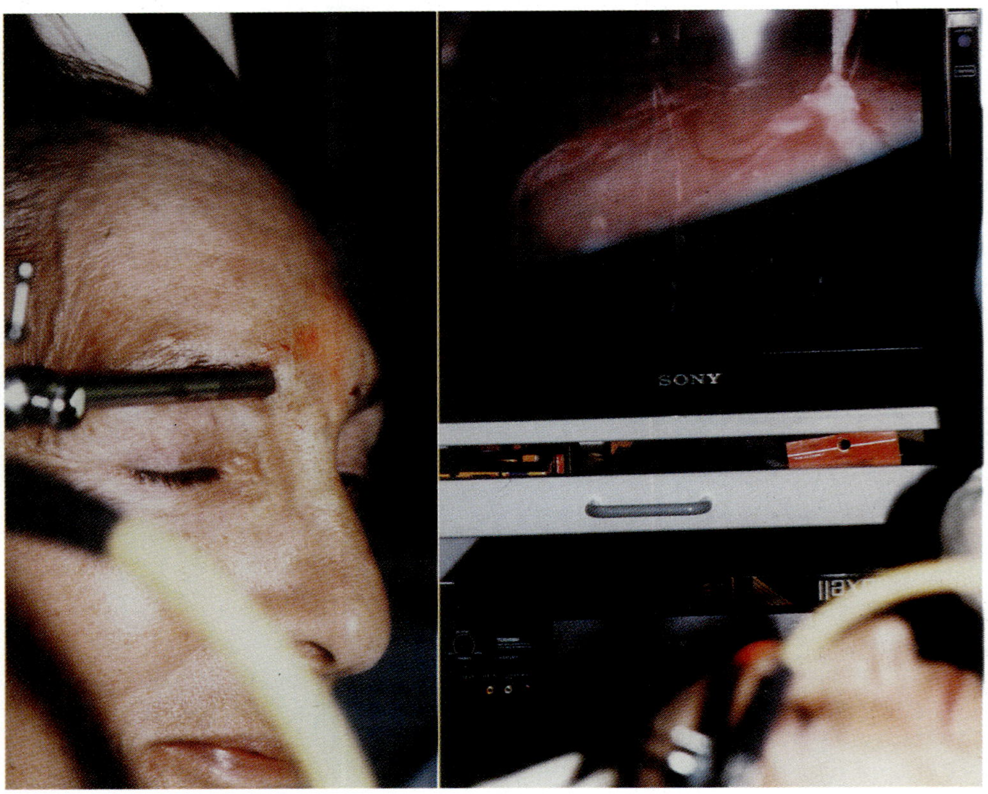

FIG. 8.7. Subperiosteal dissection of the musculature is performed, and an optical cavity is created with the introduction of the hooded 4-mm, 30-degree endoscope.

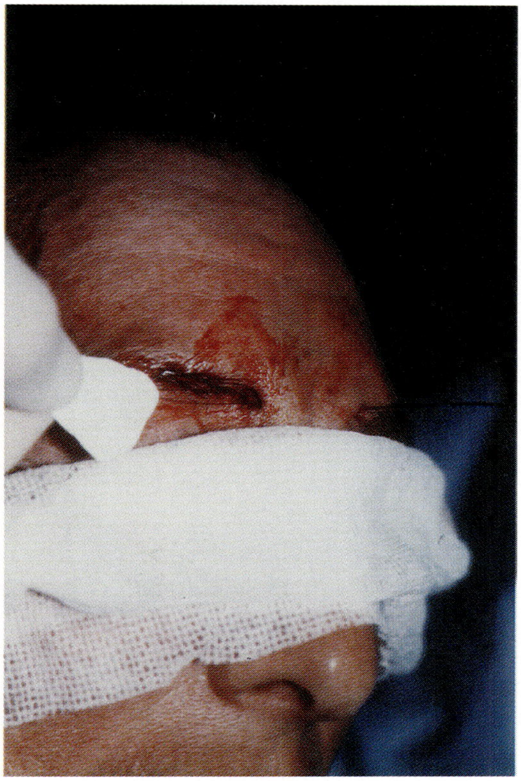

FIG. 8.8. Fixation sutures are attached to the glabellar augmentation patch.

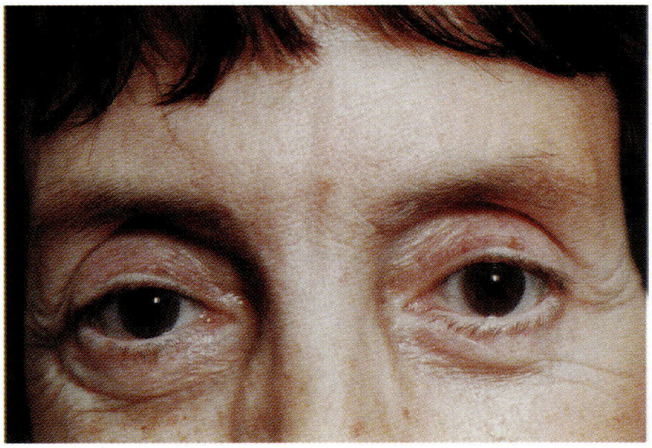

FIG. 8.9. Postoperative photograph showing improvement in the glabella furrow following myectomy and glabellar augmentation patch. The brow incisions are not visible, and there is no alopecia.

rugator and procerus muscles are easily exposed, and are resected as previously described. This approach affords enough exposure that the myectomy could also be performed as described by Guyuron et al and Knize.[5,6] The endoscope, however, allows visualization and avoidance of inadvertent nerve injury. Because GAP placement is more direct, however, the triangulation

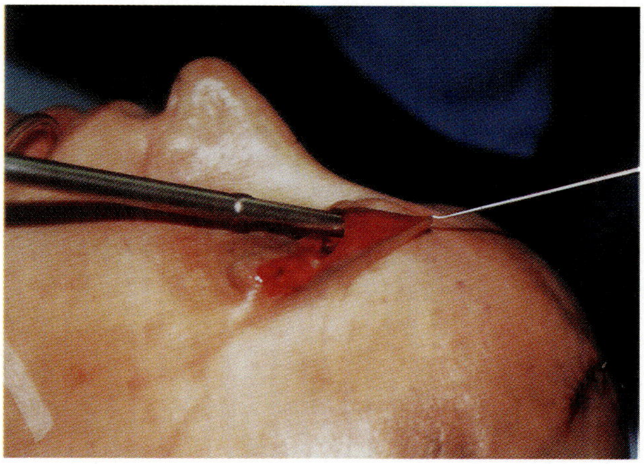

FIG. 8.10. Endoscopic dissection of the glabella via a blepharoplasty incision.

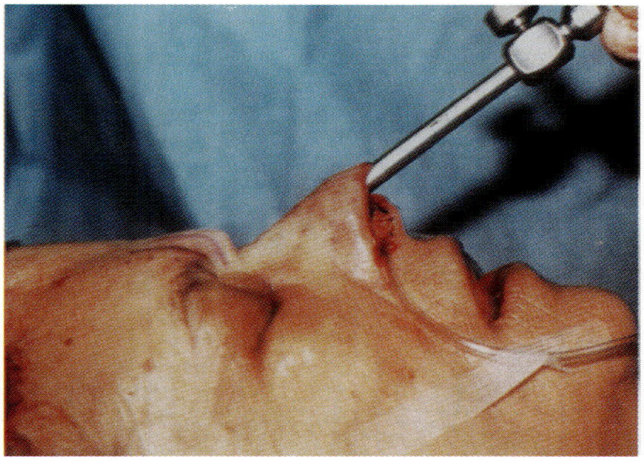

FIG. 8.11. Endonasal approach to the glabella, shown here with an open external rhinoplasty.

needs to be appropriately oriented to the approach. Completion of the upper lid blepharoplasty can then proceed in the usual manner.

External approach rhinoplasty also creates another opportunity to use the endoscopic approach to the glabella, as first described by Ramirez.[1] After the nasal-dorsal flap is created, sharp periosteal elevation over the nasion is performed to detach the procerus and corrugator muscles. The endoscope is introduced under the nasal flap to create the optical cavity (Figure 8.11). Endoscopic myectomy and placement of GAP is performed as previously described. On occasion, it may be desirable to laminate the glabellar patch with another 1- , 2- , or 4-mm strip of PTFE attached with nonabsorbable nylon suture. In patients who have nasofrontal angle, this can provide customized augmentation at the root of the nose.

COMPLICATIONS

The PTFE glabellar augmentation patch has been inserted in 90% of endoscopic brow lifts in our practice with glabellar myectomy over a 2-year period, and no complications have been encountered to date. Specifically, there have been no instances of extrusion, brow alopecia, migration, or infection. Sensory nerve hypoesthesia has not been encountered.

CONCLUSION

Technical advances in endoscopic instrumentation and techniques have allowed surgeons to expand their means of treating glabellar frown lines. Although the long-term statistical improvement in glabellar paresis and contour is yet to be determined, we find that the PTFE custom glabellar augmentation patch enhances our results when used in conjunction with endoscopic glabellar myectomy. The PTFE material serves to efface and reduce the deep glabellar furrow, and to inhibit corrugator and procerus reactivation. In addition to the standard retrohairline endoscopic approach, we have successfully used alternative approaches via the brows, blepharoplasty, and nose to perform endoscopic glabellar myectomy and placement of PTFE GAP. These alternative approaches offer an advantage when a conventional brow lift is not a concurrent option, with the instrumentation being more direct and requiring less dissection. These modalities can be useful options to offer the client who seeks facial rejuvenation.

REFERENCES

1. Ramirez O: Endoscopic techniques in facial rejuvenation: an overview. Part 1, Aesthetic Plast Surg 18:141-147, 1994.
2. Guyuron B and Davies B: Subcutaneous anterior hairline forehead rhytidectomy, Aesthetic Plast Surg 12:77-83, 1988.
3. Schoenrock L and Chernoff W: Subcutaneous implantation of Gore-Tex for facial reconstruction, Otorhinol Clin North Am 28(2):325-340, 1995.
4. Schoenrock LD and Reppuci AD: Gore-Tex in facial plastic surgery, Int J ARS 1:63-68, 1993.
5. Guyuron B, Michelow BJ, and Thomas T: Corrugator supercilii muscle resection through blepharoplasty incision, Plast Reconstr Surg 4:691-696, 1995.
6. Knize DM: Transpalpebral approach to the corrugator supercilii and procerus muscles, Plast Reconstr Surg 95(1):52-60, 1995.

chapter nine

Endoscopic Malar Pad Lift and Subperiosteal Midface Lift

M. Sean Freeman

Aesthetic facial rejuvenation has gained widespread acceptance in the general public. As more and younger patients seek facial rejuvenation, surgeons have been searching for improved techniques—improved in the sense of providing longer-lasting, natural-appearing results while at the same time decreasing the perioperative and postoperative sequelae. It is with these goals in mind that the endoscope was adapted to forehead and face-lift surgery.

The intent of this chapter is to provide the author's bias as it relates to the subperiosteal brow lift and to provide an in-depth review of how the endoscope can be useful for selective rejuvenation of the midface. Two approaches to the midface will be discussed. The first is the endoscopic subperiosteal midface lift as popularized by Ramirez and others.[1-3] This approach is an interesting procedure from a theoretical viewpoint, but from my point of view, this approach has limited applications. The other approach is the endoscopic malar pad lift, which is a technique developed by the author to selectively lift the midface while at the same time circumventing many of the disadvantages of the subperiosteal midface lift. This technique can also be used in conjunction with a subperiosteal brow lift and/or a face-lift.

INDICATIONS/CONTRAINDICATIONS

Browplasty

Endoscopic browplasty or forehead lift can be performed for glabellar frown lines alone as well as in association with brow ptosis. Any patient who is a candidate for forehead surgery can have this procedure performed endoscopically; however, there are some relative contraindications.

In general, patients who require bone recontouring should have an open approach. Although a small amount of recontouring of the supraorbital ridge can be done endoscopically, it is more difficult and potentially more dangerous. For a similar reason, patients who have had previous surgery and/or trauma of the forehead area may be better approached via conventional means.

Midface

The endoscopic subperiosteal midface lift basically provides the same rejuvenation that an open subperiosteal approach obtains without the need for a preauricular incision. The approach provides an excellent way of repositioning the soft tissues of the midface that yields a well-rested look. I have found this approach particularly useful in the occasional patient who is seen with cicatricial hemifacial deformity, due to the ability of subperiosteal undermining of the face to reposition tissue in mass more effectively than extraperiosteal approaches.

For cosmetic patients who are heavy smokers and who are seen to have a down-turned commissura labiorum, the subperiosteal approach should be considered. The technique provides an exceptional blood supply, and because of the elevation of the zygomaticus major and minor the technique helps restore the commissura of the mouth.

The endoscopic malar pad lift is in general applicable to any patient who wishes improvement in their nasolabial fold. The procedure can be used either by itself or in conjunction with a subperiosteal endoscopic brow lift. A variation of this technique can be useful in patients who are intent on a face-lift: the surgeon can use a variation of the technique originally described by Owsley.[4]

The endoscopic malar pad lift is contraindicated in patients who are noted on examination to have little to no malar fat pad. In addition, the patient must be able to tolerate an incision in a lateral crow's-foot wrinkle line. As with the endoscopic subperiosteal midface lift, patients will experience prolonged edema lateral to the orbit when this procedure is performed without a browplasty and/or face-lift, although to a lesser extent. However, unlike an endoscopic subperiosteal midface lift, this periorbital edema will be minimized when an endoscopic subperiosteal browplasty and/or face-lift are added to the procedure.

ADVANTAGES/DISADVANTAGES

Browplasty

There are many advantages to the endoscopic approach to browplasty, particularly when applied or approached subperiosteally. First is the avoidance of injury to the supraorbital and supratrochlear nerves. Not only does this approach minimize numbness of the scalp, but it also helps to prevent the occasional neuralgia or neuroma that can occur following open browplasty. The exact incidence of this latter complication is not well reported, but in my experience unpleasant or even painful neuralgias are not uncommon following transection of the supraorbital nerve.[5,6] Although these neuralgias are usually transient in nature, they are not always so.

For the most part, incisional alopecia can be prevented or at least minimized. At times, the incisional alopecia that exists with coronal forehead lifting can be difficult for a patient to hide, especially if alopecia occurs in a patient with already thinning hair.

In addition, the minimization of incisions provides for a decreased possibility of unsightly scar formation, particularly in men, because the incisions are smaller and better hidden in areas affected by male pattern baldness. This has increased acceptance of the procedure by men.

Another important advantage is the minimal change in the distance from the eyebrow to the hairline with the endoscopic subperiosteal approach. In general, a 3:1 relationship exists between scalp and brow elevation when one performs a classical coronal brow lift. For most patients, this results in an unacceptable elevation of the frontal hairline. Elevation of the frontal hairline can be circumvented by use of a trichophilic incision, but then the surgeon risks a visible hairline incision. There are patients, however, who benefit from a trichophilic approach in combination with an endoscopic brow lift. When the distance between the hairline and nasion significantly exceeds the distance from nasion to caudal columella nasi, then an excision of superior forehead skin sufficient to align the hairline should be considered.

Hemostasis using a subperiosteal endoscopic approach is significantly better than a full incisional approach. This is true despite the need for more undermining with endoscopic browplasty. The reason for this is the propensity of any scalp incision to bleed due to the scalp's rich vascular supply. An understandable corollary is that endoscopic browplasty patients tend to bruise less and look better faster than classical coronal lift patients.

The biggest disadvantage of an endoscopic approach is the cost of the equipment and the time involved in learning how to use it. This is a disadvantage for each of the endoscopic procedures described in this chapter. Physicians who are already versed in the use of the endoscope will be able to adapt to these procedures with greater ease. Despite one's background, a thorough training course that includes extensive didactic and cadaver dissection should be attended before attempting these procedures. Following this, further cadaver dissection should be performed until one feels competent with the procedure. As a further precaution, the first few brow lifts done on a patient should include a consent for both open and endoscopic approaches.

Endoscopic Subperiosteal Midface Lift

The main advantage of the endoscopic subperiosteal midface lift is the ability to lift the midface without the need for a preauricular incision. In addition, the motion attained in the malar area with this approach allows for the excision of lower lid skin with less risk of ectropion.

As a result of the repositioning of the midface soft tissue in a subperiosteal plane, the zygomaticus major and minor muscles are lifted in a superior-lateral direction, which leads to an upturning of the commissures of the mouth (Figure 9.1). It must be pointed out, however, that many patients are seen by the physician with complaints other than the position of their commissura labiorum. As with endoscopic browplasty, this procedure has good hemostasis and yields a flap of superior vascularity.

The main disadvantage of the endoscopic subperiosteal midface lift and the open subperiosteal face-lift is the inability of these approaches to improve the nasolabial fold. The reason for this can be found by reviewing the anatomy of the fold.[7,8] The nasolabial fold is formed by the fascial fiber connections between the dermis and the underlying superficial muscles of facial expression, which with repeated animation actually pull in on the fold. In addition, over time the malar fat pad rotates in a medial-inferior direction, which further deepens the fold.[4,9] The repositioning of the muscles of facial expression along with the malar pad en mass via a subperiosteal approach produces little to no improvement in the fold. Because there is no relative change in the position of the malar pad with respect to the underlying facial muscles, a positive effect on the depth of the nasolabial fold is not produced.

There are other points that must be considered before selecting the subperiosteal approach. Most of these patients experience significant postoperative periorbital swelling, which can take up to 3 months to resolve. In addition, it has been my experience that minimal improvement in jowling can be expected, with little to no change in neck laxity. This later problem can be circumvented by adding a neck suspension, which is described in Chapter 10.

The need for appropriate didactic and cadaver training cannot be overemphasized with regard to the subperiosteal midface procedure. In addition to locating and successfully dissecting the supraorbital and supratrochlear nerves, which will be described later, it is also necessary to dissect the zygomatic arch safely. This is a danger zone with regard to the frontal branch of the facial nerve, and careful attention to detail must be observed to avoid inadvertent injury to this nerve (Figure 9.2). A thorough understanding of the planes necessary to achieve a safe yet effective lift can be obtained only in the anatomy laboratory following successful completion of an accredited course.

Endoscopic Malar Pad Lift

The main advantage of this approach is its versatility and effectiveness in improving the nasolabial fold.

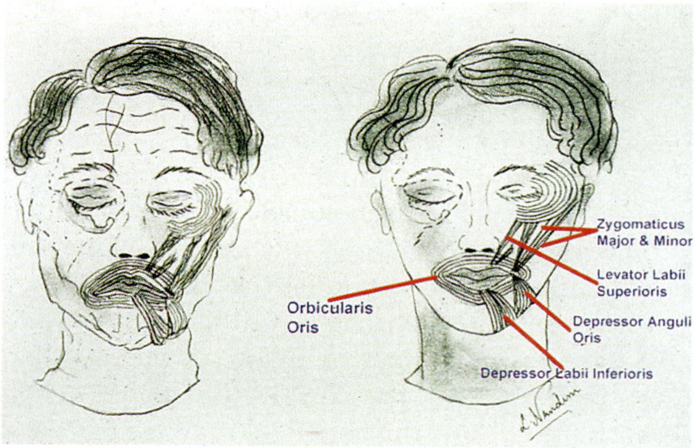

FIG. 9.1. Detachment of the zygomaticus muscle in a subperiosteal plane from its insertion onto the malar eminence, followed by repositioning in a posterior-superior vector, lifts the corner of the mouth.

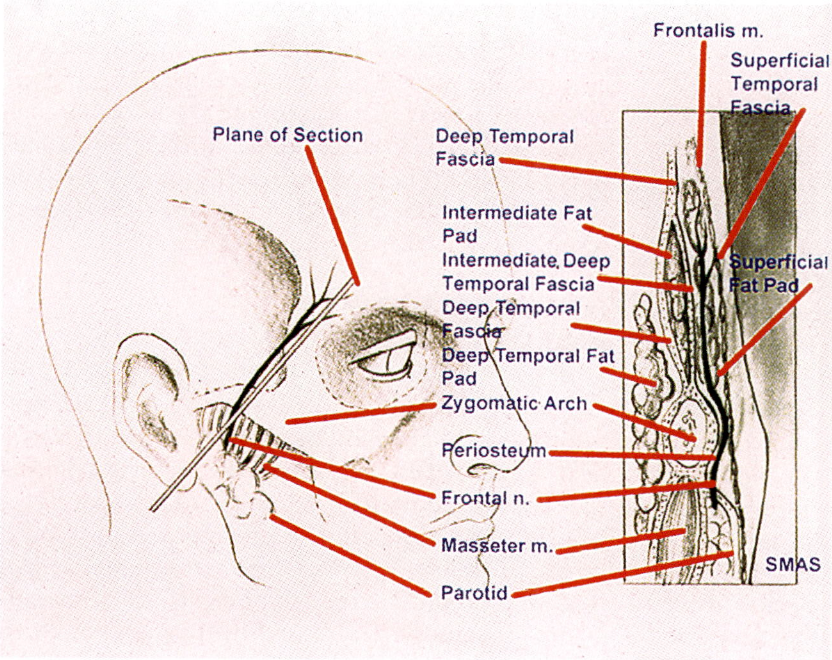

FIG. 9.2. Cross-sectional view of the zygomatic arch following the vector of the frontal branch of the facial nerve. Note that the periosteum of the arch protects the nerve at this level. Careful dissection is needed.

A,B

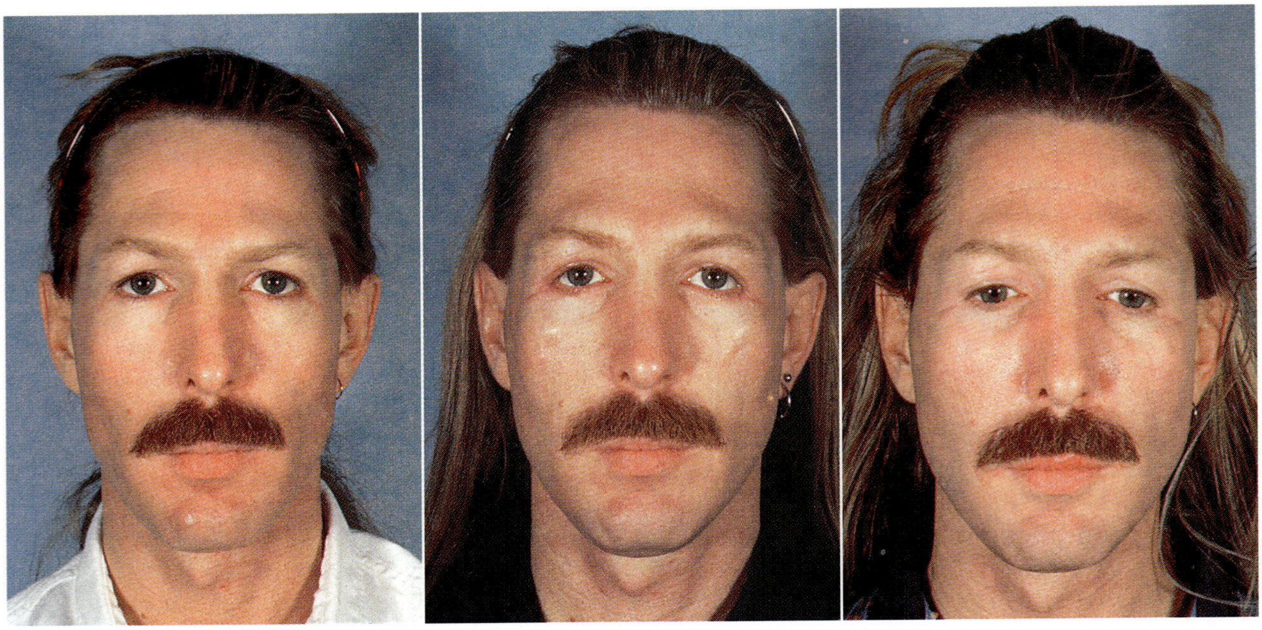

C

FIG. 9.3. **A,** Preoperative picture of ectomorphic man before undergoing malar pad lift. Note absence of fullness in malar pad area as well as lack of nasolabial fold. **B,** Postoperative crease of skin noted due to lack of malar pad noted at time of surgery. **C,** Pleating of skin was corrected by subcutaneous undermining of the area.

For patients who are seen with midface ptosis without significant brow ptosis, a selective midface lift can be offered. For patients who require a browplasty and a midface lift, the endoscopic malar pad lift may be used in conjunction with a subperiosteal browplasty. A preauricular face-lift incision will not be required in either of these scenarios. As alluded to before, an endoscopic malar pad lift can also be used during a face-lift, with or without a browplasty, to provide midface rejuvenation in place of a deep plane or composite lift. When used with a face-lift, an incision lateral to the orbit would not be required.

The efficacy of this approach as it relates to the nasolabial fold can be understood if we again look at the regional anatomy involved in the dynamics of midface laxity. The progressive deepening of the nasolabial fold occurs over time by the combination of repeated pulling on the dermis by the fascial fiber connections between the dermis and the underlying muscles of facial expression and by the inferior-to-medial rotation of the malar pad. The net effect of the endoscopic malar pad lift is to reposition this fibrofatty tissue along a posterior-to-superior vector and to provide a pull on the epidermis lateral to the fold. The effect is an improvement in the depth of the nasolabial fold as well as of the contour of the malar area.

The main disadvantage of this approach is that when it is done without a brow lift and/or face-lift, a moderate amount of swelling lateral to the orbit can persist for up to 6 weeks. In addition, redundancy of the lower lid skin can occur, which will at times require removal using a pinch technique.

One must be wary of applying this technique universally. As noted previously, there are patients who are so ectomorphic that the tissue in the malar pad has atrophied to the point that lifting this area would result in dimpling of the skin (Figure 9.3). Although the inability of using this technique for every patient is certainly a disadvantage, it has been my experience that few patients fall into this category.

As with the previously mentioned endoscopic procedures, adequate didactic and cadaver training are required. There is risk of injury to the buccal branch of the facial nerve, which lies below the zygomaticus major muscle (Figure 9.4). In addition, suture fixation must be done properly to obtain a satisfactory result and to avoid indentation of the epidermis.

OPERATIVE SETUP AND INSTRUMENTATION

For each procedure, it is best to have an anatomically shaped bed to allow better access to the operative field. It also is best to position the monitor opposite the surgeon's dominant hand; for example, a right-handed surgeon should have the monitor positioned on his or her left. The nurse anesthetist or monitoring nurse is positioned at the end of the bed, with the surgeon's assistant to the left and the operative nurse to

A

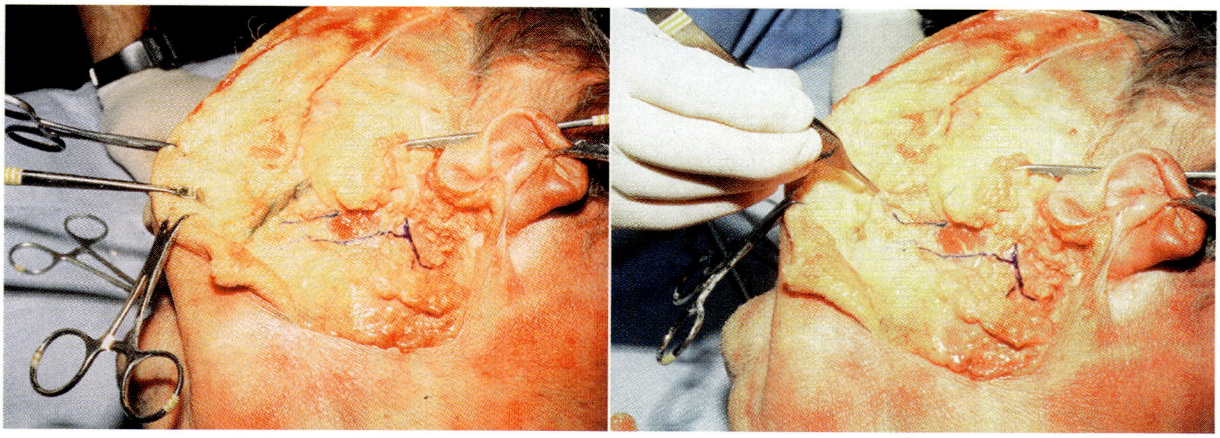

B

FIG. 9.4. **A,** Relationship of the buccal branch of the facial nerve (blue) to the zygomaticus muscle (green). Parotid gland has been split to show the underlying anatomy. **B,** Zygomaticus muscle is being held up by the forceps to show the buccal branch of the facial nerve entering underneath.

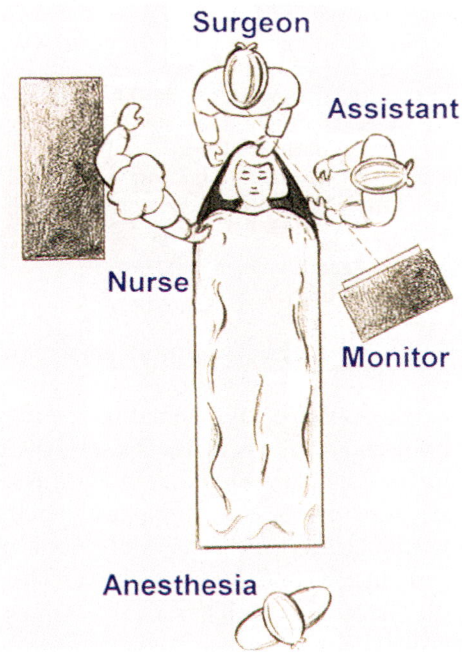

FIG. 9.5. Setup for a right-handed surgeon. Note that monitor is normally positioned over the bed. Left-handed surgeon would be set up in a mirror image.

the right. Careful preoperative positioning will increase efficiency (Figure 9.5).

Instrumentation does not need to be extensive. Several special instruments can be used for these procedures, including a 30-degree, 5-mm endoplastic scope and cannula, which deliver better optics and visual cavity than a 4-mm scope, various soft-tissue elevators, and an insulated alligator instrument for cauterizing and muscle debulking. Only the endoscope and its sheath are required for the endoscopic malar pad lift.

INCISIONS/MARKINGS

Endoscopic Subperiosteal Browplasty

The markings for an endoscopic subperiosteal browplasty are described in other chapters in this book. There is one point concerning the preoperative markings for this procedure that I would like to review. A fairly precise lift can be attained by this procedure, individualized by side in relation to the midbrow, when the surgeon uses the two medial incisions versus a single incision in the midline. The reason for individualizing the lift in the midbrow is that in many patients asymmetry of the brow can be improved. To estimate the amount of lift needed in the midbrow, the patient is put in a sitting position with his or her eyes closed, and the position of the brow is marked. Next, the physician marks the point where he or she wants the midbrow to be after the surgery. The difference between these two points is recorded and will be used later when fixating the inferior edge of the periosteum to the screw above the midbrow incision (Figure 9.6). If it is decided during the patient's consultation that a high arched brow is preferable, then the same process is used in deciding the amount of lift required via the middle of the three forehead incisions.

For patients who do not want a high arched brow, two screw fixations of the midbrow will suffice, with the lateral lift provided by suture fixation of the superficial temporal fascia to the deep temporal fascia (see discussion later in this chapter). For patients who desire a higher arch to their brow, screw fixation via the middle brow incision above the lateral canthus will need to be added.

The incisions needed depend on two variables: the patient's sex and whether the patient requires brow

A

B

C

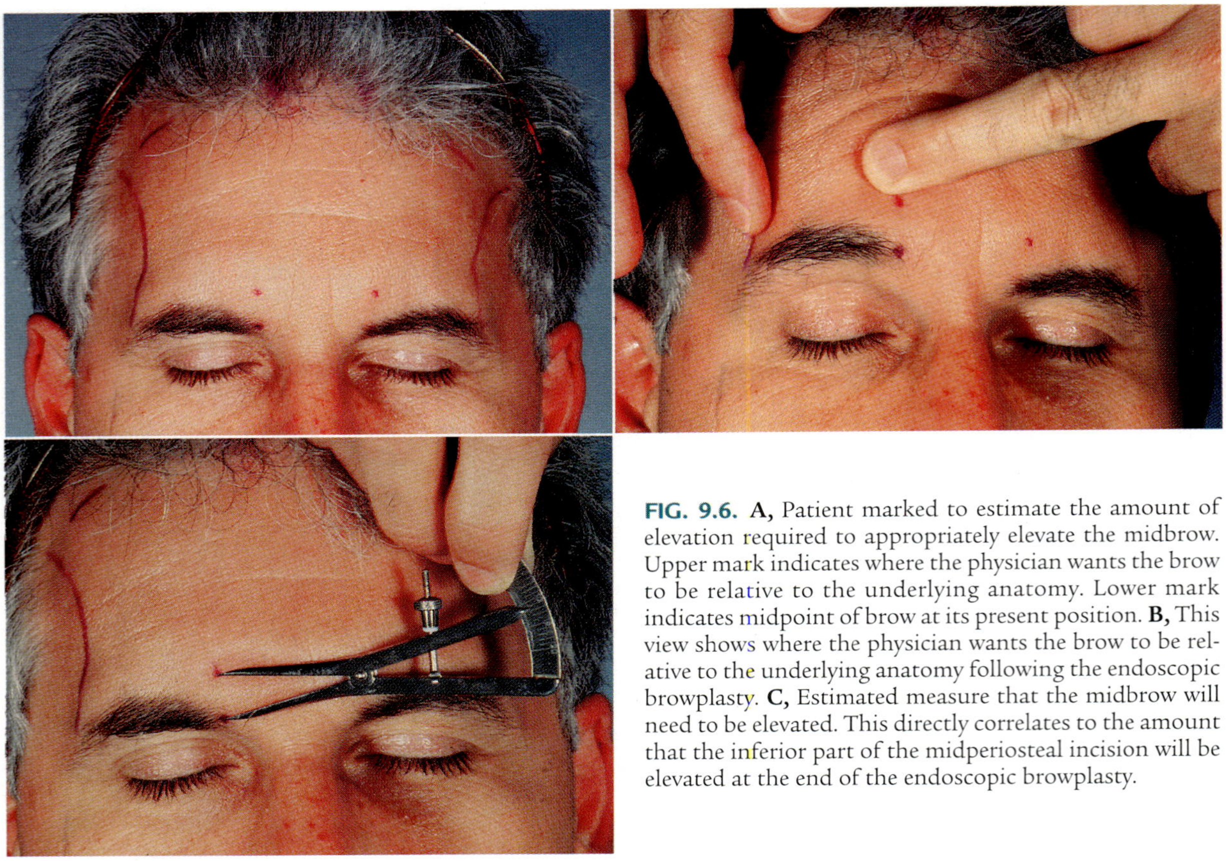

FIG. 9.6. **A,** Patient marked to estimate the amount of elevation required to appropriately elevate the midbrow. Upper mark indicates where the physician wants the brow to be relative to the underlying anatomy. Lower mark indicates midpoint of brow at its present position. **B,** This view shows where the physician wants the brow to be relative to the underlying anatomy following the endoscopic browplasty. **C,** Estimated measure that the midbrow will need to be elevated. This directly correlates to the amount that the inferior part of the midperiosteal incision will be elevated at the end of the endoscopic browplasty.

elevation or simply improvement in the glabellar lines. For the few patients who desire only glabellar line improvement, three incisions are needed: two incisions just lateral to the supraorbital nerve, and one incision in the midline. Each incision is approximately 2 cm in length.

For women, vertical incisions at the caudal edge of the hairline are appropriate and heal very well. For men, however, vertically placed incisions in a thinning hairline can be undesirable. I have found that horizontal incisions in the patient's most superior forehead wrinkle line are a good alternative. The surgeon must be careful not to transect the supraorbital nerve with these incisions.

For the majority of patients, however, brow elevation will be requested in addition to improvement of glabellar frown lines. These patients will need six separate incisions, approximately 2 cm in length. One incision is made above the medial head of each brow. The reason for using two incisions here rather than one sagittal incision is twofold. First, these incisions are used to elevate the right and left medial brows individually. Second, the means of brow suspension in the area requires drilling into the external cortex of the frontal bone to a depth of 4 to 5 mm, and drilling lateral to the sagittal suture eliminates the possibility of inadvertent injury to the superior sagittal sinus.

The incisions placed just medial to the temporal line are done to allow easier dissection of the lateral canthal area and for precise separation of the periosteal and fascial attachments at the temporal line. In addition, these middle brow incisions will be used to selectively elevate the arch of the brow if a high arched brow is the goal. The supra-auricular incisions can be made separately or in conjunction with an incisional face-lift. These incisions are needed to dissect the lateral temporal area and help to suspend the lateral brow.

For women patients, vertically oriented hairline incisions are made in the middle brow, with the lateral incisions placed in the hairline approximately on a line that connects the lateral canthus to the lateral alar groove. For men, I prefer using horizontal incisions similarly placed (Figure 9.7).

The only exception to the preceding is in a female patient who has an abnormally high forehead, which is in general a hairline higher than 6 cm. For these patients, consideration of excision of a necessary amount of forehead skin at the level of a trichophilic incision should be considered. The skin is removed above the level of the frontalis muscle. Vertical incisions are then made as before, but now through the frontalis muscle.

A

B

C

D

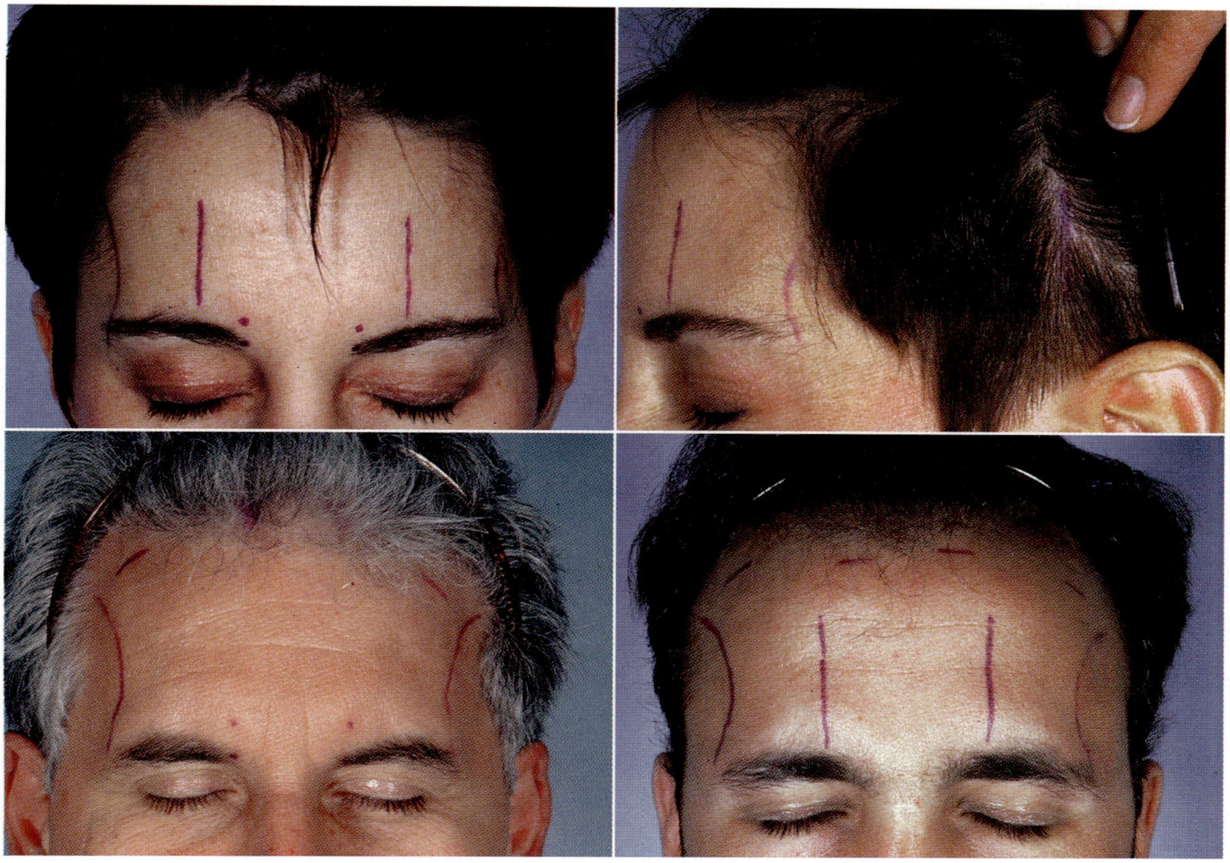

FIG. 9.7. **A** and **B,** These views demonstrate the four medial incisions for a woman. The two incisions placed directly above the midbrow are used to selectively elevate each midbrow. The two incisions placed medial to the temporal line are used to selectively elevate the lateral brow in those women wishing a high arched brow as well as to facilitate dissection of the lateral canthal area. The two lateral incisions are made above the helix just inferior to the temporal line. **C,** This view demonstrates the four medial incisions for a man without male pattern baldness. For men, the lateral incision above helix is made more caudal to the temporal line than in women. **D,** This view demonstrates the four medial incisions for a man with male pattern baldness.

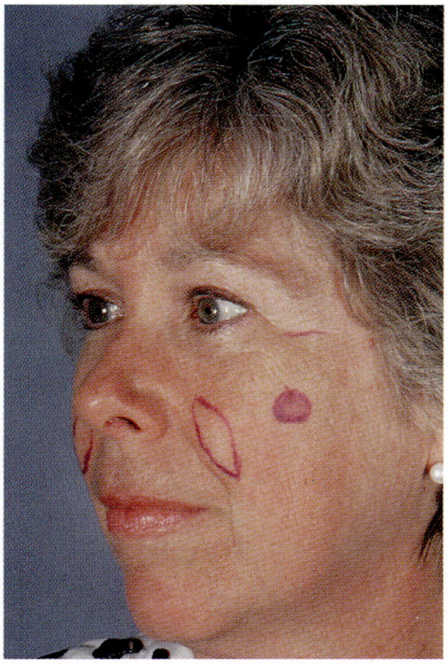

FIG. 9.8. Incision is made in the predominate wrinkle line. Insertion point of the zygomaticus muscle is palpated and marked. Inserts are at the most anterior lateral eminence of the malar bone. Malar pad can be found lateral to the nasal alae.

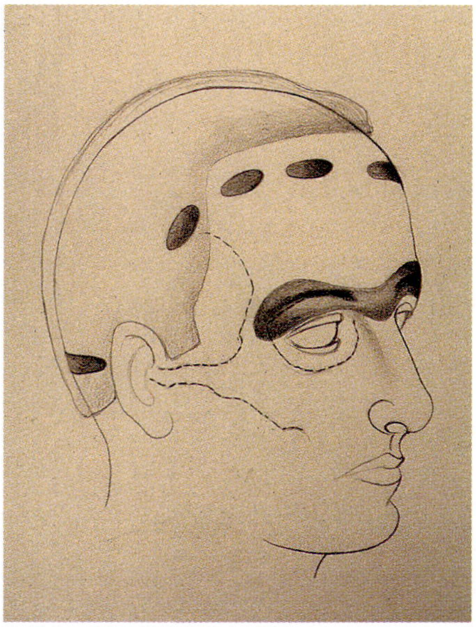

FIG. 9.9. Injection sites for endoscopic browplasty.

Endoscopic Subperiosteal Midface Lift

The incisions in the brow for endoscopic subperiosteal midface lift are the same as for endoscopic subperiosteal browplasty. In addition, a lower eyelid incision is made so that a skin muscle flap can be raised. Finally, bilateral Caldwell-Luc incisions are made.

Endoscopic Malar Pad Lift

When performing an endoscopic malar pad lift, the insertion point of the zygomaticus major muscle is palpated and marked. The insertion point can be found by asking the patient to widely smile while palpating the inferior aspect of the malar eminence just lateral to the lateral canthus. A deep crow's-foot wrinkle below the lateral canthus is selected and marked in patients who are not having a face-lift as part of their procedure (Figure 9.8).

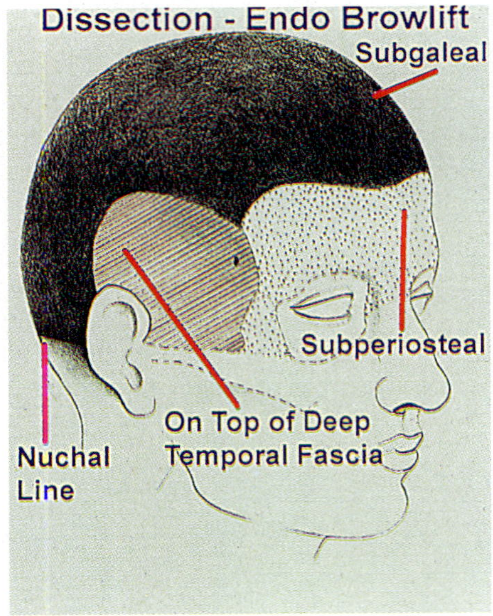

FIG. 9.10. Author's preferred dissection planes for endoscopic browplasty.

ANESTHESIA/INJECTIONS

Endoscopic Browplasty

Endoscopic browplasty can be done under IV sedation or general anesthesia. Patients operated on under IV sedation need to be appropriately prepared and blocked because they will hear much of the dissection.

The supraorbital and nuchal line blocks are done using 1% lidocaine (to block supraorbital/supratrochlear nerves) with 1:1,000,000 epinephrine (to block the greater/lesser occipital nerves). These two lines are then connected with spot injections of 0.25% lidocaine, 1:400,000. In addition, the incision sites are injected with 1% lidocaine with epinephrine (Figure 9.9).

Endoscopic Subperiosteal Midface Lift

Endoscopic subperiosteal midface lift should be done under general anesthesia and all incision sites are injected with 1% lidocaine with epinephrine.

Endoscopic Malar Pad Lift

When the endoscopic malar pad lift is being done by itself, the physician can use oral versus IV/IM sedation. The infraorbital and the zygomaticotemporal nerves are blocked using 1% lidocaine with epinephrine and augmented with local injection as needed.

PROCEDURE

Endoscopic Browplasty

The four medial incisions of endoscopic browplasty are made down to the cranium. The two lateral incisions are made down to the deep temporal fascia. A drill is used to mark the starting point at the inferior edge of the two midperiosteal incisions as well as the middle incisions in those patients where a high arched brow is the goal. Similarly, a small cut is made to mark the starting point of the dissection in the deep temporal fascia. The four medial incisions are connected in a subperiosteal plane. The lateral incision is connected to the medial dissection by following the top of the deep temporal fascia.

The posterior and lateral scalp are dissected without the use of the endoscope. From the medial incisions to the temporal line, the dissection plane is subgaleal, whereas from the lateral incisions to the temporal line, the dissection plane is on top of the deep temporal fascia. The posterior extent of the dissection is to the nuchal line, the level of attachment of the occipitalis muscle. The lateral and medial dissections are connected through the temporal line from lateral to medial.

The forehead and anterior temporal areas are dissected next. Again, the initial dissection is done without the use of the endoscope. The forehead area medial to the temporal line is dissected in a subperiosteal plane. Medially, the dissection is carried out down to the glabellar area, avoiding the supratrochlear nerve. At the level of the supraorbital nerve, the dissection is done to within 2 cm of the supraorbital ridge. Lateral to the supraorbital nerve, the dissection is carried out to the supraorbital ridge down to the lateral orbital rim lateral to Whitnall's tubercle (Figure 9.10).

The temporal dissection is then done up to, but not through, the forehead part of the temporal line and inferiorly to within 2 cm of the zygomatic arch and lateral orbital rim; the surgeon must stay in the plane immediately above the deep temporal fascia.

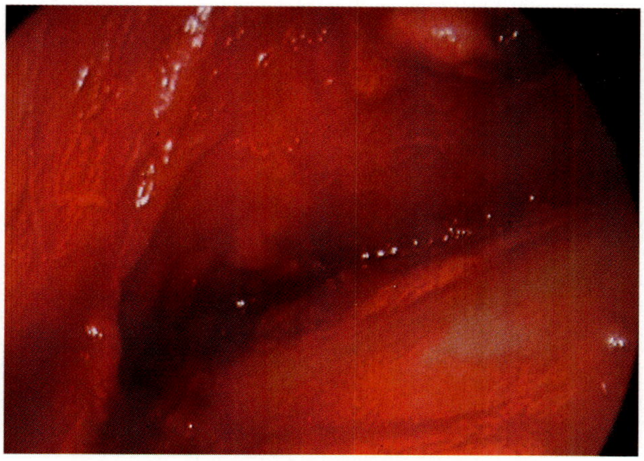

FIG. 9.11. View of lateral orbital rim fully dissected, as pictured through the endoscope.

A 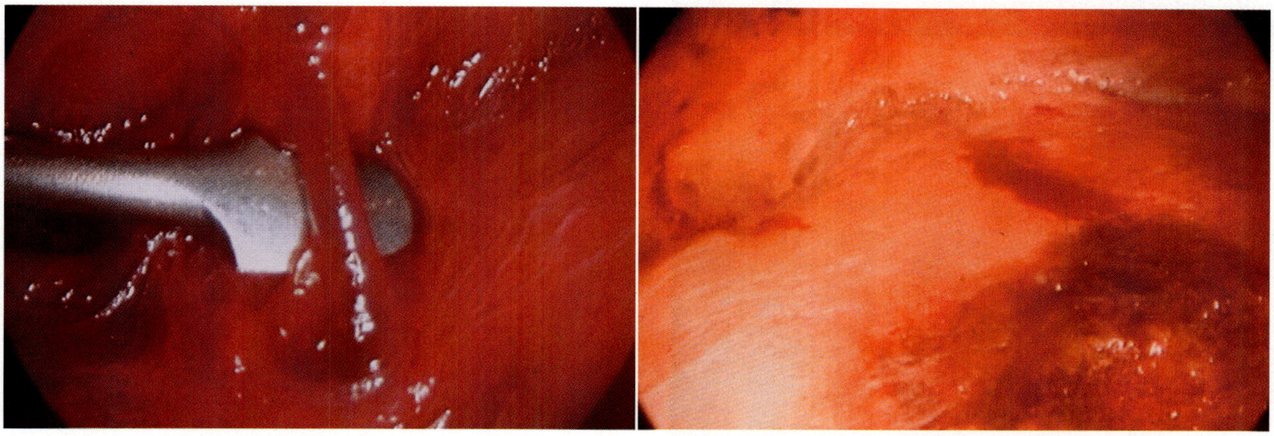 B

FIG. 9.12. **A,** Several small zygomaticotemporal veins will be encountered during temporal dissection. They can easily be cauterized using a bipolar cautery. **B,** Fat pad that has been elevated is the superficial temporal fat pad investing the temporoparietal fascia. The fat pad noted below is the intermediate fat pad covered by the superficial division of the deep temporal fascia. The frontal division of cranial nerve VII lies within the superficial temporal fat pad.

The endoscope is used for the rest of the temporal dissection. The fascial attachments to the forehead component of the temporal line are sharply severed under endoscopic control from lateral to medial; the blade is pointed toward the frontal bone. The inferior medial part is then dissected under endoscopic control down to, but not through, the zygomatic arch. The dissection is then carried medially, where it is connected to the subperiosteal dissection of the lateral orbital rim (Figure 9.11). This step is key because it provides the release needed to satisfactorily pull the lateral brow and improve lateral hooding. Again, the lateral dissection should be done sharply from lateral to medial, with the surgeon keeping the blade pointing toward the lateral orbital rim. Several small, lateral zygomaticotemporal veins are normally dissected, cauterized, and transected. The surgeon also will note the superficial temporal fascia investing the superficial temporal fat during this dissection. This fat envelops the frontal nerve and must be elevated to avoid injury to the nerve. Care must be taken in this area to elevate all of the tissue superficial to the deep temporal fascia (Figure 9.12). All cauterization should be done with the vessel fully dissected and the insulated alligator forceps held toward the deep temporal fascia.

The endoscope is then used to complete the supraorbital ridge dissection around the supraorbital nerve (Figure 9.13). The supraorbital and supratrochlear nerves are terminal sensory branches of the ophthalmic branch of the trigeminal nerve VI. This nerve enters the orbit via the superior orbital fissure, with the frontal branch then dividing into the above-named nerves. These nerves remain extraperiosteal throughout their course so that by staying subperiosteal during the dissection, the surgeon is simply dissecting the nerves inferiorly. The surgeon must be careful, however, because approximately 20% of the time the nerve enters the forehead via a foramen (Figure 9.14). Once the supraorbital nerve is reflected, the orbital rim is dissected from Whitnall's tubercle to the nasion under endoscopic control.

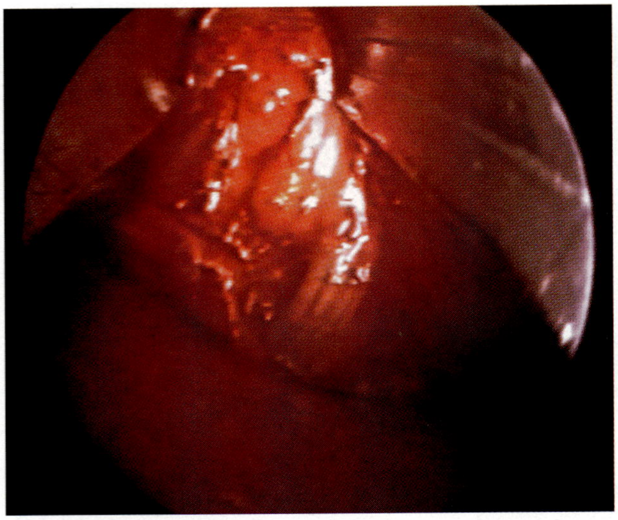

FIG. 9.13. Endoscopic view of supraorbital nerve reflected below supraorbital rim. This occurs in approximately 80% of patients.

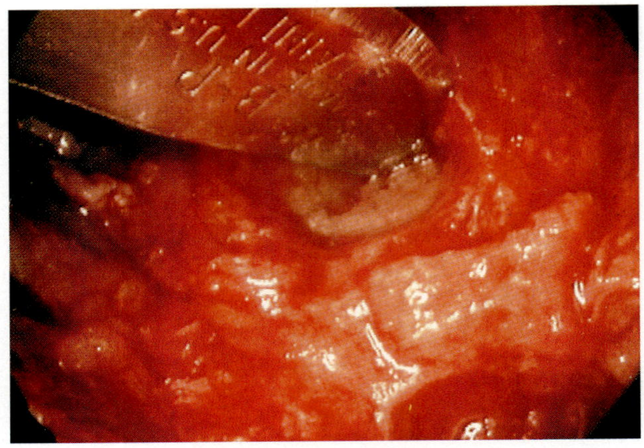

FIG. 9.15. Endoscopic view of the periorbital release. Release is done at or below the level of the brow from the supraorbital nerve to Whitnall's tubercle and is done through the periosteum as well as the periorbital fascia until one sees the fat layer (the retro-orbicularis oculi fat [ROOF]) immediately beneath the orbicularis oculi.

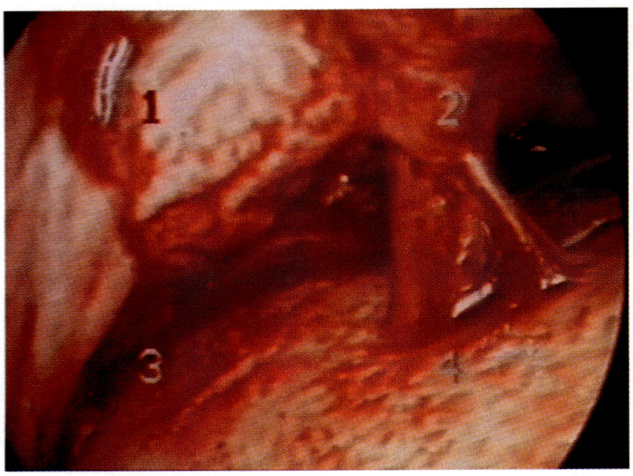

FIG. 9.14. Endoscopic view of supraorbital nerve entering the forehead via a foramen. This occurs in approximately 20% of patients.

The periorbita immediately inferior to the eyebrow is then separated with an alligator forceps, and the separation points are connected sharply under endoscopic control; the surgeon is careful not to injure the branches of trigeminal nerve VI. As long as this procedure is done at or immediately below the level of the brow, the frontal nerve should be untouched (Figure 9.15). Using a nerve hook to protect the supraorbital nerve, the corrugator, procerus, and depressor supercilii muscles are debulked using an insulated alligator forceps and cautery, scissors, or a CO_2 laser.

When a midface suspension is being performed, the brow suspension is done last. The two procedures will be discussed in that order here. Before brow suspension and fixation is done, a Penrose drain may be inserted. The midbrow is suspended first. From the preoperative estimate, 10% is added to the number of millimeters of lift desired on each side. A 1.5-mm diameter drill hole is made that many millimeters superior to the initial mark made in the frontal bone at the beginning of the procedure to a depth of 4 mm. A 2.0-mm diameter, 4.0-mm long screw is partially inserted into the hole. A 2-0 PDS is tied from the periosteum at the inferior edge of the medial incision to around the screw, lifted, and tied. The screw is then tightened (Figure 9.16). For patients who desire a high arch at the level of the lateral canthus, a similar procedure will need to be followed via the middle forehead incision.

Lateral suspension is then performed with a 2-0 Prolene suture. I believe that it would be difficult to oversuspend the lateral brow. With this in mind, the suture is run in a figure-eight fashion from the temporoparietal fascia medial from the lateral temporal incision to the deep temporal fascia, with a mainly posterior yet slightly superior pull as far as technically feasible. The temporoparietal fascia used should be just medial to the temporal incision and within the hairline to prevent notching of the skin. The superior level of the lateral brow can be altered by observing what effects different degrees of superior pull have on brow position and then placing the vector accordingly. The skin is then closed appropriately, and a face-lift-type dressing is applied. During this procedure, the surgeon ensures that pressure is applied from the nuchal line to the supraorbital ridge.

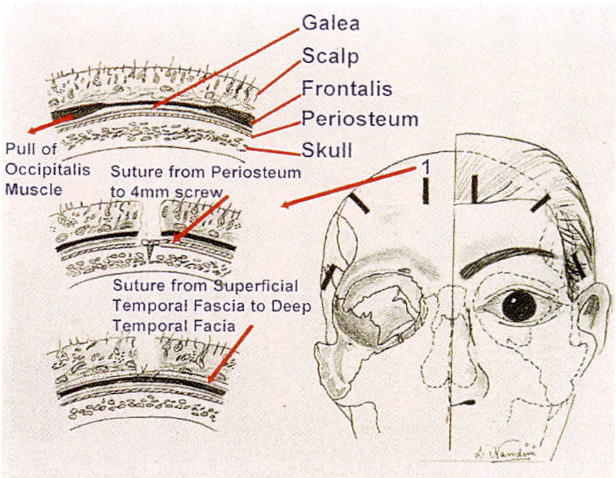

FIG. 9.16. Suture fixation of midbrow involves lifting the periosteum directly above the head of the brow to the screw fixed at a predetermined point above the notch made at the start of the periosteal dissection. Similar fixation can be done via the middle incision to yield a high arched brow. Lateral lift for the majority of patients can be adequately obtained via suture suspension of the temporoparietal fascia to the deep temporal fascia.

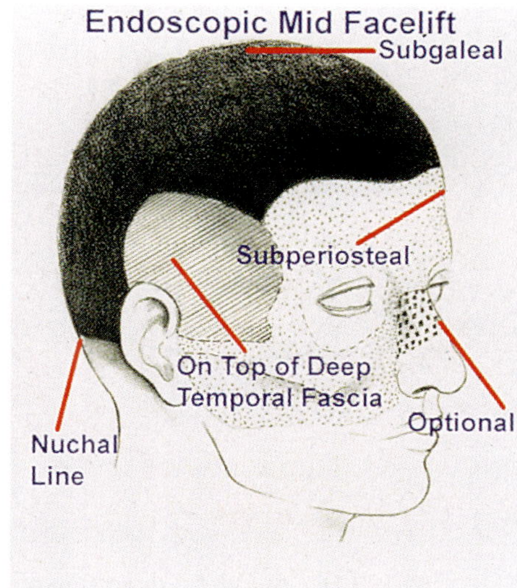

FIG. 9.17. Schematic showing dissection planes for the endoscopic subperiosteal midface lift.

Endoscopic Subperiosteal Midface Lift

This procedure is started following completion of the brow dissection but before brow suspension. A skin-muscle flap is dissected, preserving the orbicularis sling over the tarsal thickening. Subperiosteal dissection of the orbital rim and zygomatic arch is performed (Figure 9.17). To prevent injury to the frontal nerve, the periosteal elevator is brought over the superior edge of the zygomatic arch and then, under endoscopic control, the elevator is pushed into the previously dissected pocket over the deep temporal fascia (Figure 9.18). The surgeon should endeavor to stay out of the pocket between the intermediate deep temporal fascia and the deep temporal fascia where the intermediate fat pad resides. If the intermediate fat pad is elevated out of its pocket it can atrophy, which results in a depression in this area.

A Caldwell-Luc incision is then made, and the maxilla is dissected, with preservation of the infraorbital nerve. Dissection is carried out laterally over the masseter muscle. All dissected areas should connect.

The midface suspension suture is placed in the lateral malar pad just medial to the area of insertion of the zygomaticus major muscle. The suspension suture is carried over the zygomatic arch and secured to the deep temporal fascia. The right and left suspension sutures are secured at the same time; the surgeon should be careful to avoid asymmetry and pleating of the skin.

The skin-muscle flap is then redraped, trimmed, and closed appropriately. The Caldwell-Luc incision is closed. Brow suspension is carried out as previously described. A routine face-lift dressing is applied, with the surgeon being careful to apply pressure in back of the nuchal line. The patient should receive intraoperative IV antibiotics as well as postoperative oral antibiotics.

Endoscopic Malar Pad Lift

When performed by itself or in conjunction with an endoscopic browplasty, an incision in a lateral wrinkle line will be required (a crow's-foot). Dissection is carried down through the orbicularis (Figure 9.19). The orbicularis oculi is then retracted, and dissection is carried out underneath this muscle until the head of the zygomaticus major muscle is identified at its attachment to the malar eminence (Figure 9.20). Recall the spatial anatomy in this area: the orbicularis oculi overlies the zygomaticus major muscle, and the buccal branch of the facial nerve comes in underneath the zygomaticus major muscle (Figure 9.21). Being careful to stay superficial to the fascial layer investing the zygomaticus, the head is dissected to the point that a finger can be inserted. The endoscope is useful in identifying the zygomaticus muscle. Confirmation that you are looking at the zygomaticus can be made by observing contraction of the muscle when the patient smiles.

Using a combination of finger dissection and endoscopic controlled blunt dissection, the surgeon creates a pocket between the underlying zygomaticus muscle and the overlying fascia fat and skin. The direction of the dissection is parallel to the zygo-

A

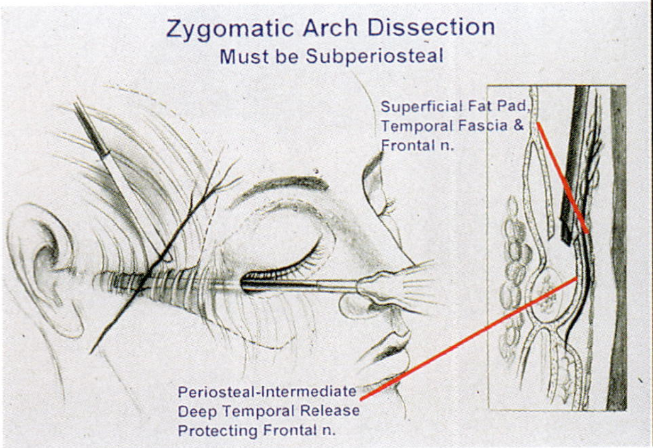

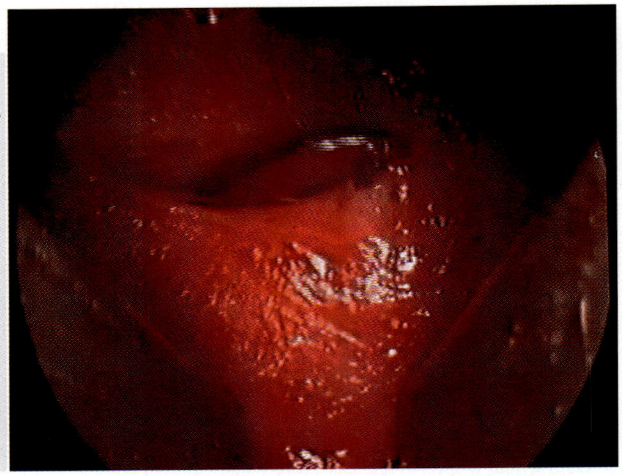

B

FIG. 9.18. **A,** Careful dissection of the zygomatic arch must be performed to prevent injury to the frontal branch of the facial nerve, which is protected from injury only by the periosteum. **B,** Endoscopic view of the periosteal elevator connecting from the zygomatic arch to the temporal pocket on top of the deep temporal fascia.

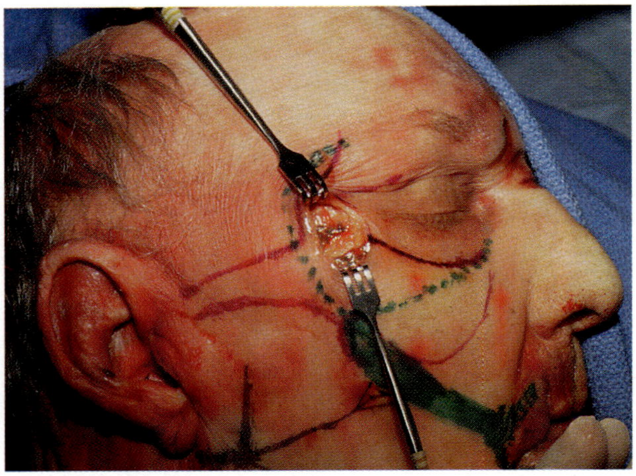

FIG. 9.19. Incision has been made through orbicularis oculi muscle (colored green). The zygomatic muscle has been drawn on the skin in green, and the outline of the zygoma has been drawn in purple. The buccal branch has been drawn in blue.

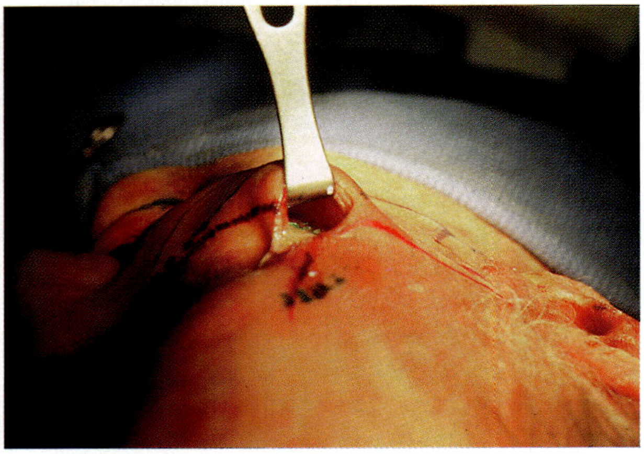

FIG. 9.20. Dissection is carried out underneath the orbicularis oculi muscle toward the previously marked zygomaticus muscle until the head of the muscle is identified (colored green).

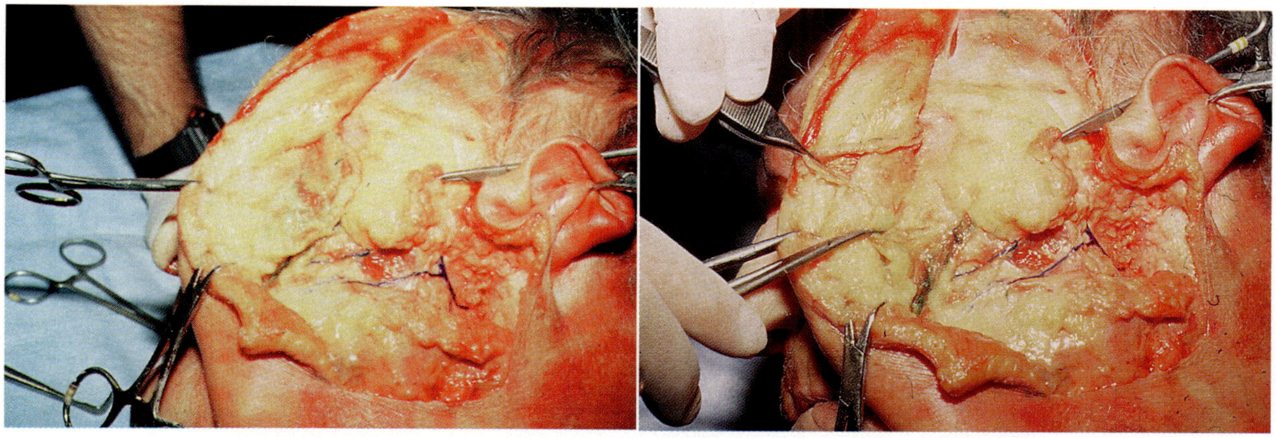

FIG. 9.21. **A,** The circular-shaped orbicularis oculi muscle can be seen overlying the zygomaticus muscle. The parotid has been split, and the facial nerve outlined in blue. **B,** The orbicularis oculi muscle has been elevated, revealing the zygomaticus muscle (colored green). The buccal nerve can be seen penetrating underneath the muscle.

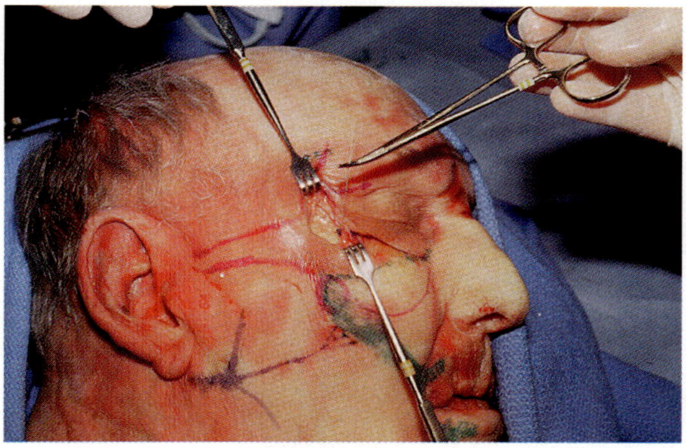

FIG. 9.22. Suture fixated to periosteum and fibrous tissue lateral to orbital rim when procedure is done by itself. When accomplished with a face-lift and/or a browplasty the fixation suture is passed to the deep temporal fascia.

maticus or toward the commissura labiorum. The depth of the dissection proceeds from deep on top of the fibromuscular layer of the zygomaticus to superficial, and the dissection ends before crossing the melolabial line. At this point, the fibrofatty malar pad is identified just medial to the dissection pocket, and 4-0 clear Prolene is used to suture the malar pad in a superior-lateral direction. When the endoscopic malar pad lift procedure is done by itself, the suture is secured to the periosteum lateral to the orbital rim (Figure 9.22). When the endoscopic malar pad lift procedure is done with an endoscopic browplasty, the suture is secured to the deep temporal fascia. This suture is passed from the temporal dissection to the midface dissection via a clamp that can be safely punched through from the temporal dissection side on top of the lateral orbital rim. The malar pad lift should be done before the actual browlift is done.

The surgeon must be careful about the level at which the malar pad is suture-fixated. A suture secured in a superficial plane may produce an indentation of the epidermis, whereas a suture fixated at the level of or through some of the fibers of the zygomaticus may actually deepen the fold while at the same time elevating the commissure of the lips. It is not infrequent to have to repeatedly suture-fixate the malar pad before an adequate lift is obtained.

POSTOPERATIVE CARE

No matter which procedure is done, if an endoscopic browplasty is included, then the postoperative care is basically the same. On day 1, the dressing is removed, and a 3-inch elastic dressing is applied. The dressing is removed on the third to fourth postoperative day, and the patient may then wash his or her hair. The patient is instructed to wear a 3-inch-wide elastic headband at home (and at night) for the next 10 days. For patients who have an endoscopic malar pad lift without another procedure, no special dressings are needed.

Text continued on p. 129.

A B C D

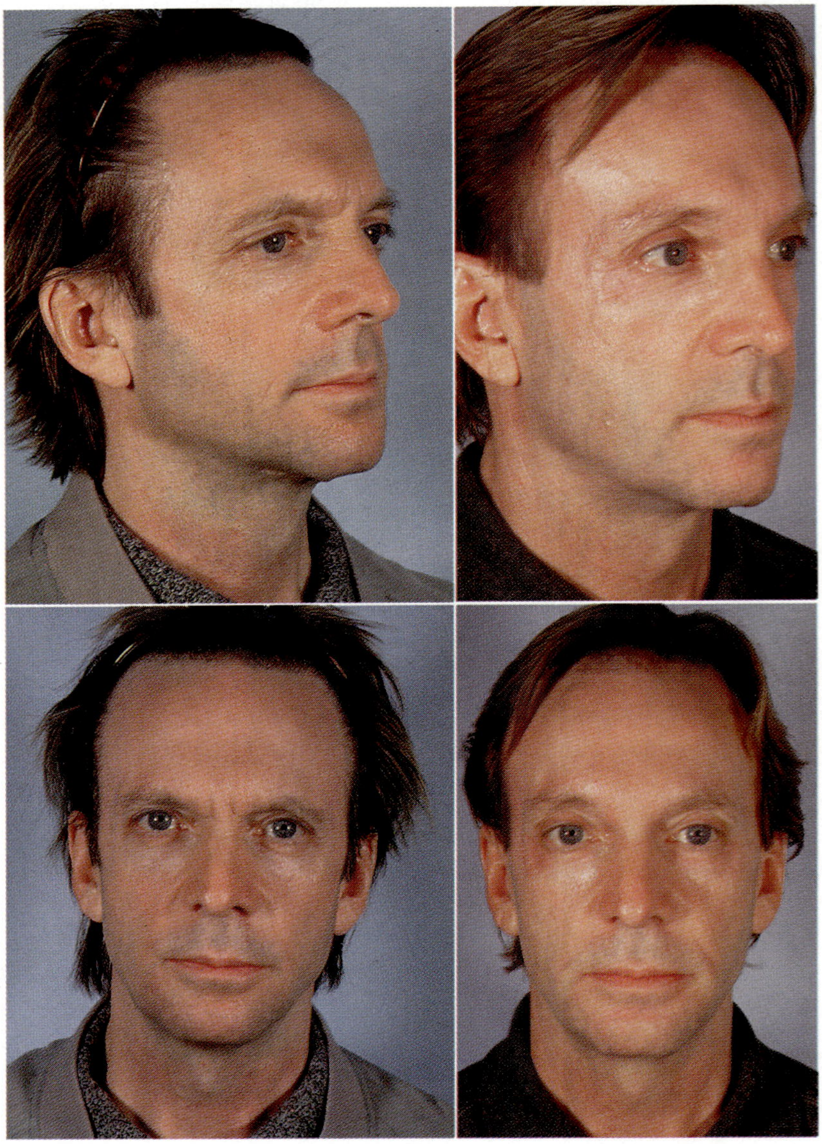

FIG. 9.23. **A, C,** Male patient preoperatively. **B, D,** Six-month result from endoscopic browplasty. Note difficulty in finding scars.

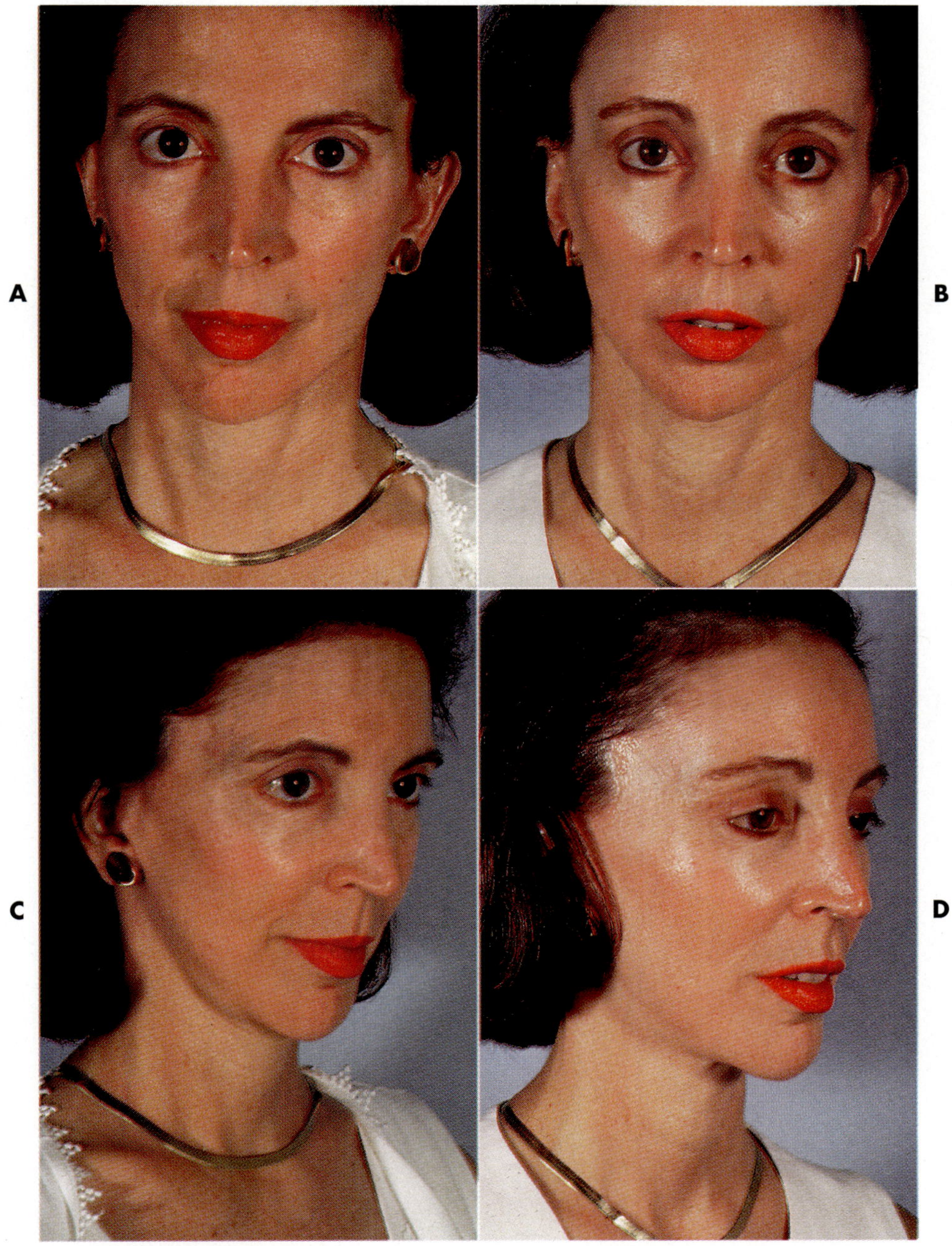

FIG. 9.24. **A, C,** Female patient who had undergone previous coronal lift 1 year previously at another facility and was unhappy with result. **B, D,** Six-month result from endoscopic subperiosteal browplasty.

A B C D

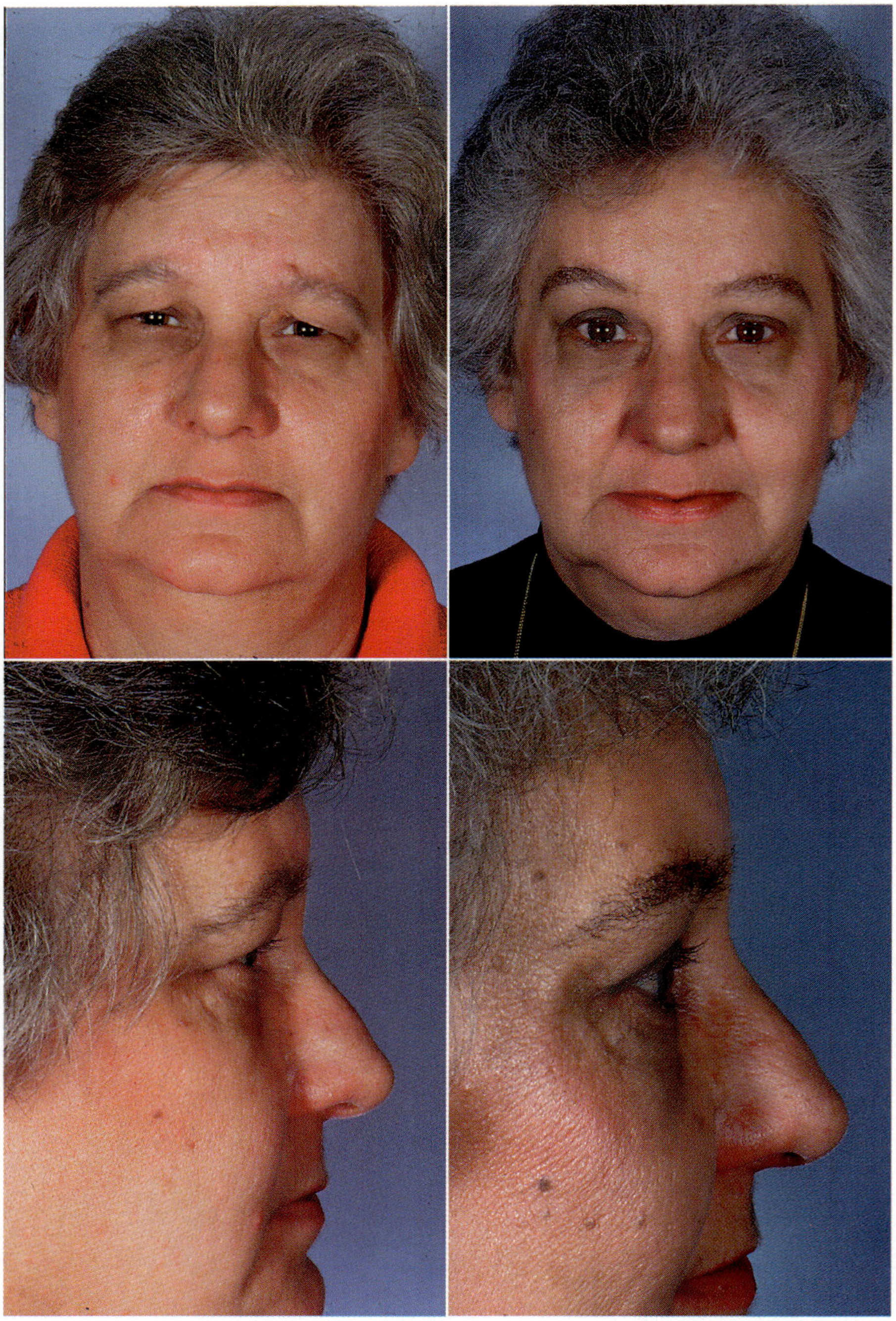

FIG. 9.25. **A, C,** Patient with significant brow ptosis. **B, D,** Patient following functional endoscopic subperiosteal browplasty. Note good improvement in lateral hooding.

A,B

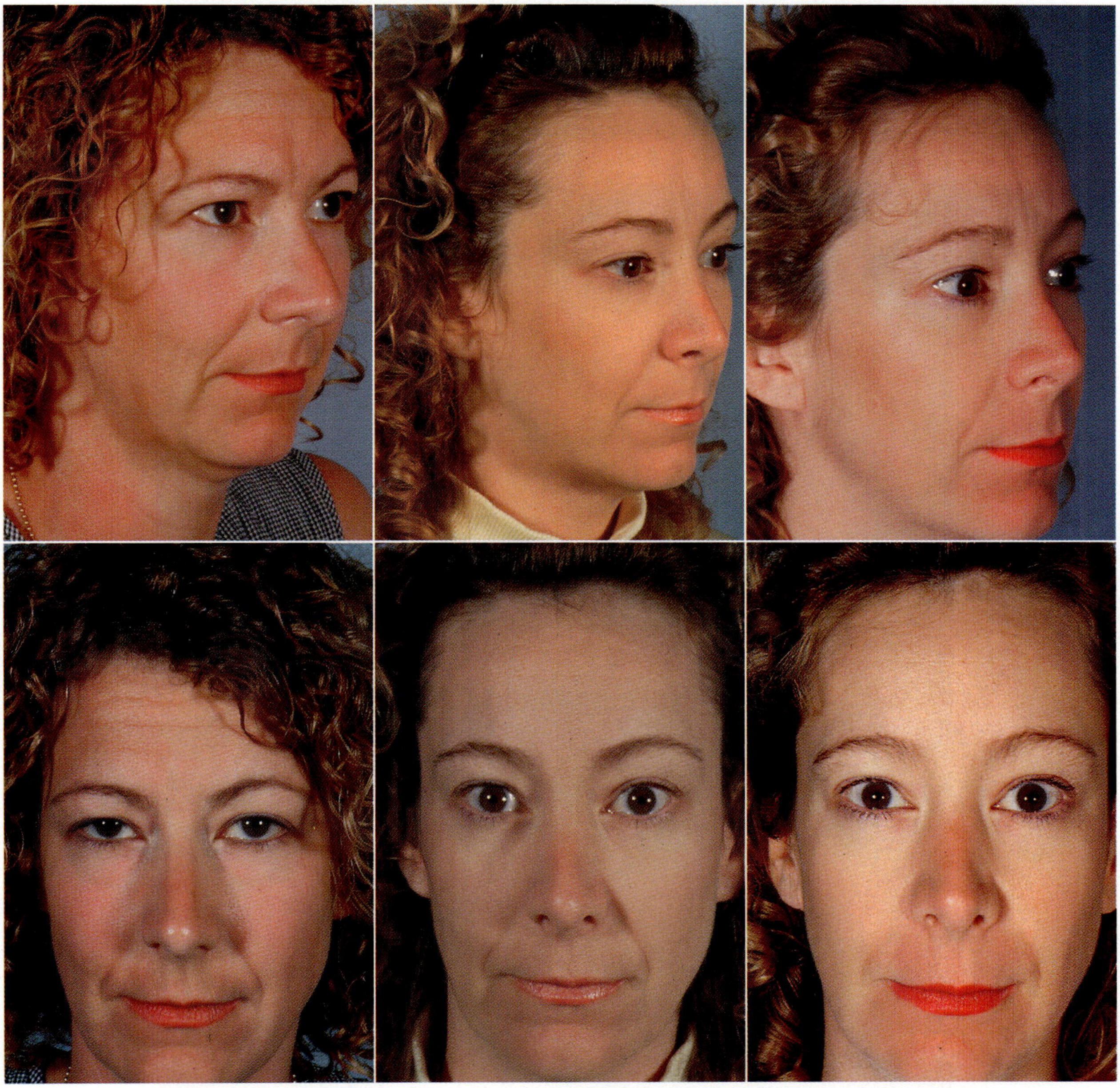

C

D,E

F

FIG. 9.26. **A, D,** Young patient with significant brow ptosis who underwent endoscopic subperiosteal browplasty and rhinoplasty as well as subconjunctival blepharoplasty. Note good maintenance of brow position at 1- (**B, E**) and 2- (**C, F**) year postoperative visits.

A B C D

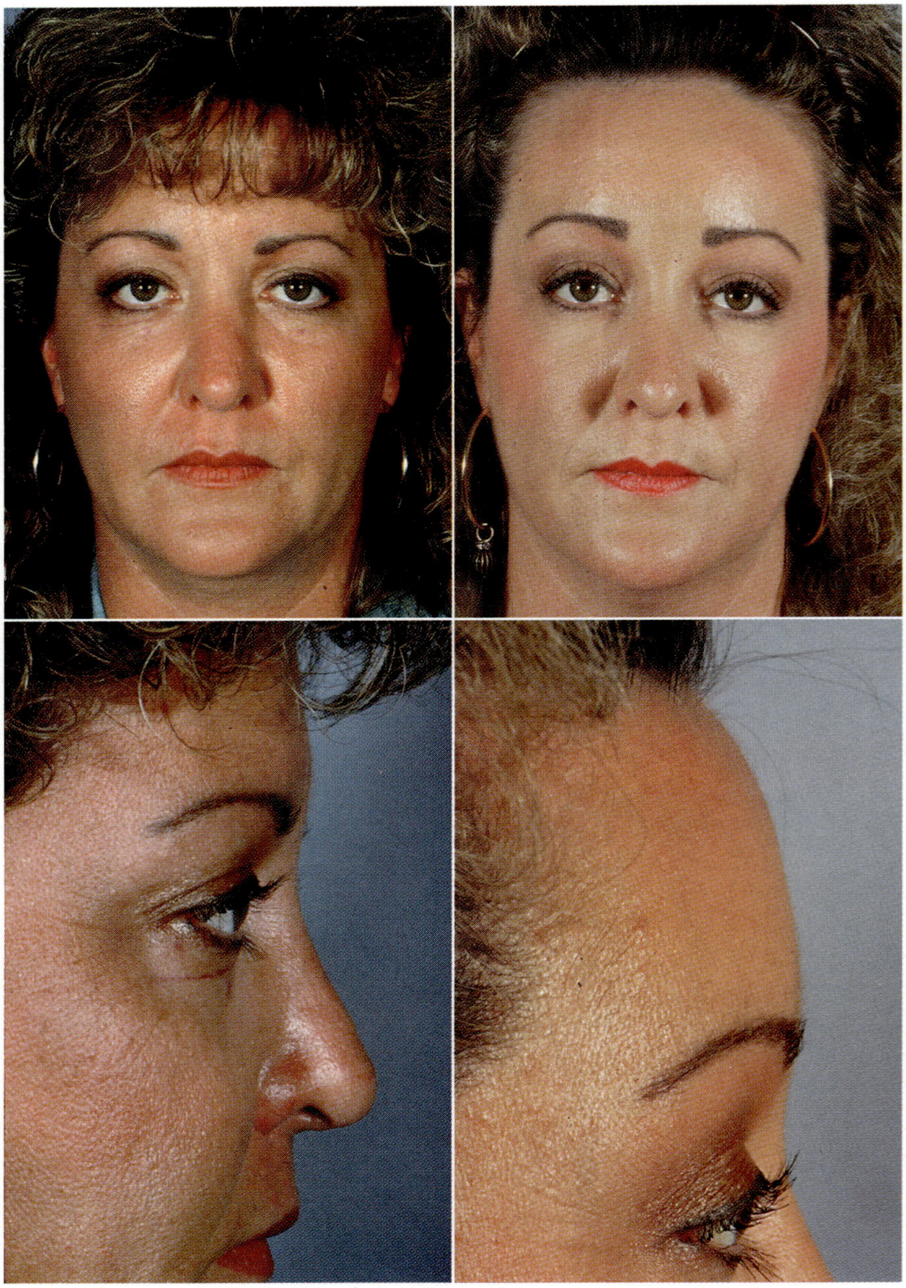

FIG. 9.27. A, C, Patient preoperatively. **B, D,** Patient 1 year following endoscopic subperiosteal browplasty. Note good maintenance of improvement in lateral hooding.

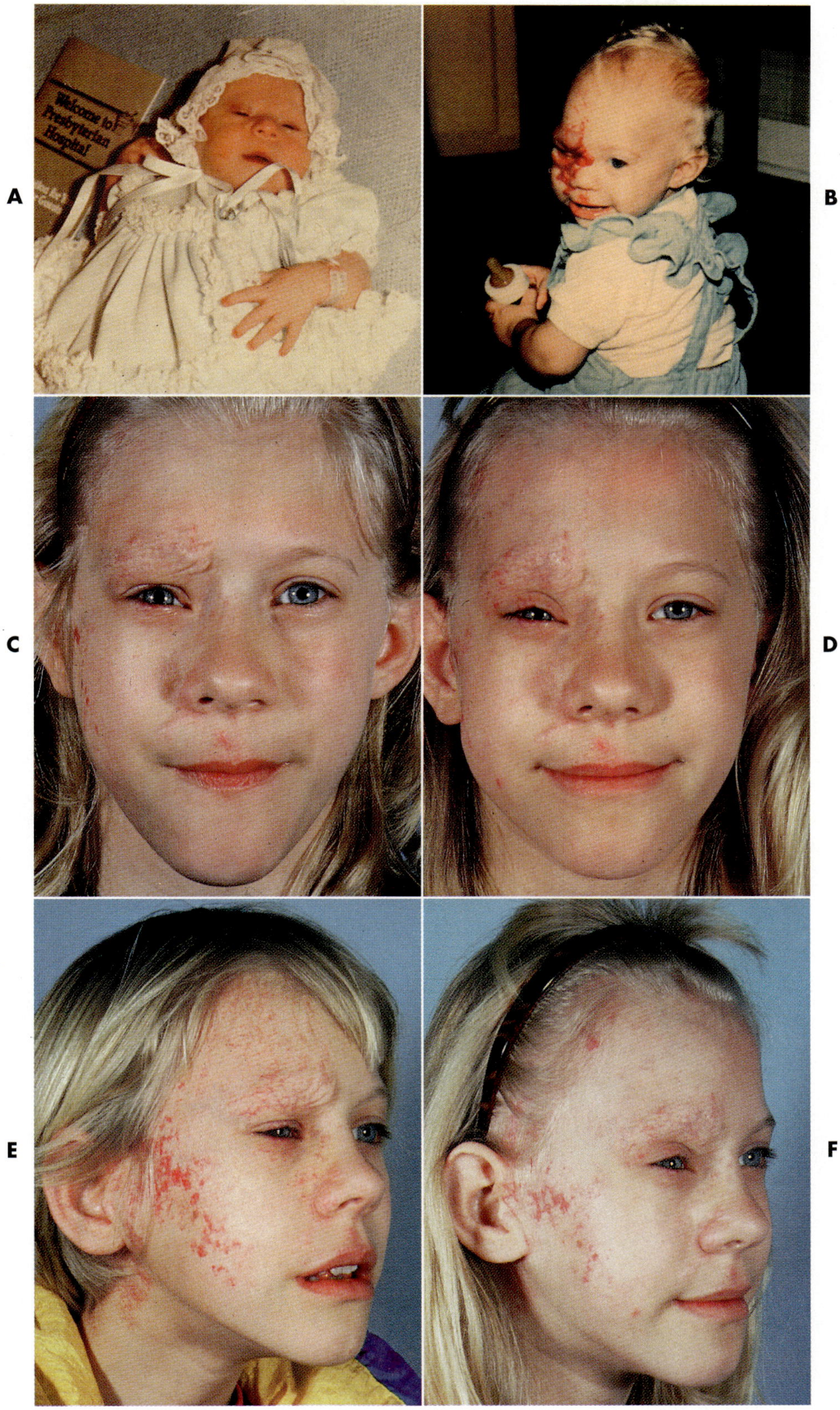

FIG. 9.28. **A, B,** Patient born with congenital vascular lesion classified as transcutaneous hemangioma, which left her with redundant brow skin. Patient underwent unilateral endoscopic subgaleal browplasty, which smoothed the redundant skin. **C, E,** Preoperative. **D, F,** Postoperative.

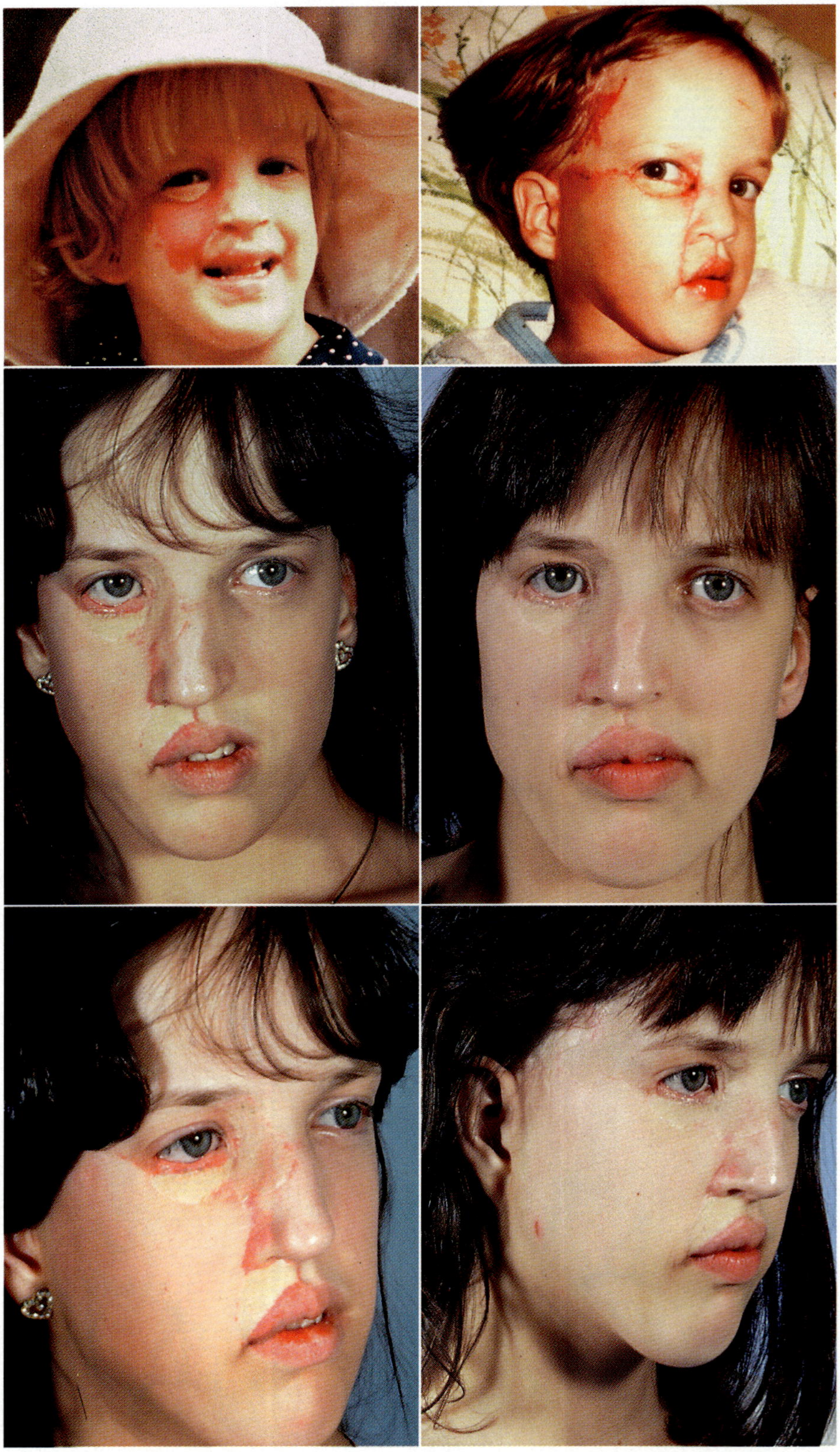

FIG. 9.29. **A, B,** Patient born with congenital vascular lesion classified as a venular malformation. Surgeon performed serial excision as well as full-thickness skin graft to lower lid at another institution resulting in cicatricial hemifacial deformity. **C, E,** Preoperative views. **D, F,** A unilateral subperiosteal midface lift was achieved, which provided good mass movement of tissue and improvement in her facial distortion.

DISCUSSION

Since learning the endoscopic subperiosteal browplasty, I have found that, for all intents and purposes, it has replaced the incisional browplasty. The results have been good to exceptional in my series of more than 80 patients dating from June 1993 through September 1995 (Figures 9.23 to 9.25). For those patients who are followed for more than 1 year, good resiliency has been noted (Figures 9.26 and 9.27). After trying both the subperiosteal and subgaleal approach to browplasty, I believe the former is superior for the majority of cosmetic patients, although at times the subgaleal approach may be useful (Figure 9.28). The subperiosteal approach is faster because there is less blood loss, which results in less time needed to clean the endoscope. The main reason this approach is better for cosmetic browplasty is because of the stiffness of the periosteum relative to the galea. In my experience, this gives a more predictable elevation of the brow and a ratio close to 1 between hairline elevation and brow elevation.

The endoscopic subperiosteal midface lift has in general been replaced by the endoscopic malar pad lift for most cosmetic patients because of the ability of the malar pad lift to reduce the nasolabial fold. There are, however, some patients who remain candidates for the subperiosteal approach (Figure 9.29), and I would consider this approach as an option for a cosmetic patient who is a heavy smoker, has redundancy of the lower eyelid skin, or has complaints of a downturned corner of the mouth, as long as the patient understands that the nasolabial fold will not be significantly improved (Figure 9.30).

I developed the endoscopic malar pad lift to selectively improve the nasolabial fold either by itself, in conjunction with an endoscopic subperiosteal brow lift, and/or with a face-lift. The main disadvantage of this approach is the need for a lateral orbital incision when this procedure is performed by itself or in combination with a browplasty. This problem has been largely overcome by counseling patients at their initial visit that they will require a laserbrasion 6 weeks to 2 months postoperatively to blend in the incision and tighten the lower lid skin (Figure 9.31).

The versatility of the approach has been an advantage and will allow the physician to offer segmental rejuvenation to the patient. When done alone, swelling lateral to the orbit can be anticipated for 4 to 6 weeks. This problem has been relatively well

Text continued on p. 136.

A

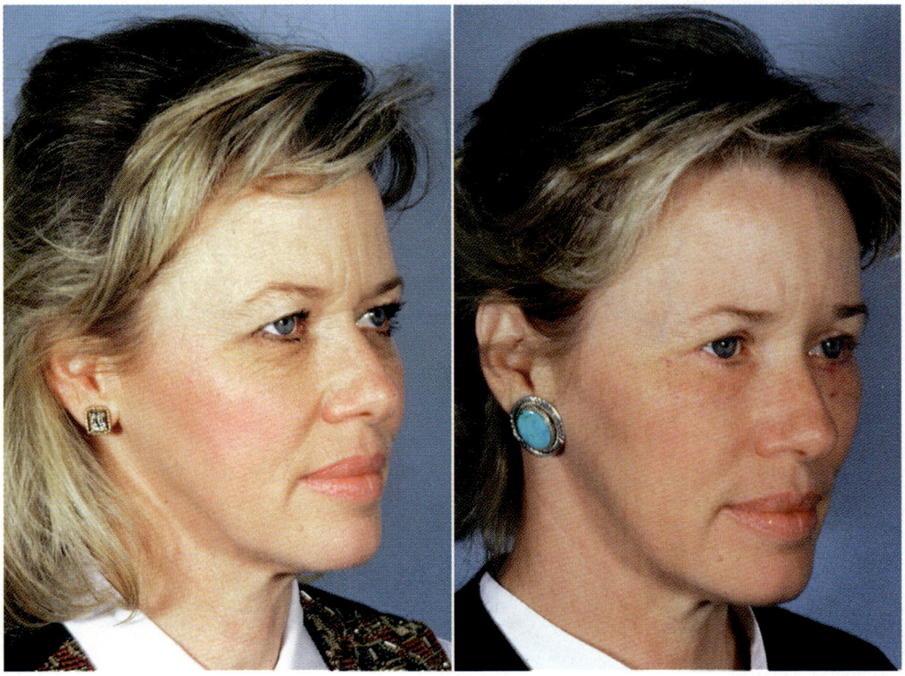

B

FIG. 9.30. **A,** Patient before a subperiosteal midface lift. **B,** Note good improvement in overall rested appearance after 1 year, but little improvement in the appearance of the nasolabial fold.

A B C

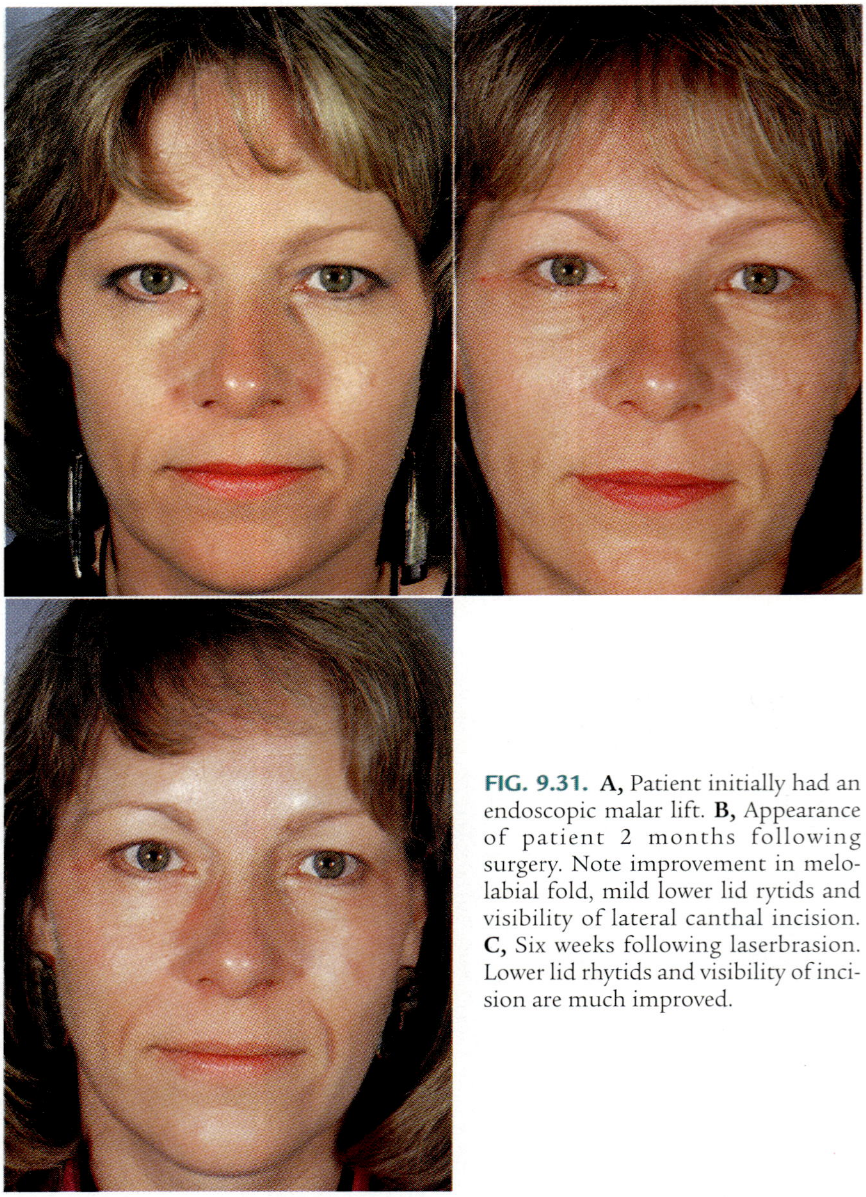

FIG. 9.31. **A,** Patient initially had an endoscopic malar lift. **B,** Appearance of patient 2 months following surgery. Note improvement in melolabial fold, mild lower lid rytids and visibility of lateral canthal incision. **C,** Six weeks following laserbrasion. Lower lid rhytids and visibility of incision are much improved.

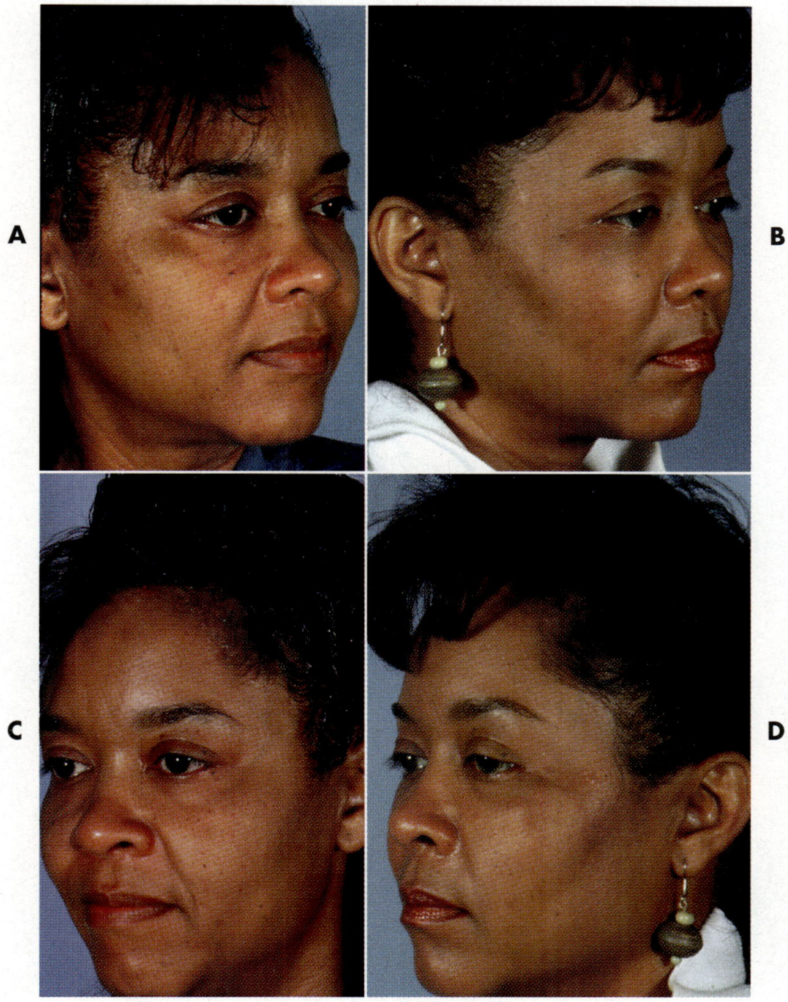

FIG. 9.32. **A, C,** Preoperative appearance. **B, D,** Patient 6 months following an endoscopic malar pad lift, with good improvement in the position of her malar pad and the depth of her nasolabial fold.

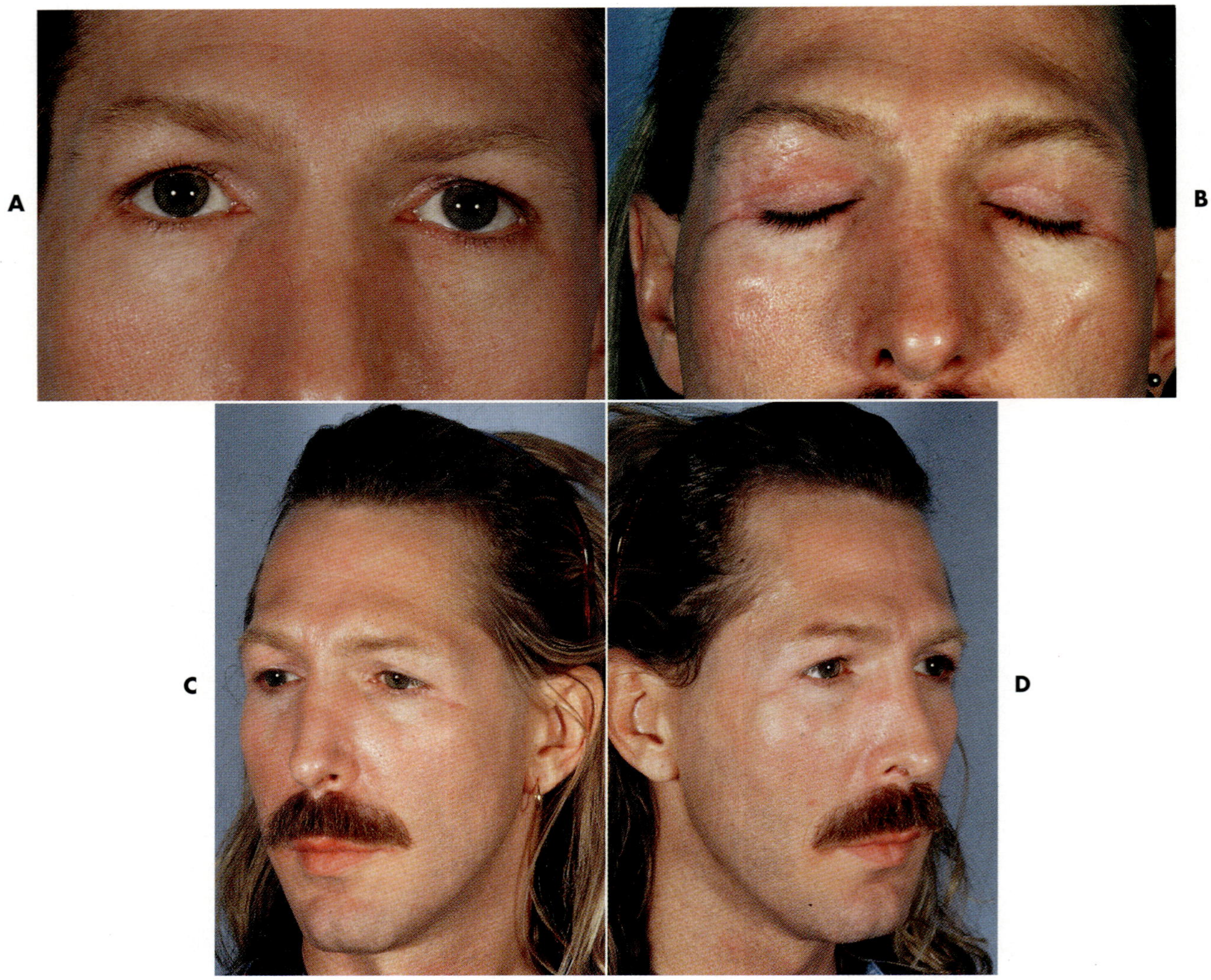

FIG. 9.33. **A,** Preoperative picture shows an ectomorphic man with little to no malar pad or nasolabial fold. Patients with this finding are not good candidates for this procedure; this was an early case. **B,** After the procedure, dimpling of the skin was noted. **C, D,** Subcutaneous undermining in the area of the pleat reversed this problem.

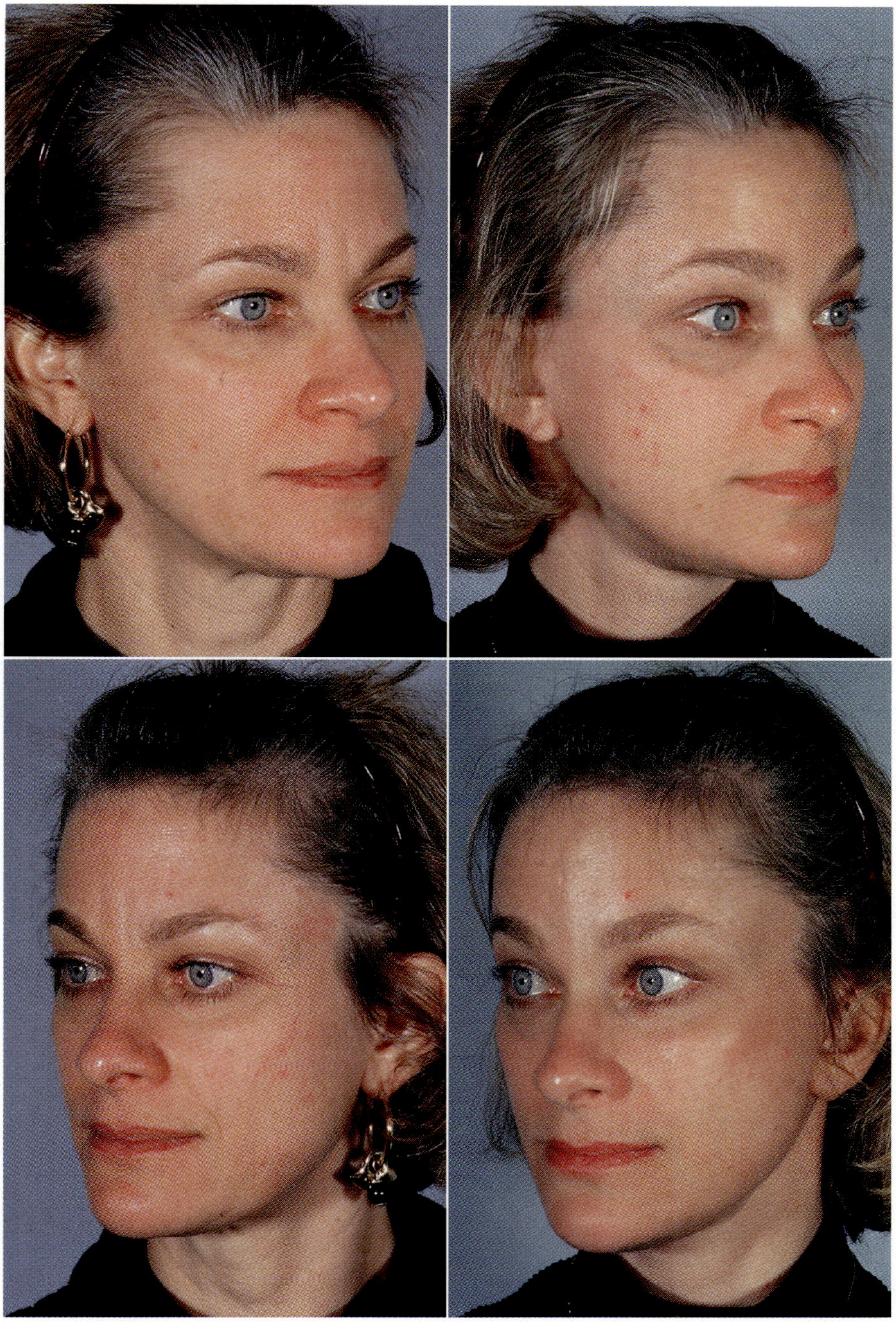

A B C D

FIG. 9.34. **A, C,** Preoperative appearance. **B, D,** Patient 6 months following an endoscopic subperiosteal browplasty with an endoscopic malar pad lift. Note progress in the position of the malar pad as well as the pitch of the nasolabial fold.

A B C D

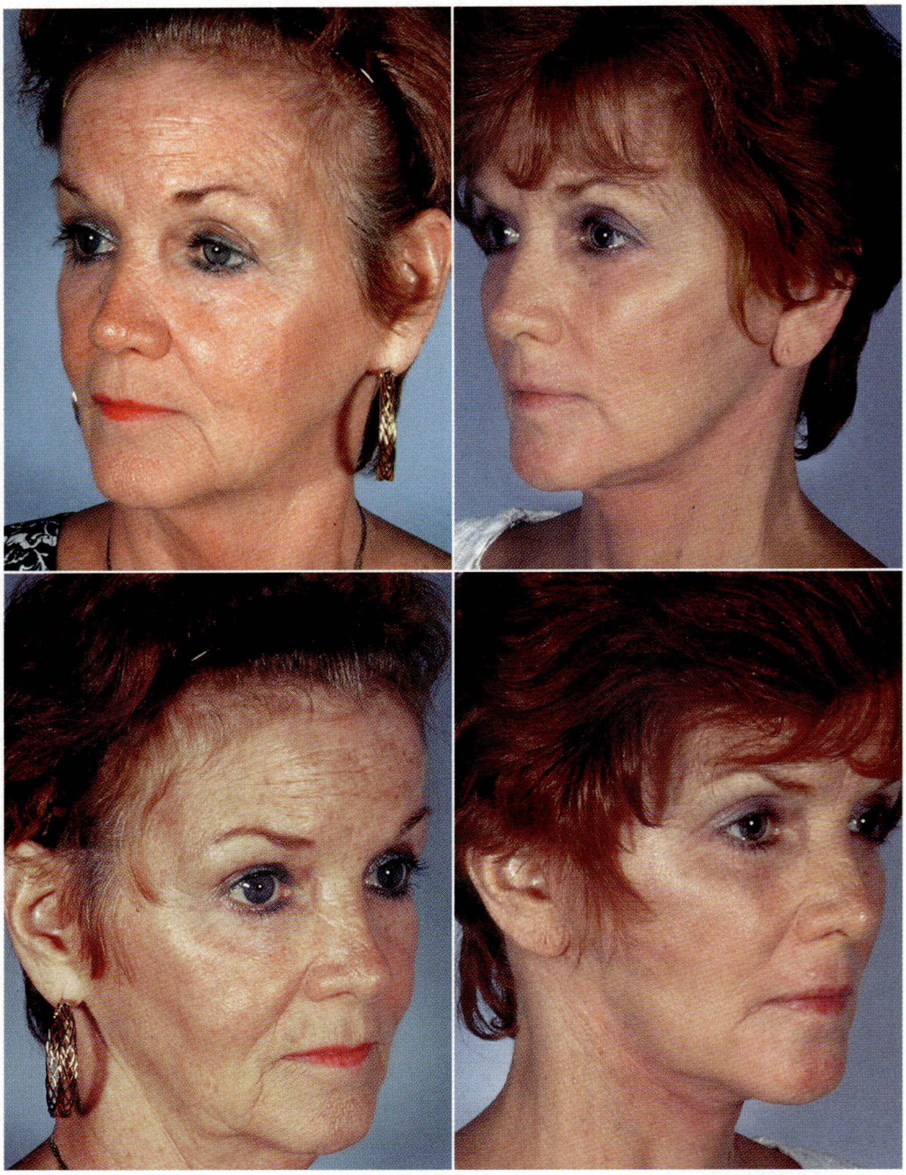

FIG. 9.35. **A, C,** Preoperative appearance. **B, D,** Patient 6 months following a face-lift with an endoscopic malar pad lift. Note good improvement in the position of the malar pad as well as the depth of the nasolabial fold.

A B C D

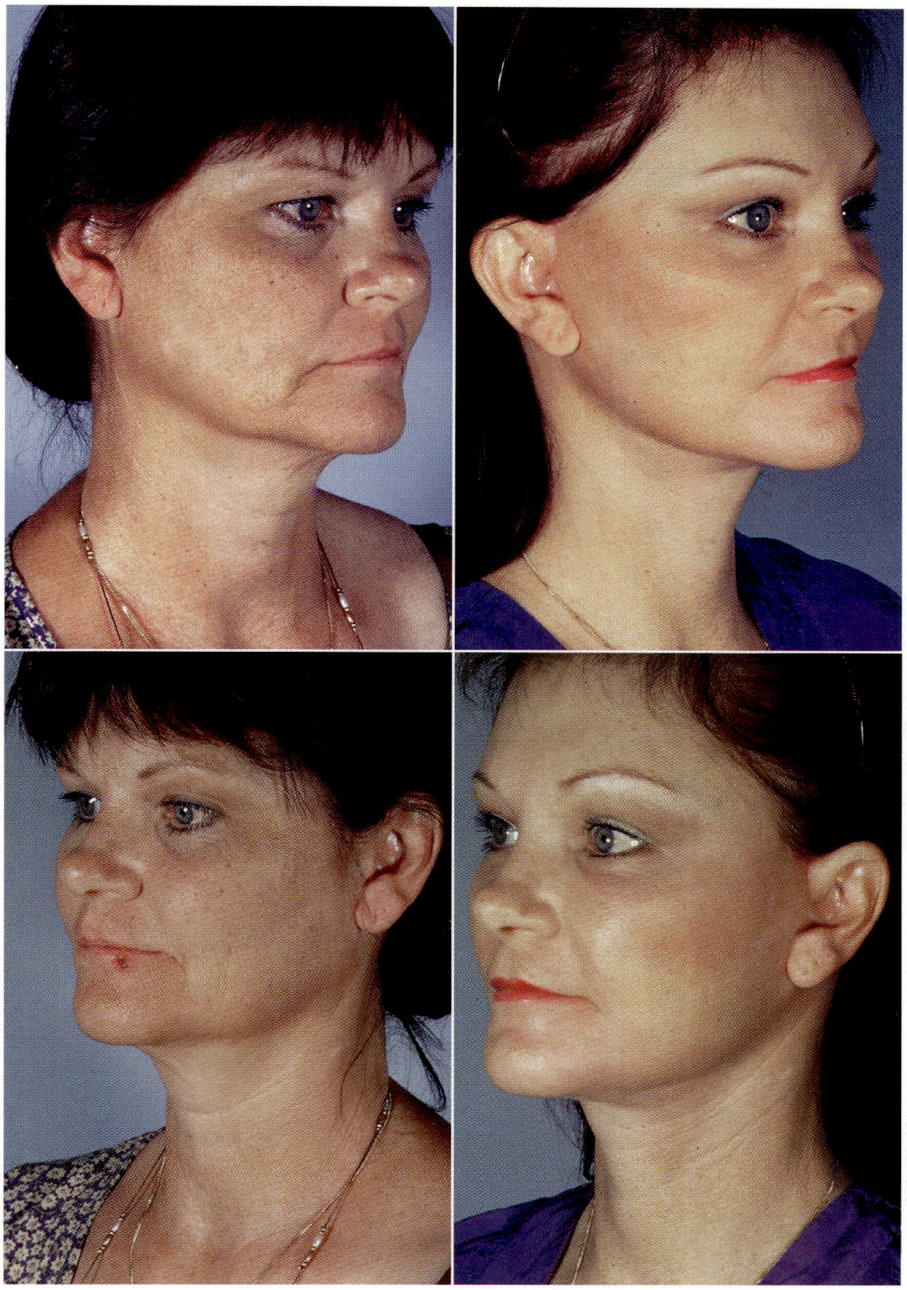

FIG. 9.36. **A, C,** Preoperative appearance. **B, D,** Patient 6 months following an endoscopic subperiosteal browplasty, an endoscopic malar pad lift, and a face-lift. Note that this patient had four point fixation of her brow to enable the surgeon to provide a higher arch to her lateral brow. Note improvement in her nasolabial fold and position of her malar pad.

accepted in the informed and motivated patient. The results have been good (Figure 9.32), and patient satisfaction has been high. In my series of patients who have undergone this approach, one of the initial patients had persistent dimpling of the skin that required reversal of the lift (Figure 9.33). This patient was felt to be ectomorphic to the point that his malar pad was effectively nonexistent. Careful patient selection has eliminated this problem. Patients who fit into this category may be better suited to a malar or submalar augmentation and/or a deep plane or composite face-lift.

The majority of patients have had an endoscopic malar pad lift applied either with an endoscopic browplasty, face-lift, or both (Figures 9.34, 9.35, and 9.36). Results have been gratifying. There have been no cases of postoperative facial nerve paralysis noted, although two cases of mild midface dyskinesia have been observed in the more than 30 cases completed, both of which cleared in less than 6 weeks. These two cases were early in the series and were believed to be the result of excessive pressure exerted on the zygomaticus and/or violation of the fibrous sheath of the muscle during the initial dissection. These particular maneuvers have been avoided over the past several months, with good results.

CONCLUSION

Endoscopic browplasty using a subperiosteal approach has supplanted incisional browplasty in the majority of cosmetic patients. The endoscopic subperiosteal midface lift is a procedure that in my opinion has limited applications but does provide for good soft-tissue repositioning for patients who have cicatricial deformities. The endoscopic malar pad lift has many advantages, and initial results are encouraging. In the future, techniques such as this may become more commonplace in the quest to find procedures that offer good, reliable results with minimal chance of significant morbidity and result in segmental targeted facial rejuvenation.

REFERENCES

1. Ramirez OM, Maillard GF, and Musolas A: The extended subperiosteal face-lift: A definitive soft tissue remodeling for facial rejuvenation, Plast Reconstr Surg 88:227, 1991.
2. Del Campo AF: Face-lift without preauricular scars, Plast Reconstr Surg 92:642, 1993.
3. Ramirez OM: Endoscopic full face-lift, Aesthetic Plast Surg 18(14):363, 1994.
4. Owsley JQ: Lifting the malar fat pad for correction of prominent nasolabial folds, Plast Reconstr Surg 91:463, 1993.
5. Riefkohl R, Kosanin R, and Georgiade GS: Complications of the forehead-brow lift, Aesthetic Plast Surg 7(3):135, 1983.
6. Beeson WH and McCollough EG: Complications of the forehead lift, Ear Nose Throat J 64(12):575, 1985.
7. Rubin LR, Mishriki Y, and Lee G: Anatomy of the nasolabial fold: the keystone of the smiling mechanism, Plast Reconstr Surg 83:1, 1989.
8. Zufferey J: Anatomic variation of the nasolabial fold, Plast Reconstr Surg 89:225, 1992.
9. Wassef M: Superficial facial and muscular layers in the face and neck, Aesthetic Plast Surg 11:171, 1987.

chapter ten

Percutaneous Video-Endoscopic Necklift with Suture Suspension Platysmaplasty

Gregory S. Keller and Julene E. Cray

One of the most common reasons that patients of all ages seek facial cosmetic surgery is for the amelioration of neck sagging. Until relatively recently, the treatment of this condition was limited to submental lipectomy, direct excision of the neck waddle with a variety of closures, and standard rhytidectomy procedures.

Contemporary techniques for reduction of the hanging neck include liposuction, subdermal liposuction, corset platysmaplasty, interlocking mattress suture platysmaplasty, hyoid drop, and platysma incision and/or rotation. Although these procedures are successful and reduce the neck waddle, they have limitations.

New endoscopic techniques, as illustrated in this chapter, provide an opportunity to diminish the size of the incision used in necklifts. Submental incisions may be omitted entirely in the absence of platysmal "bands" and postauricular incisions of less than 2 cm are often possible when endoscopy is part of the surgeon's repertoire. These minimally invasive endoscopic procedures have the advantage of a quick recovery, usually allowing the patient to return to work in 4 or 5 days.

For younger patients who have elastic skin and localized neck lipodystrophies, many surgeons use liposuction. The elastic skin in patients who are younger or who have darker skin will contract to fill the void created by the removed fat.

Although uniformly successful in patients who have isolated lipodystrophies of the submental area as well as elastic skin, liposuction is less reliable as a technique for middle-aged patients with skin of less elasticity, patients of any age with platysma sagging or banding, male patients with heavier skin or beards, and patients with any degree of submaxillary gland ptosis or soft-tissue structure collapse. Removal of the fat from the neck can, at times, accentuate these underlying disorders, because the presence of the fat in the neck had previously camouflaged them.

Subdermal liposuction has been advocated by some surgeons as a method of extending the use of liposuction to older patients. These surgeons rationalize that the injury to the skin caused by the subdermal liposuction causes it to contract sufficiently to duplicate the results seen in younger patients. Other surgeons believe that the results of subdermal liposuction are not predictable (with regard to the degree of skin contraction) and that the underlying problems of soft-tissue and muscle ptosis are not addressed by this procedure.

Although many techniques for tightening the neck's underlying muscle and soft-tissue structures have been advocated, Feldman's[1] corset platysmaplasty was the first to achieve a wide degree of acceptance as an isolated procedure for the fallen neck. By bringing the anterior edges of the two platysma muscles together in the midline with plication or imbrication sutures and removing varying amounts of subplatysmal fat, Feldman fashions the underlying platysma into a "corset," which is laced up in the midline, forcing the neck to come together and, at the same time, to be cinched as reinforcement to the "corset." A degree of inward movement to the submaxillary gland can also be achieved.

Although Feldman's operation represents a major advance, instruments currently available do not allow it to be readily adapted to a video-endoscopic technique. Giampapa's interlocking suture suspension platysmaplasty[2] provides an easier technique for the video-endoscopic surgeon to reliably achieve correction of neck ptosis. Giampapa's procedure uses two crossed interlocking mattress sutures to pull the platysma muscle together and upward (Figure 10.1).

These two sutures, in essence, pull the right platysma toward the left mastoid and the left platysma toward the right mastoid. Because the platysma is sutured in the midline at a relatively inferior position (the desired break point of the neck) and posteriorly in a more superior position (the mastoid eminence), the suture suspension platysmaplasty not only pulls the platysma muscles together in the midline, but also pulls the anterior neck upward and defines the angle of the neck at the break point. The submaxillary gland and other soft tissues are also pushed inward, defining the mandible from the mental area to the angle (Figure 10.2).

Our current endoscopic procedure, which is a modification of a previous small incision procedure,[3] uses liposuction and Giampapa's suture as a basis. Portions of Feldman's corset procedure, older platysma band division procedures, and, in some instances, a hyoid drop, as described by Giunta and others,[4-6] are used when necessary.

Although imperfect (as all face-lifting procedures are), video-endoscope necklift can usually define and refine the aging neck without a superior face-lift. It is not adequate for individuals who want full resolution of their jowling, nor does it ameliorate midfacial sagging above the mandible. By its nature, the procedure cannot provide the "up" directional lift of the platysma of a full rhytidectomy. Elements of skin irregularity or contracture of the submentum, usually temporary, can

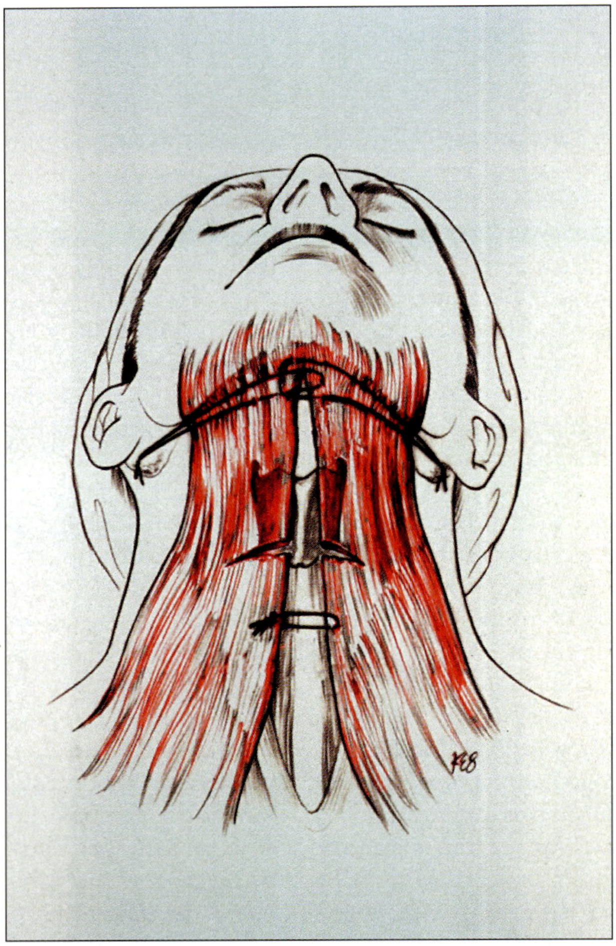

FIG. 10.1. Interlocking mattress suture platysmaplasty. A horizontal mattress suture is placed from the patient's right side, and a vertical mattress suture is placed from the left. These sutures are fastened to the mastoid fascia. Incisions in the platysma below the mattress suture may be made to break up platysmal bands. The bands may be sutured together below the incision, if they extend below the thyroid cartilage.

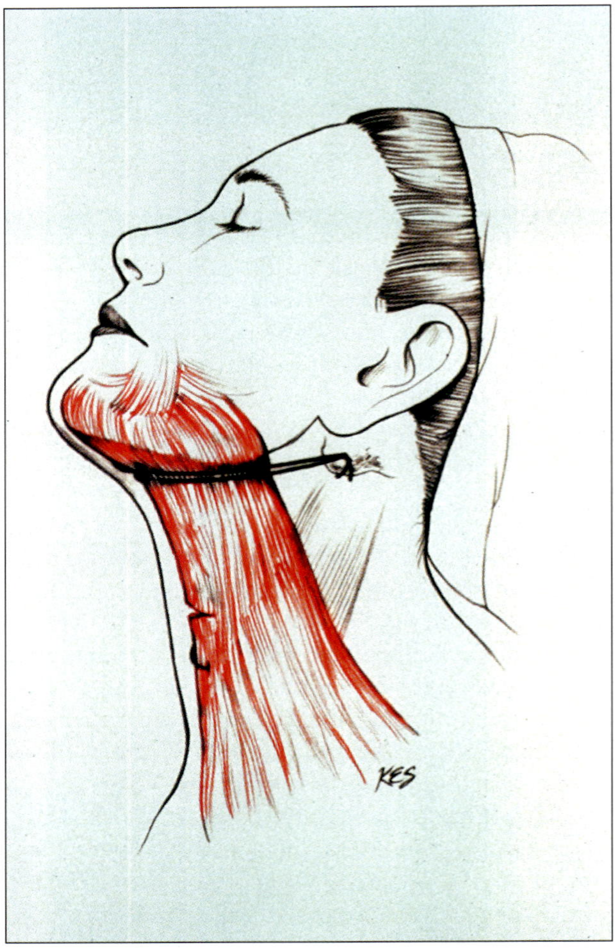

FIG. 10.2. From the side, it can be seen that the direction of pull is from inferior to superior (break point of the neck to mastoid). The vertical platysmal bands reorientate into a horizontal position, accentuating the neckline. The entire mandible is accentuated along its length, and the submaxillary gland is pushed inward.

also rarely occur. These usually resolve with ultrasound treatments.

Nonetheless, the procedure appears to be acceptable to both male and female patients. It can lend improvement to the younger patient who wished early correction of aging, as well as the older patient who wishes only a "cleanup" of a "turkey waddle." Men, in particular, accept the limitations of the procedure, because they want to avoid an anterior auricular incision that removes the hairless areas forming the sideburns.

Because of special endoscopic and suturing techniques, the submental incision can usually be avoided or limited in size to less than 1 cm in length. Occasionally, the submental incision may need to be lengthened to handle a bleeder or to perform more involved surgery, although this lengthening has, in recent times, become quite rare.

For the younger individual, the postauricular incision can be limited to 2 cm in length. For the middle-aged individual, this may have to be extended to the top of the ear, and, for the older individual who has loose skin, the incision may have to be brought into the posterior hairline.

The diminution of these incisions and the control afforded by endoscopic and laser surgery have made necklifts more acceptable to patients. The control afforded by endoscopic and laser surgery allow the surgeon, under direct vision, to stop bleeders and to remain precisely in tissue planes. This control usually avoids the prolonged bruising that can be seen with blind undermining techniques.

TECHNIQUE

Liposuction of the anterior neck and submandibular area is first performed. A tumescent technique is used to diminish bruising.[7,8]

Through a 1-cm incision in the submental area, an optical cavity in the anterior neck is created, using either a video-endoscopic dissector or laser attached to the endoscopic sheath (Figures 10.3, 10.4, and 10.5). This incision may be larger if extensive work is required in the neck. Performing this maneuver with endoscopic or direct vision, especially with the laser, allows the surgeon to avoid bleeders, especially the emissary veins near the mandible (Figures 10.6 and 10.7).

If there are no platysmal bands, the submental incision is not constructed. In this event, dissection of the submentum is accomplished from the postauricular incisor.

A 2-cm postauricular incision is then created. Although rare, this incision may be larger and may extend into the hairline if skin resection is required (Figures 10.8 and 10.9). Through this incision, dissection posteriorly over the mastoid fascia to the hairline and then anterior over the sternocleidomastoid and platysma to the anterior pocket is then performed under direct vision and with the 30-degree endoscope (Figures 10.10 to 10.13).

The endoscopic sheath, with the 70-degree endoscope in place, is then placed in the 1-cm submental incision so that the platysma muscles can be visualized. A long Keith needle is then placed subcutaneously

Text continued on p. 146.

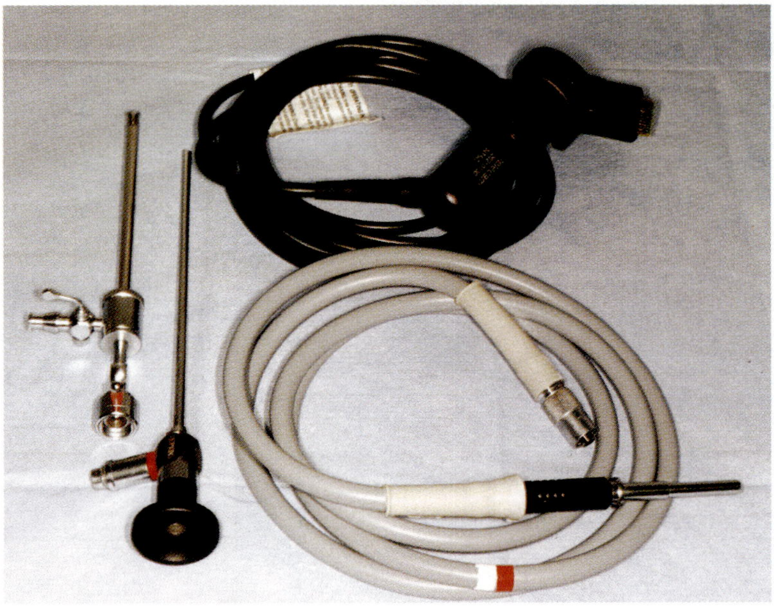

FIG. 10.3. Video-endoscopic dissector with camera, endoscope, and dissecting sheath (Karl Storz, Culver City, Calif).

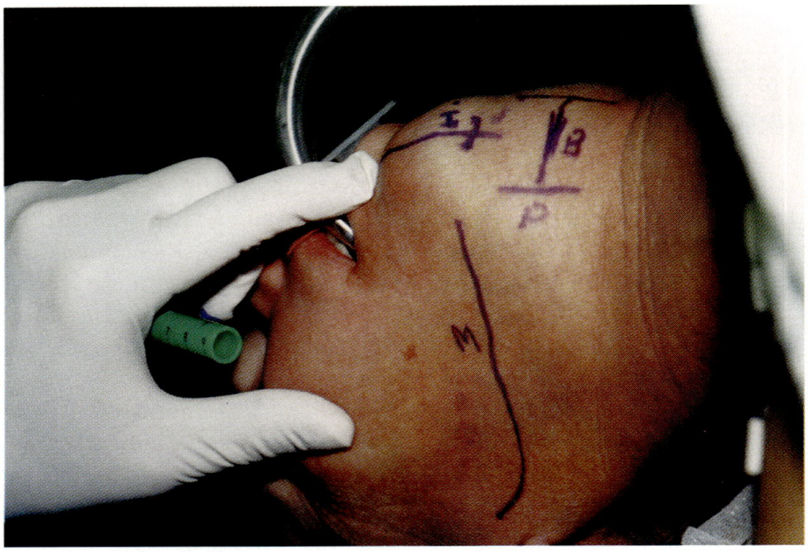

FIG. 10.4. Markings: I = incision, P = platysmal bands, M = mandible, and B = break point of neck.

A

B

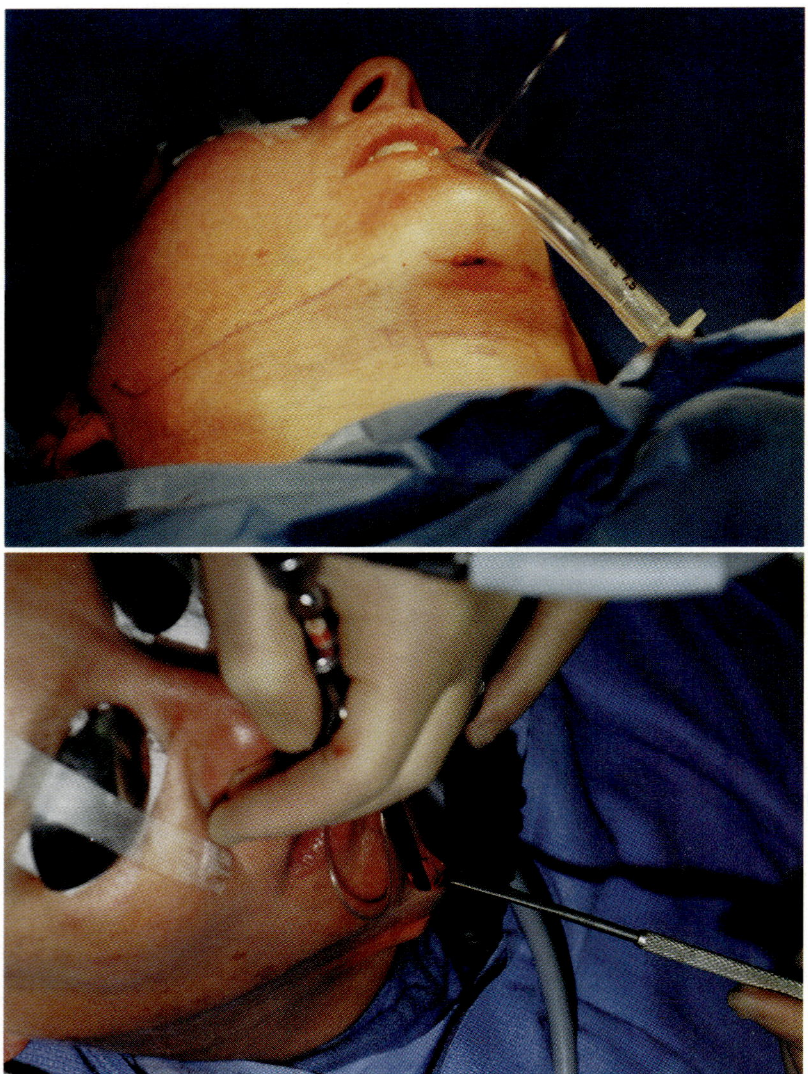

FIG. 10.5. A, After liposuction, a 1-cm curvilinear submental incision is performed. **B,** 30-degree 4-mm endoscope (Karl Storz, Culver City, Calif) is inserted.

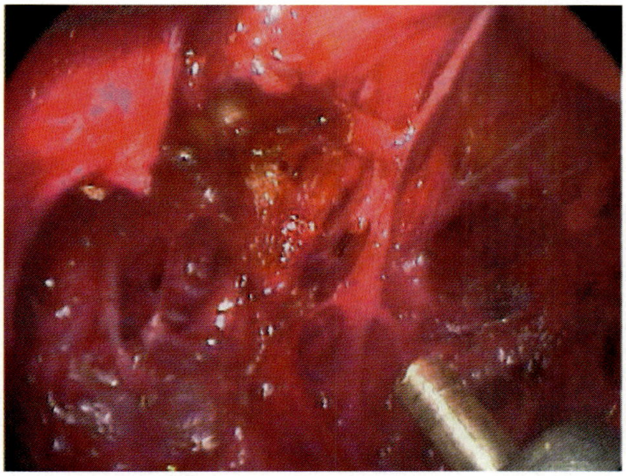

FIG. 10.6. View through the video-endoscope showing liposuction tunnels. The connecting bands often contain vessels.

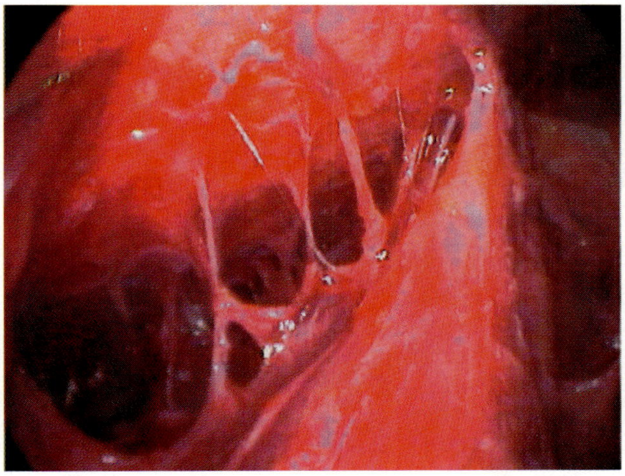

FIG. 10.7. Connecting bands between the liposuction tunnels are lysed with the laser to avoid bleeding. (Alternatively, the video-endoscopic dissector or endoscopic scissors may be used to separate the bands, although more bleeding is seen.) Care is taken to avoid the emissary veins.

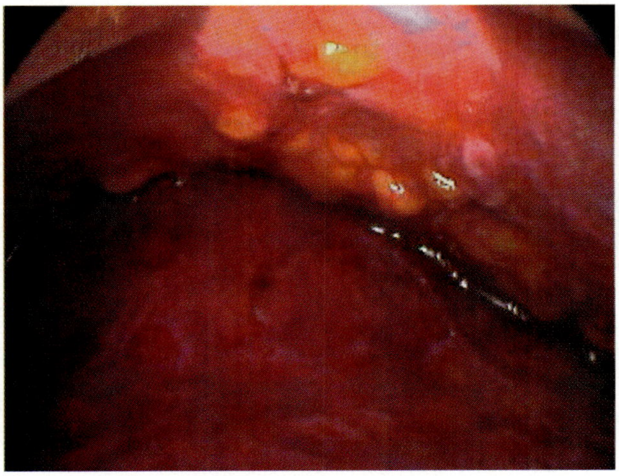

FIG. 10.8. Dissection creates an anterior pocket, which is carried laterally as far as is possible. A 4×4 is then inserted.

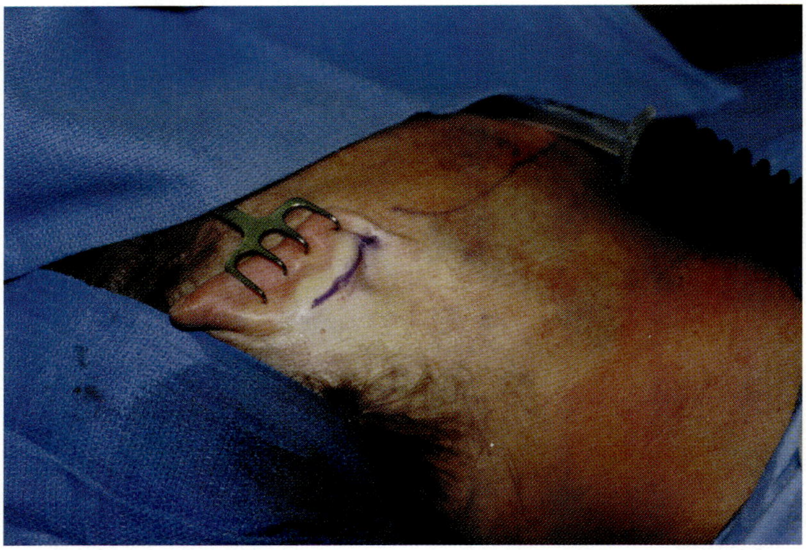

FIG. 10.9. A 2-cm postauricular incision is then constructed just above the fold. This may be elongated, if needed.

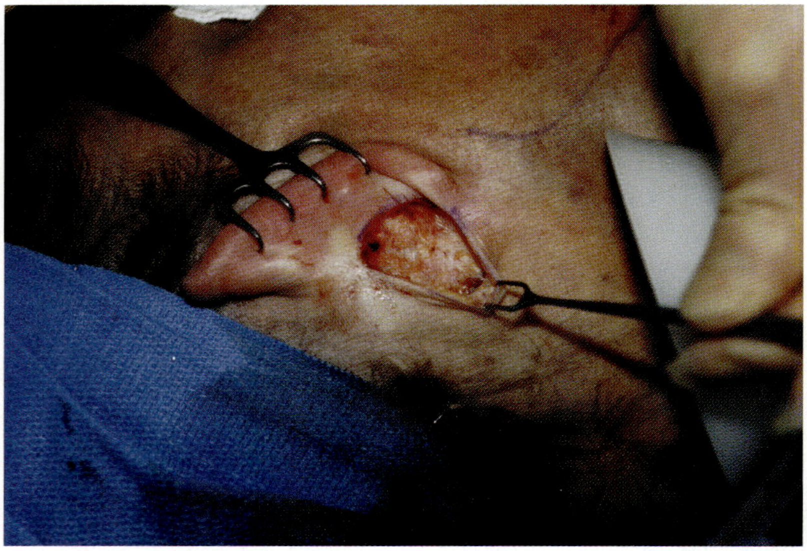

FIG. 10.10. Dissection is carried posteriorly under direct vision over the mastoid to the hairline. In this view, the laser with flexible waveguide (model 150 XJ, Sharplan, Warick, R.I.) has created a bloodless dissection.

A

B

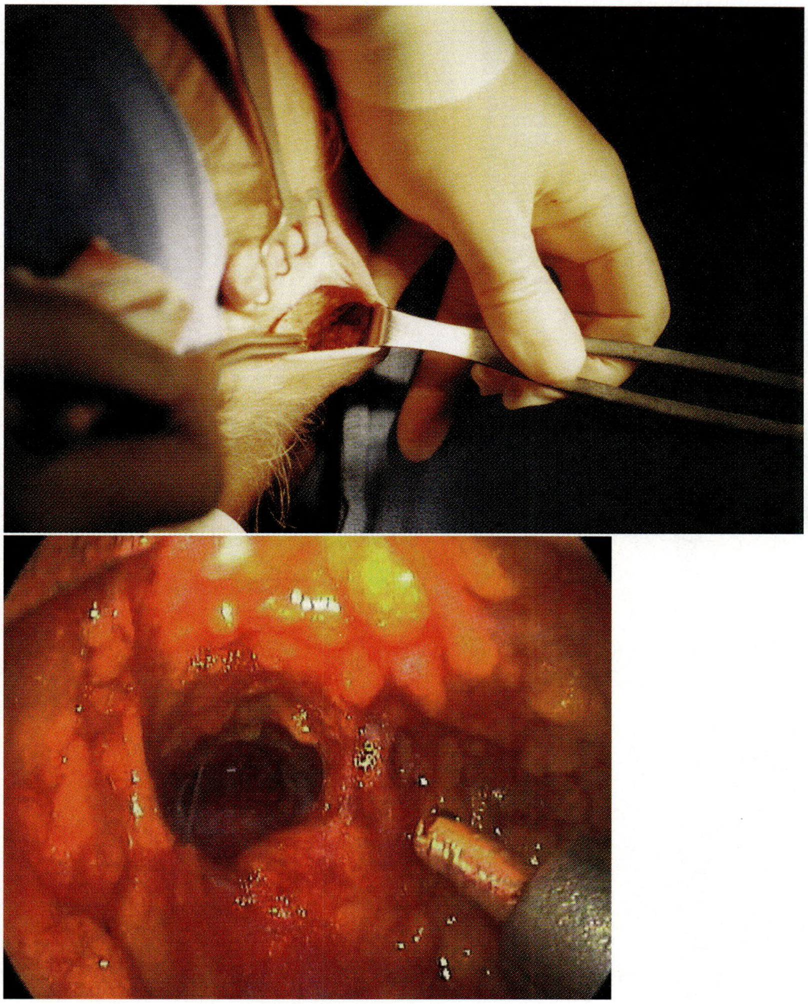

FIG. 10.11. **A,** Dissection is then carried inferiorly and anteriorly over the sternocleidomastoid fascia. Most of this dissection is accomplished under direct vision, but the video-endoscope may be used. **B,** Endoscopic view.

A

B

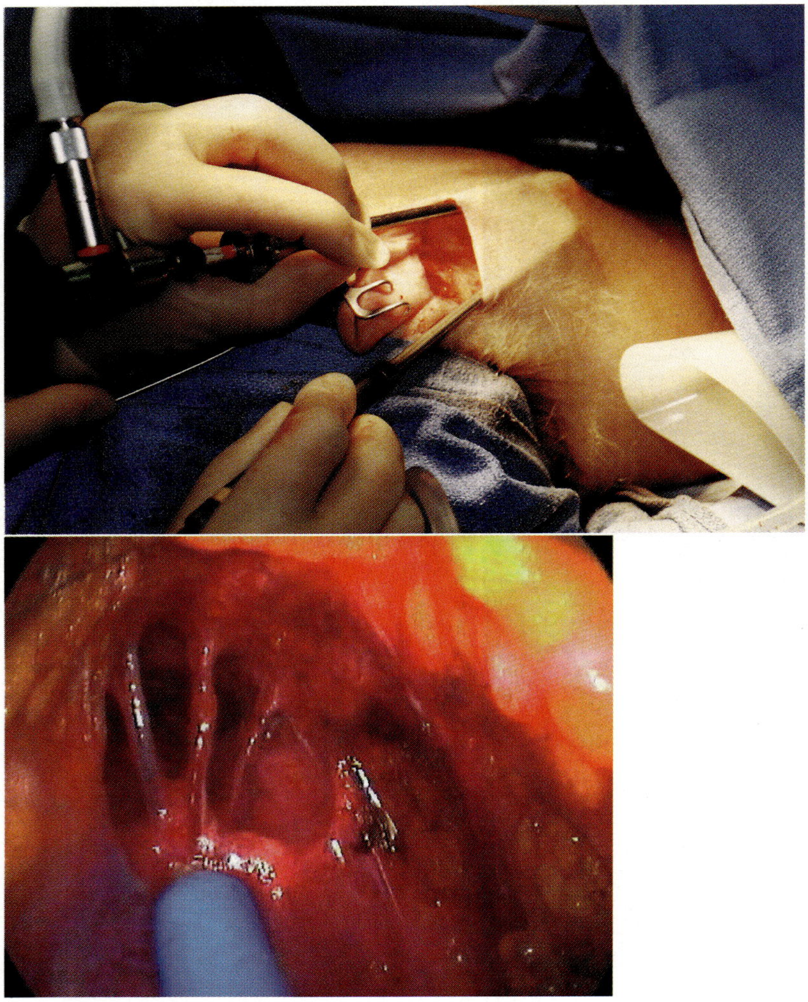

FIG. 10.12. **A,** Liposuction tunnels are visualized over the platysma muscle at the anterior edge of the sternocleidomastoid. Videoendoscope is used at this point to visualize the surgical field and any bleeding points. Dissection is performed with the laser or with endoscopic scissors (Karl Storz, Culver City, Calif). **B,** Endoscopic view.

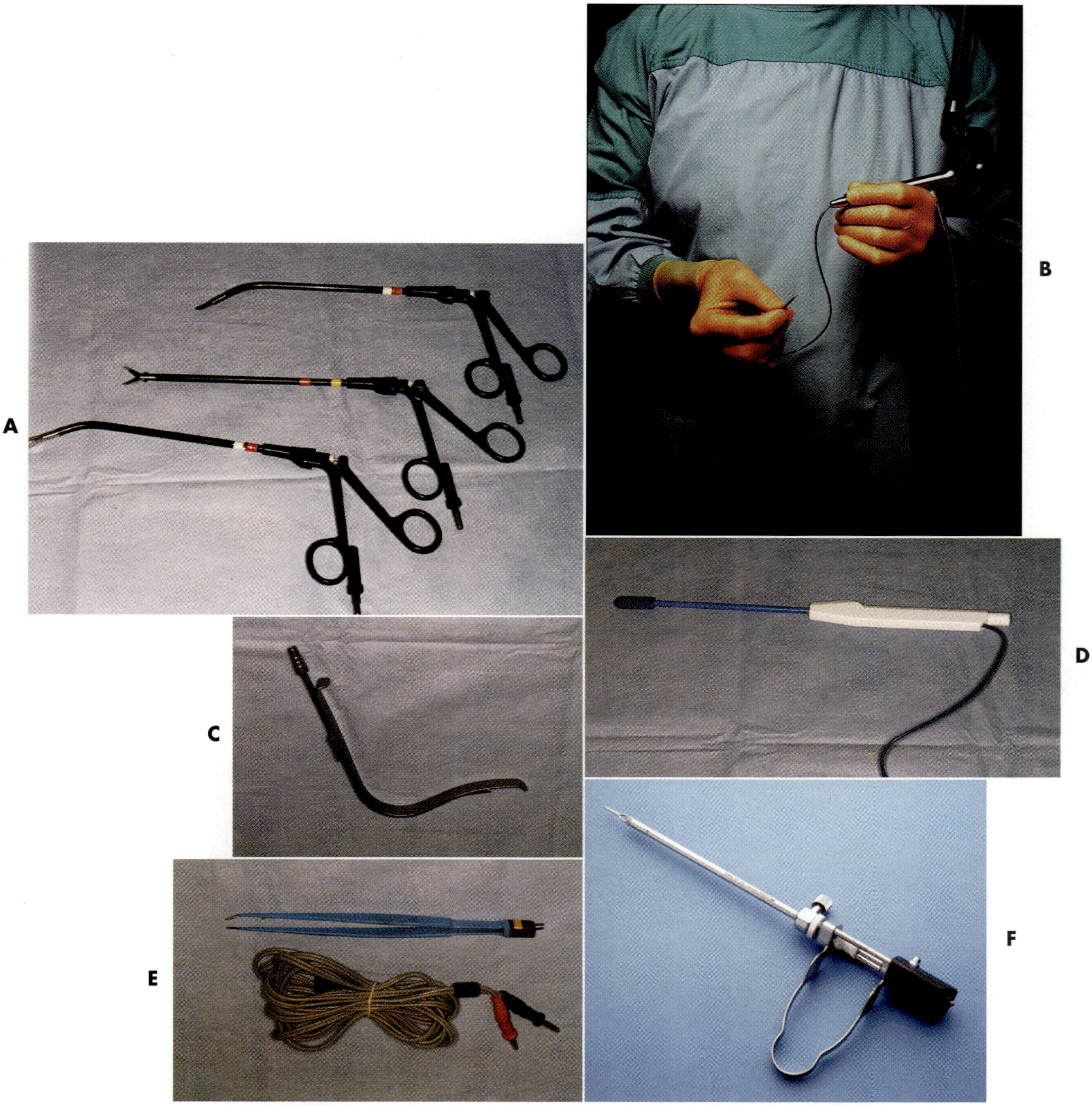

FIG. 10.13. Equipment for the posterior dissection: **A,** Endoscopic scissors. **B,** Flexible wave-guide for laser in handpiece (Sharplan, Warwick, R.I.). **C,** Smoke suction evacuator/retractor. **D,** Disposable (Weck) tonsil suction cautery. **E,** Standard bipolar forceps. **F,** Endoscopic bipolar cautery forceps (Karl Storz, Culver City, Calif).

through the skin and platysma muscle to place a horizontal mattress suture from the right side and a vertical mattress suture from the left (Figures 10.14 to 10.27). It is important to place the sutures higher on the neck than where the break point of the neck might appear to be. Currently a second set of mattress sutures is also placed. The first set of mattress sutures is placed one third of the distance from the hyoid to the submental incision (or submental crease if an incision has not been made). The second set of sutures is placed immediately below the submental incision (or crease). Two sets of sutures avoids a "pooching" forward of submental tissues.

These sutures are then retrieved from the posterior incision and sutured to the mastoid fascia. They are pulled only tight enough to define the mandibular border and to pull the platysma muscles together (Figures 10.28 to 10.36). If there is platysma banding inferior to the hyoid, incisions in the platysma and/or platysmal excision and suturing may be performed.

Text continued on p. 154.

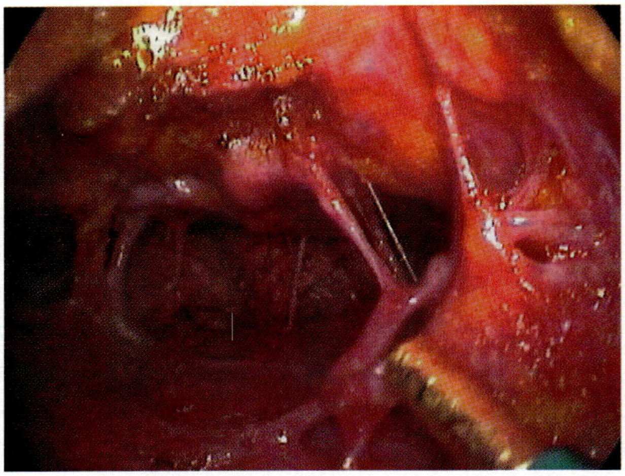

FIG. 10.14. Liposuction bands are lysed, and the dissection is carried forward to connect it to the anterior pocket. A 4×4 can be seen.

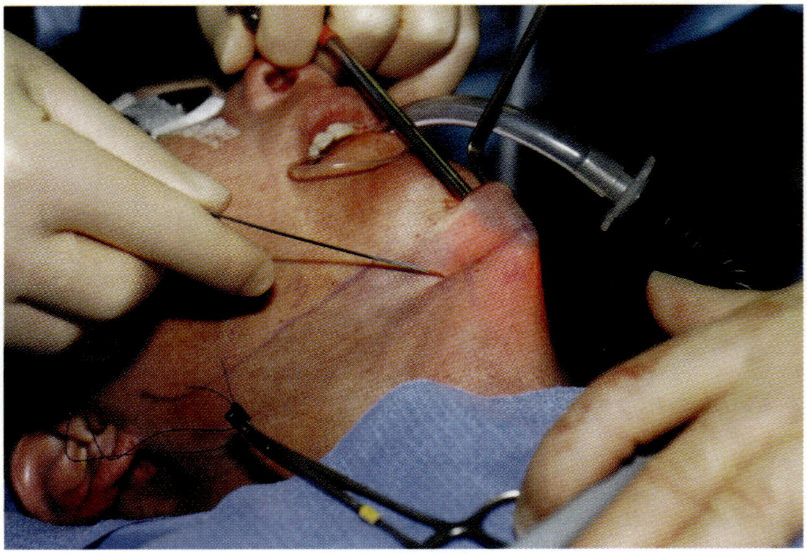

FIG. 10.15. Video-endoscope is then again placed through the anterior incision, and a Keith needle is inserted subcutaneously lateral to the platysma.

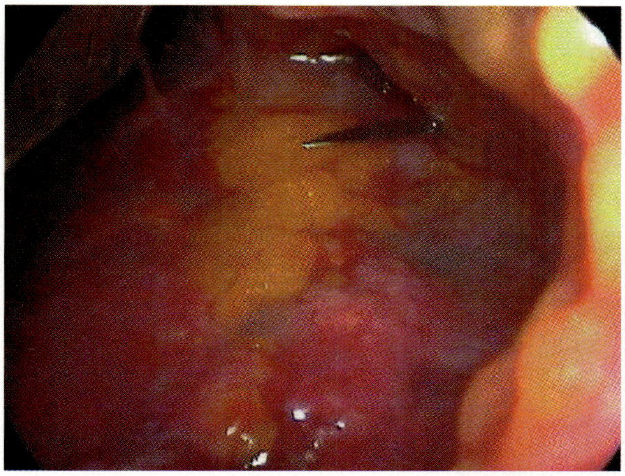

FIG. 10.16. Endoscopic view of the Keith needle placed subcutaneously.

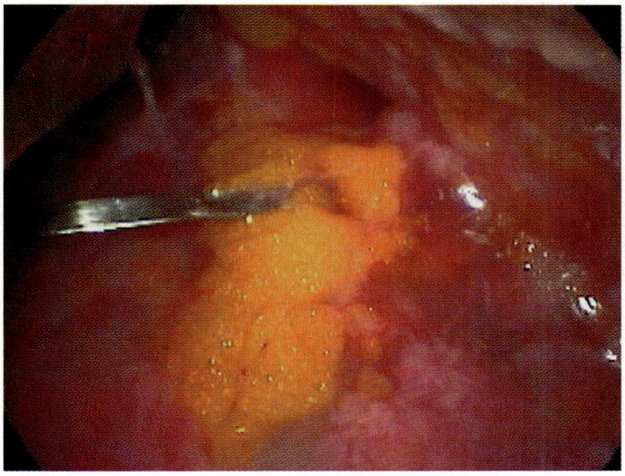

FIG. 10.17. Keith needle then penetrates the right platysma and emerges in the midline.

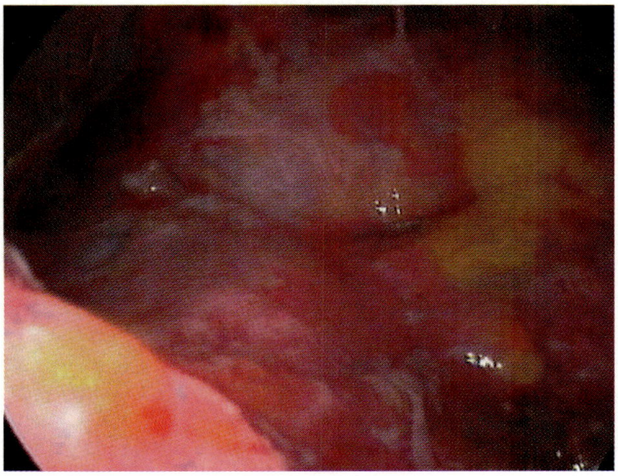

FIG. 10.18. Keith needle is then placed through the left platysma.

A

B

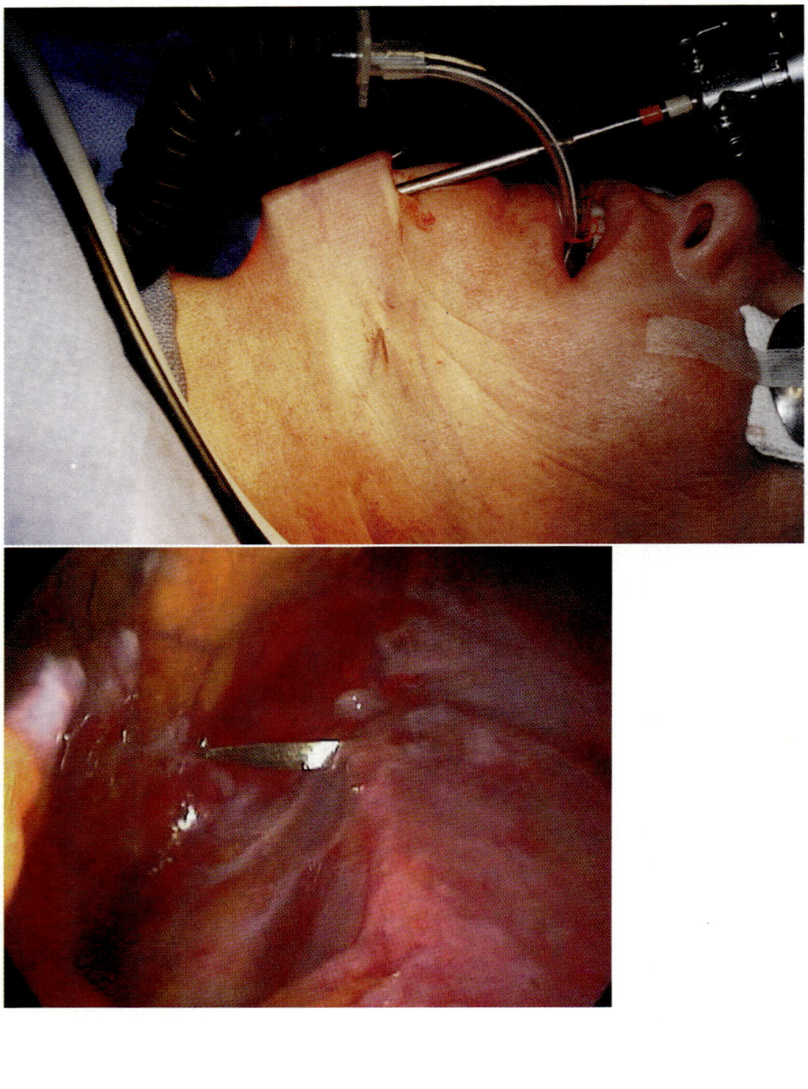

FIG. 10.19. **A,** Needle is then extended through the skin on the left side. **B,** Endoscopic view.

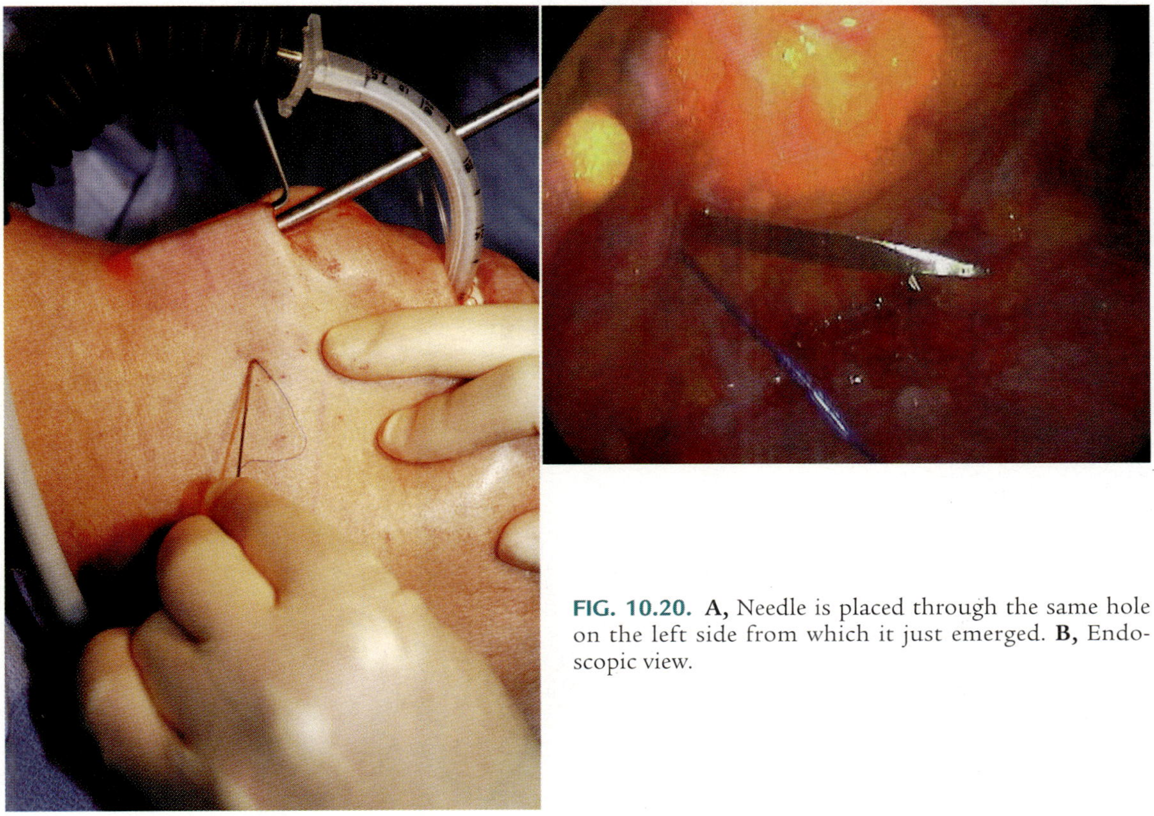

A

B

FIG. 10.20. **A,** Needle is placed through the same hole on the left side from which it just emerged. **B,** Endoscopic view.

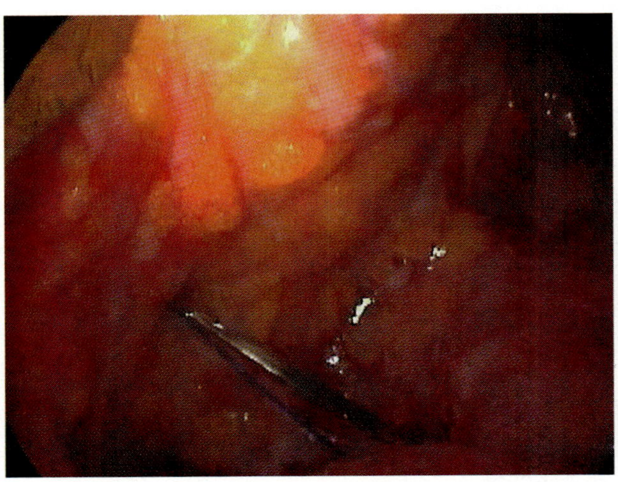

FIG. 10.21. Left platysma is then pierced superior to where it had been pierced on the previous pass.

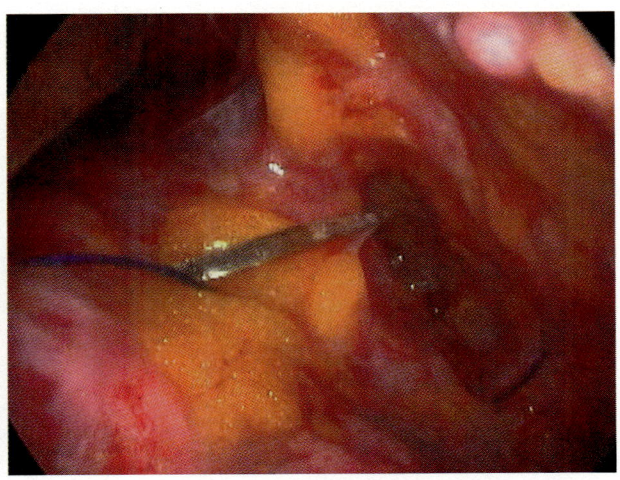

FIG. 10.22. Needle then emerges in the midline. The suture from the previous pass is seen.

A

B

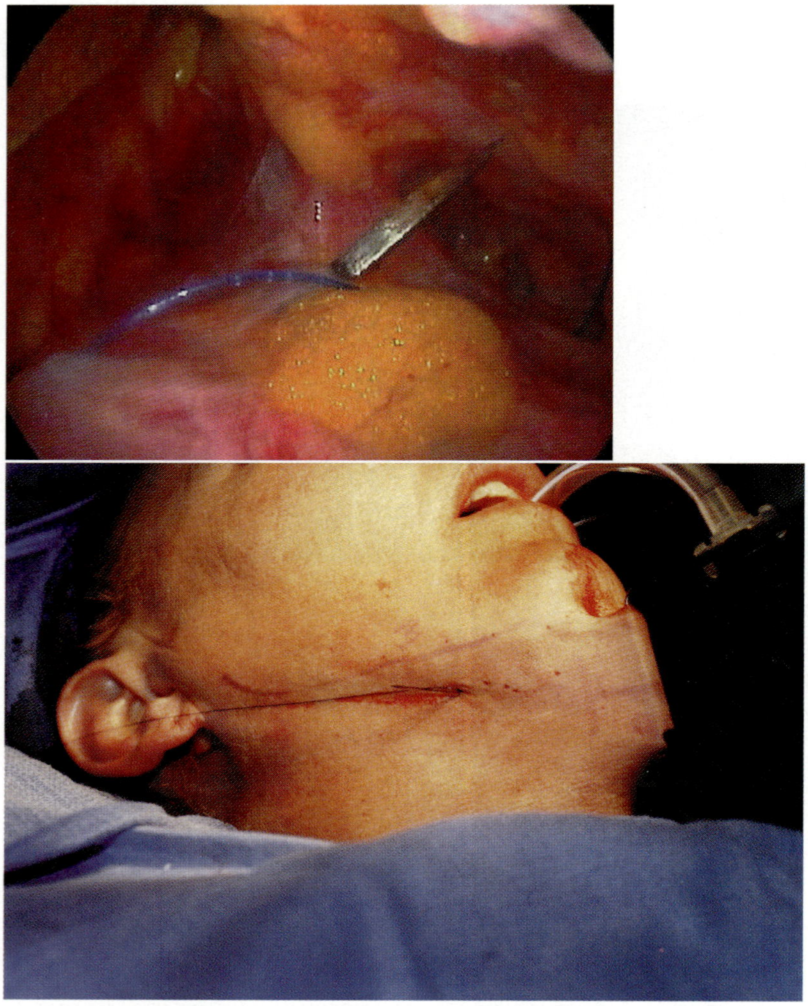

FIG. 10.23. **A,** Right platysma is then pierced. **B,** Needle then emerges from the right side, forming a horizontal mattress.

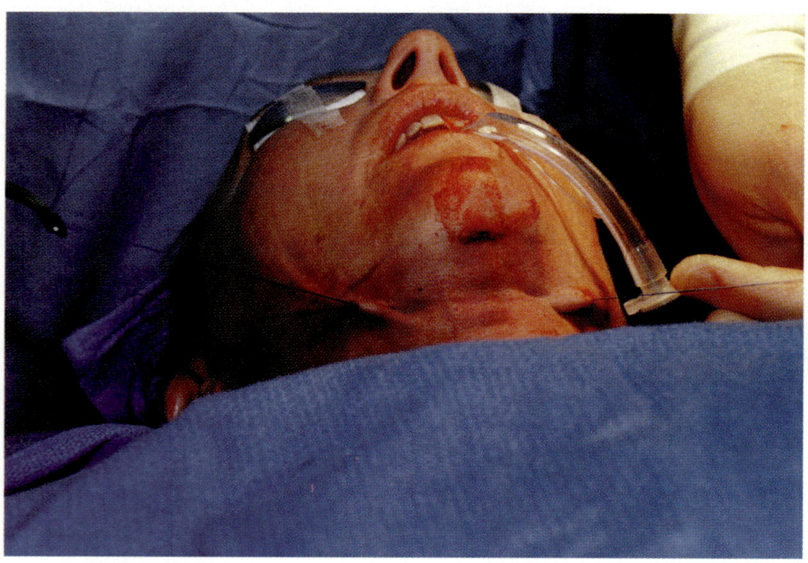

FIG. 10.24. Vertical mattress suture is then placed from the left side. Both horizontal and vertical mattress sutures are seen protruding through the skin.

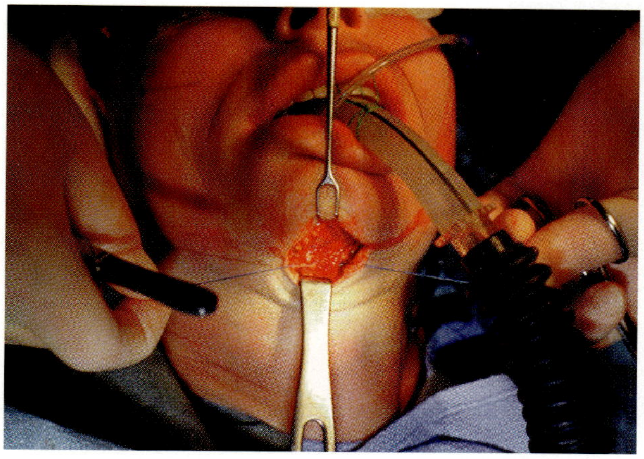

FIG. 10.25. View of the interlocking sutures through a larger incision.

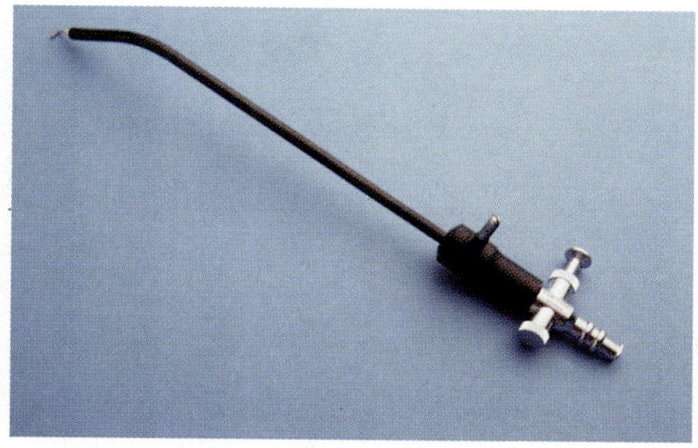

FIG. 10.28. Endoscopic nerve hook (Karl Storz, Culver City, Calif).

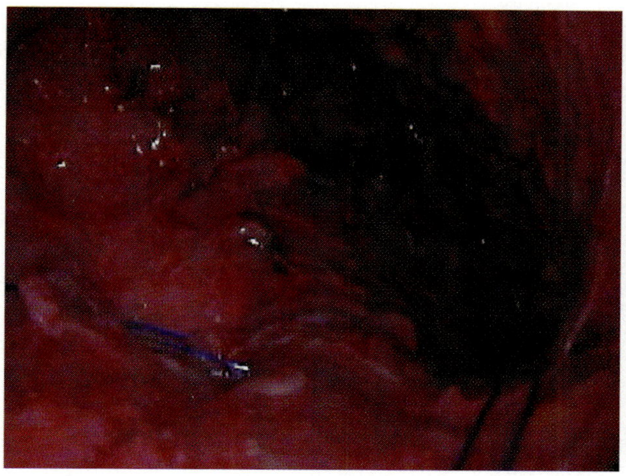

FIG. 10.26. Endoscopic view of the interlocking sutures between the platysma muscles.

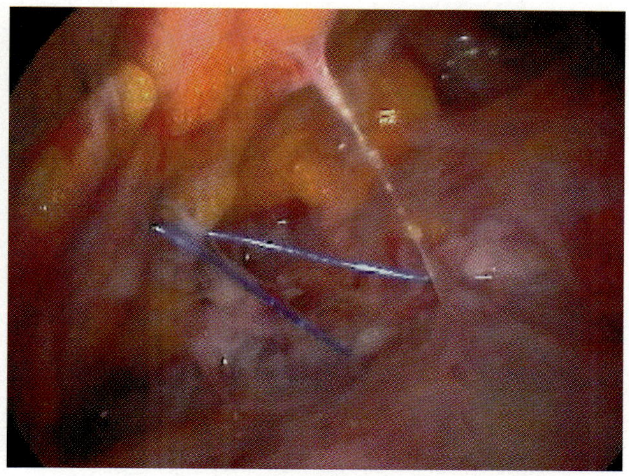

FIG. 10.29. Endoscopic view of the sutures as they emerge from the optical cavity through the skin.

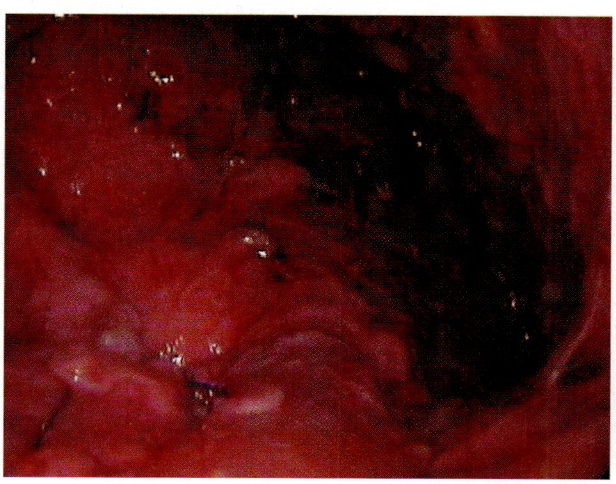

FIG. 10.27. Platysma muscles pulled together.

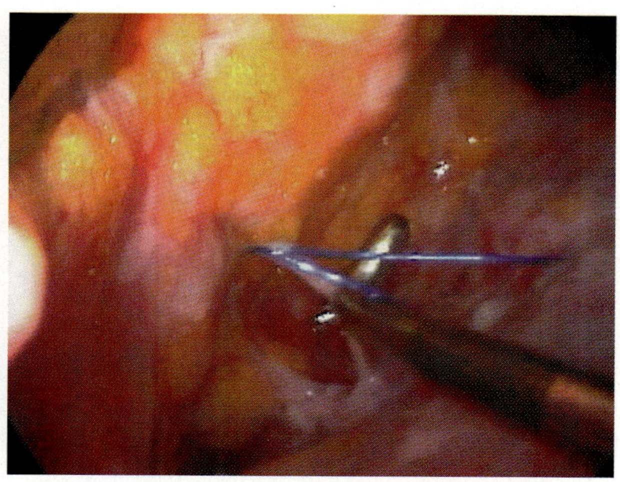

FIG. 10.30. Nerve hook, placed through the submental incision, engages the sutures.

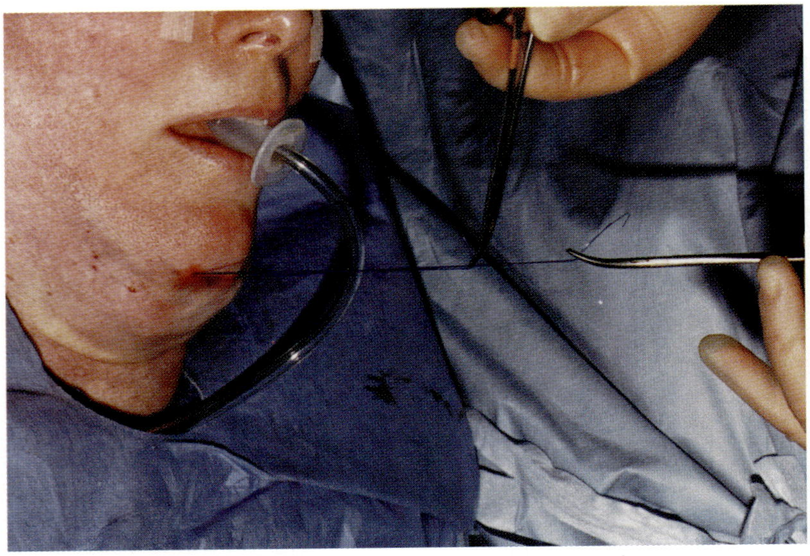

FIG. 10.31. Sutures are brought through the anterior incision.

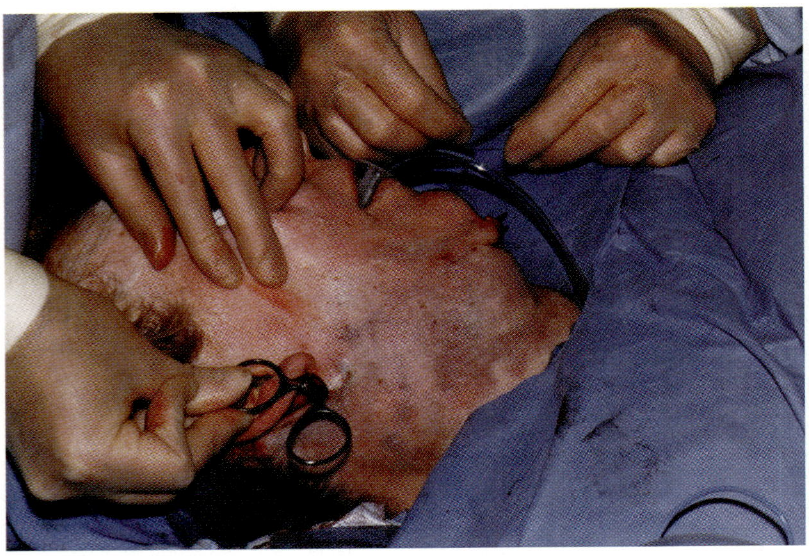

FIG. 10.32. A long needle holder is placed from the posterior incision to emerge from the anterior incision.

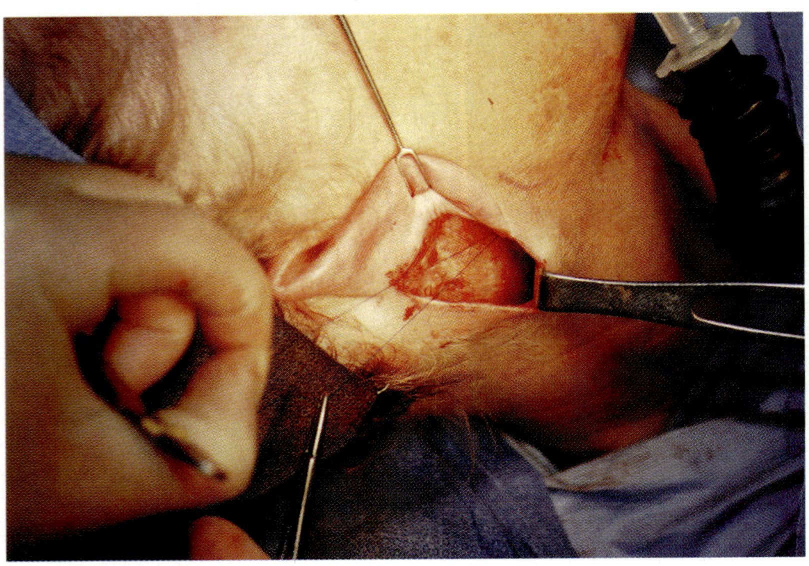

FIG. 10.33. Sutures are grasped and pulled through the posterior incision.

A

B

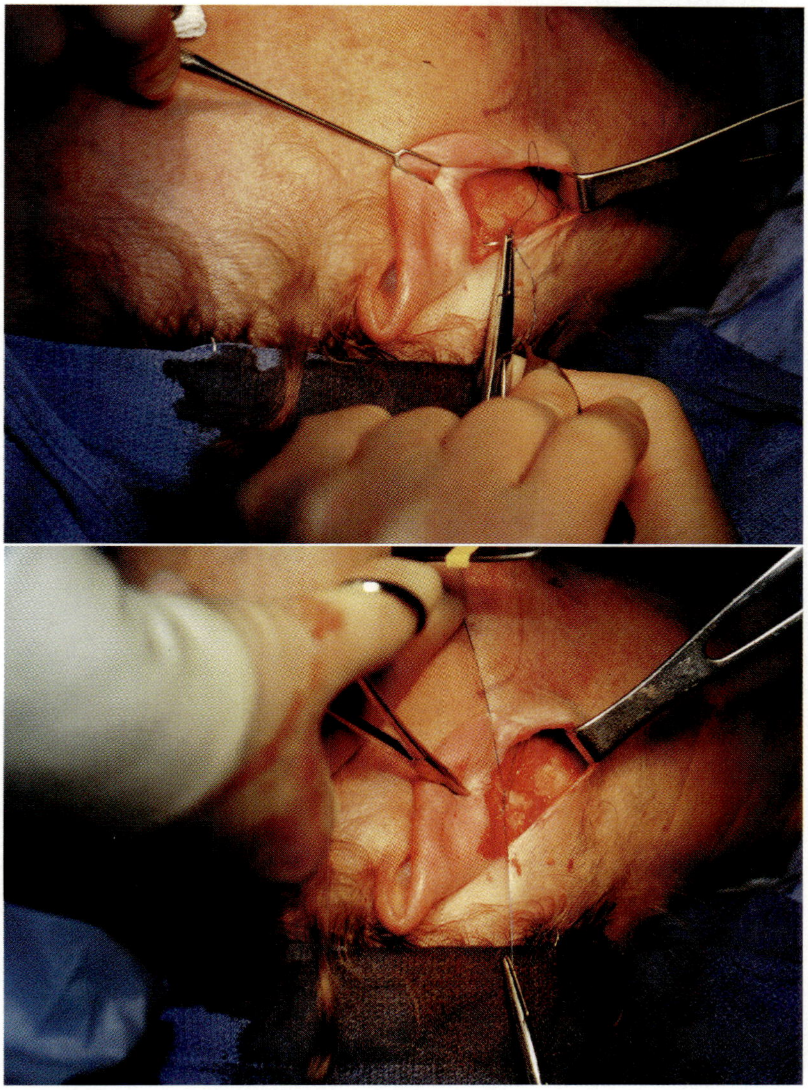

FIG. 10.34. **A,** Free needle is then used to sew the sutures to the mastoid fascia. **B,** Sutures are only tightened enough to see a neck "break."

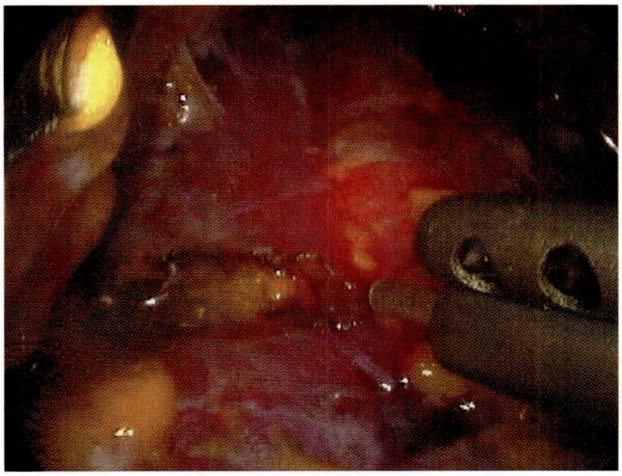

FIG. 10.35. Endoscopic view of the midportion of the platysma band incision made with the laser in the midline below the sutures.

A

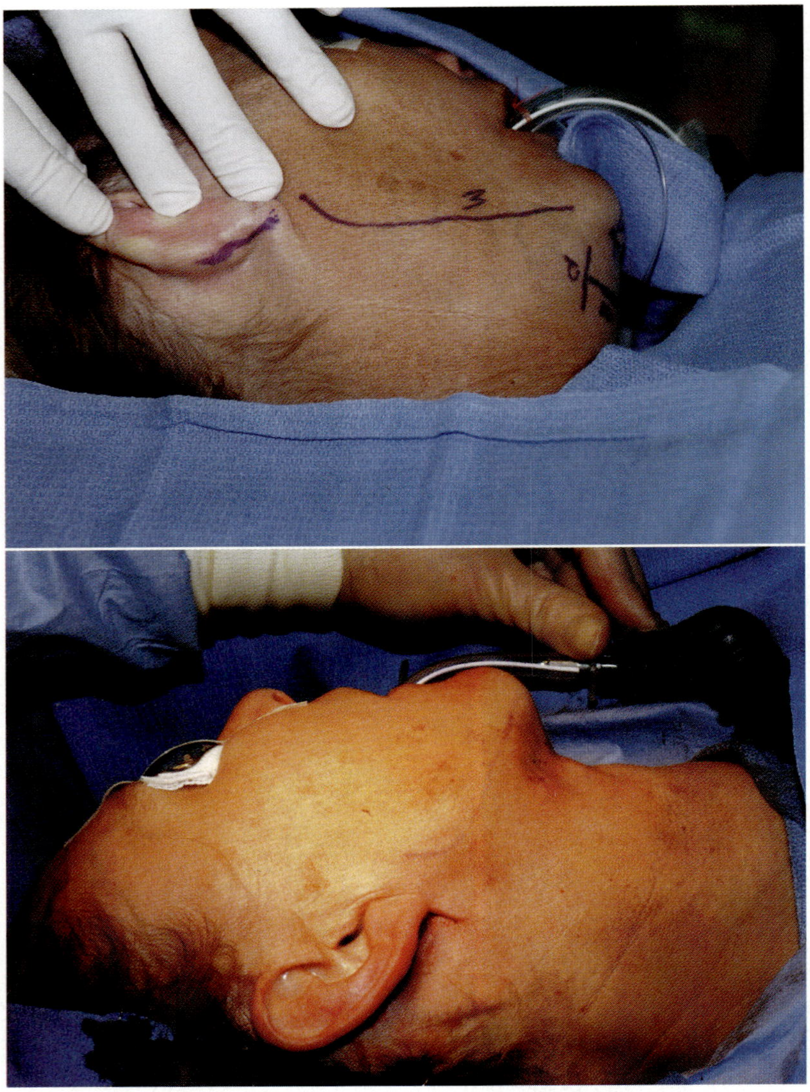

B

FIG. 10.36. With the suture placed over the skin, the inward positioning that defines the mandibular border and the elevation of the "break point" above the hyoid is appreciated. **A,** Preoperative and **B,** Postoperative.

RESULTS

This technique is capable of defining the neck contours in a variety of patients. The only element missing, when compared with a full face-lift procedure, is the small amount of upward pull, which adds to the "tautness" of the latter procedure. The procedure does not correct the midface above the mandible and gives improvement to the jowls only below the mandible (Figures 10.37 and 10.38).

The recovery period is quite short. Most patients can be out in public with a turtleneck or high collar for brief periods after the chin strap is removed. If a chin implant has been added, the recovery period is commensurate with (and limited by) the chin implant procedure. Complications in 40 patients (32 women, 8 men) who have undergone the current necklift procedure, as just described, have been limited to three cases of skin irregularities, which resolved with ultrasound treatment. Two patients had small hematomas that responded to needle aspiration. Only one of the patients experienced a seroma, a problem that occurred in our earlier nonendoscopic-technique patients who did not wear a supportive chin strap. There have been no facial nerve injuries.

CONCLUSION

The video-endoscopic necklift procedure provides a quick recovery with few complications that are usually of a "minor" nature. Although not satisfactory for the patient who desires midface improvement, the necklift can produce significant improvement in the patient whose complaints or desire for improvement are limited to the neck.

A 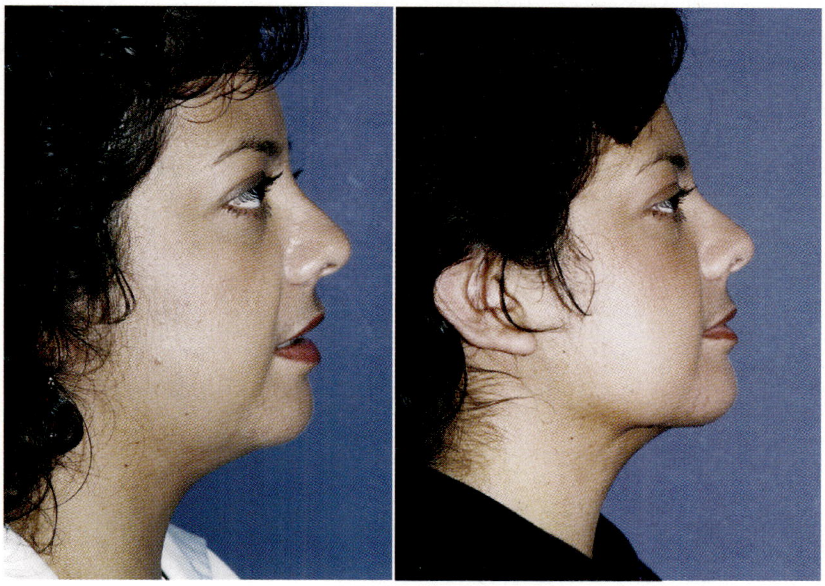 B

FIG. 10.37. **A,** Preoperative view of necklift patient. **B,** Postoperative view of patient.

A 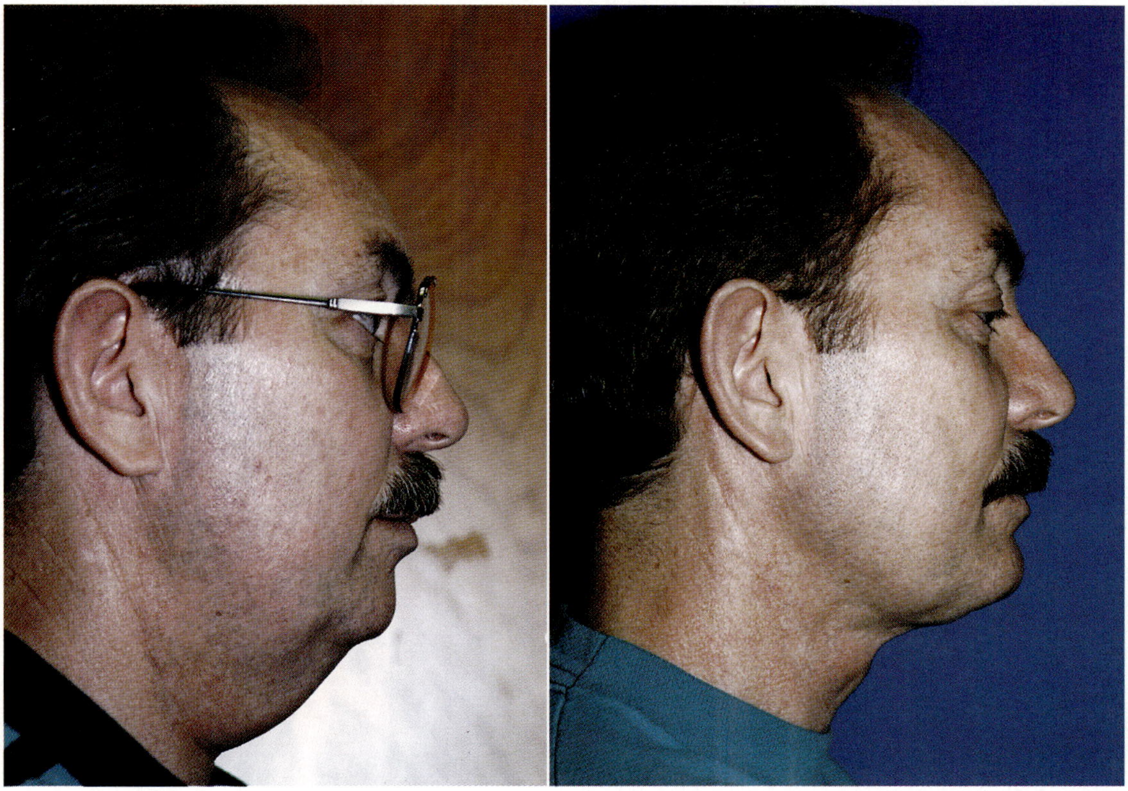 B

FIG. 10.38. **A,** Preoperative view of necklift patient. **B,** Postoperative view of patient.

REFERENCES

1. Feldman JJ: Corset platysmaplasty, Plast Reconstr Surg 86:53-61, 1990.
2. Giampapa VC, and Di Bernardo BE: Neck recontouring with suture suspension and liposuction: an alternative for the early rhytidectomy candidate, Aesthetic Plast Surg 19:217-220, 1995.
3. Keller GS, and Cray J: Laser-assisted surgery of the aging face, Facial Plast Surg Clin North Am 3:319-341, 1995.
4. Giunta S: Suprahyoid release. Abstract of a presentation at the 6th International Symposia of Facial Plastic Surgery, San Francisco, Calif, June 19, 1993, American Academy of Facial Plastic Surgery, 43.
5. Collins PC, and Epger, B: Improvement in the augmentation genioplasty via suprahyoid muscle repositioning, J Maxillofac Surg 11:116, 1983.
6. Guyuron B: The problem neck, hyoid bone, and submental myotomy, Plast Reconstr Surg 90:830-837, 1992.
7. Klein J: Tumescent technique, Dermatol Clin 8:425, 1990.
8. Hunsted JP: Tumescent and syringe liposculpture: a logical partnership, Aesthetic Plast Surg 19:321, 1995.

Index

Note: Page numbers for illustrations are in *italics.* Page numbers for tables are followed by a "t."

G

H

I

K

L

M

N

O

P

V

X

Y

Z